FROM SOLE TO SOUL

A 21ST CENTURY GUIDE TO DEEP HEALTH

BARRY MARMORSTEIN, M. D.

12/15/12

Dear Phyllis,

I am flattered that you would choose to look this over.

I hope you find enough in it to help you stay well into "old age"

Fondly,

"Dr M"

FROM SOLE TO SOUL

A 21ST CENTURY GUIDE TO DEEP HEALTH

BARRY MARMORSTEIN, M. D.

Published by:

Joshua Tree Publishing

www.JoshuaTreePublishing.com

ISBN: 0-9829803-2-9
13-Digit: 978-0-9829803-2-3

Printed in the United States of America

DEDICATION

To Lil and Eddie,
who gave me everything I needed.

To Di,
who opened the cage and set me free.

To Ella and Gracie,
who have given me so much so quickly.

CONTENTS

INTRODUCTION

A s has been stated many times before, the only thing that can be counted on is change. Those of us living at this time have become witness to the fact that change is occurring progressively more rapidly. The medical establishment is obviously embedded in society and is participating fully in rapid change. The inclination is to consider change to be beneficial, which of course it may be. However, in actuality, change is value neutral. What we do as a society with a changing landscape is what will determine whether change is ultimately beneficial or detrimental to humans, and to our earthly home.

In a description by Dave Morrison, and others, what is evolving in the future has been coined the "Second Curve," with the present time and the immediate future being termed the "First Curve." It is difficult enough to look at ourselves now and describe what we see. It is much more difficult to look at what we perceive to be a changing landscape and describe what the landscape will look like in a few years, as societal pressures relentlessly push on. It is much more difficult, yet, to predict what societal pressures will create for us in a generation or two. In fact, most historians concede the truth of Hegel's presumption that "The owl of Minerva spreads its wings only with the falling of the dusk." That is, we can only assess a culture, or historical epoch, when it is finished.

I have been witness to fundamental changes within the health care system during the time of my chosen career path. I see the emergence of problems in the delivery of health care which perhaps are still value neutral, but which I believe are trending toward negative outcomes. After all, what doctors are supposed to do is deliver health care. I am disturbed by what I see, and I wish to bring this to the awareness of you, the consumer. *Aha*! A timely example of change! Doctors are no longer termed doctors. We are now "providers." You are no longer termed "patients." You are now consumers.

So, as my career drifts relentlessly towards its dusk, I wish to share some thoughts with you and give you a distillation of what I have learned in the past forty-six years since I was anointed with an "MD" degree.

My father died when I was young, and I was raised by a mother, for whom I would do anything to make happy. Our family doctor was Maurice Goldstein, likely fifty years old at the time. He was the quintessential "GP" of the time. He took care of my grandmother's blood pressure and was the recipient of the call from my mother on an early morning in December, 1952, when Grandma was coughing relentlessly. I can still hear those coughs as I headed off to school. He met her at the hospital shortly thereafter but was unable to save her from the heart attack and heart failure which caused her to die, the same day. Prior to that, he had fixed my broken finger and made house calls to give my sister shots of penicillin. He was the obstetrician who delivered my other sister as well. He removed my tonsils, as well as a rusty nail from my butt, incurred while climbing through a basement window. He removed my mother's breast lump and fixed her hemorrhoids (at the same time!). My last contact with him was in 1962, while a freshman in medical school. I had been told by University doctors that I needed an operation to clear an infection. It seemed ghastly to me, with a proposed long recovery. I consulted Dr. Goldstein who told me to leave it alone and gave me some simple tips about prevention of complications. I followed his advice and have never had a problem with it.

My mother looked up to Dr. Goldstein with obvious great admiration. At age 12, based on his role model, I wrote to the AMA requesting information on how to proceed with becoming a doctor. I received a number of pamphlets in a large brown envelope, and I was hooked. I never looked back. In my graduation high school year book, next to "Ambition," I declared "Doctor of Medicine." I thought I was doing it for my mother, but perhaps she was doing it for me.

I considered the day that I received my acceptance to medical school to be the happiest day of my life. Medical school was very difficult, and I saw my student colleagues as all being much smarter than me. All I could do to compete with them was to work even harder than they. I loved medical school. I couldn't study too much. I loved internship and residency in Internal Medicine, and almost regretted when I had to leave the hospital and go home. After a two-year stint in the Army (drafted), I finished my training with a two-year fellowship in pulmonary medicine. It was 1974, twelve years after starting medical school, and I had literally gone as far as I could go. I was Board Certified in both Internal Medicine and Pulmonary Medicine. In other words, I was "hot!"

I entered solo private practice in 1974. I never forgot Dr. Goldstein. I had all of the credentials of the specialist and sub-specialist, but in my heart, I was still the "GP." As mentioned, Dr. Goldstein was the prototypic general practitioner, who was trained to take care of the vast majority of everyday maladies, with roots stretching back to antiquity. Perhaps the birth of modern-day medical practice began sometime in the late 19th Century, under the leadership of many great physicians, with perhaps the most towering figure of all being William Osler. Had he done nothing else but redirect the emphasis from the disease to the patient, he would have been immortalized. ("A good physician treats the disease. A great physician treats the patient.") But he did much more, being highly influential in establishing the basics of medical investigations, and of the medical establishment in general. His writings are still awe-inspiring and should be mandatory study for doctors for re-credentialing and preventing burnout.

Within the first few days of entering medical school, we were told emphatically and repeatedly that proper diagnosis is the bedrock of medical practice, and that knowledge of diagnosis comes from the medical history; that is, the story that the patient relates. As Osler put it, "Listen to the patient, he is telling you the diagnosis." Everything that comes after the history including physical examination, lab testing, imaging studies, and others were emphasized to be designed to confirm the diagnosis established in the history. Recent research has demonstrated that when a patient now speaks to a doctor, the first interruption by the doctor occurs after eighteen seconds! Medical care is now remarkably fragmented, with a plethora of medical specialists (142 listed in my county medical society roster), each one looking at their little corner of the patient. When I entered medical practice in 1974, there were a few "Dr. Goldsteins" still active in this community. Now, there are none. I am now in the thirty-eighth year of that same practice. It has been a fantastically rewarding experience. I feel myself to be "The luckiest man on the face of the Earth," after Lou Gehrig, of course.

Where do we go from here as "providers" and "consumers?" Does the medical option meet our needs? Do we need to change it? Can we afford it now, and into the future? Does the cost of it detract from other segments of society? Questions like this could go on ad infinitum. I freely admit to my own biases, and how difficult it is to look at situations with a truly open mind. We cannot help but bring our life experiences to the debate. I see deepening problems on the medical horizon. Because of this bias of mine, I see the need for each person to take much greater responsibility for their own mental and physical well-being. I say this at a time when our knowledge of disease processes is growing exponentially. Although this may have the appearance of a paradox, it is not. In fact, it may be a reflection of diverging trends in the science and the art of medicine. As the science is rapidly expanding, the art appears to be collapsing. Along the way we will learn a great deal about health and disease. We will see some sad truths, such as the beleaguered doctor being just as overwhelmed by the medical system as everyone else. You will learn the basics about how to stay well. The basic principles set forth are both deceptively simple and difficult at the same time. The keys are commitment to good health and waking up spiritually. Let's take a look.

The true "Second Curve" will involve an increasing recognition that the factors creating health have very little to do with the medical care. Evidence coming from the population health literature suggests that a person's educational level, income, and job have an enormous impact on future health status, longevity, and so forth. One of the central features in the population health literature is the recognition that people who are in positions of less authority and no control tend to have much higher death rates from cancer and other diseases than those who are in a position of some autonomy in their work environment. There will be increasing recognition that the kinds of work places we design have an impact on the future health of the population, and it will also become clear that investment in early childhood development will yield enormous benefits down the line in terms of reducing health cost and improving health status.

Although medical school, formal residency, and fellowship training is essential as a launching pad, most of what I have learned has come in my interactions with patients (or, consumers) on a day-to-day basis. I have worked in the office, in the hospital, and in the intensive care unit. I have worked in the nursing home, assisted living, and adult family home environments. I still make a few house calls. I have followed patients whenever they have wanted me to go.

I do not wish nor intend my observations to be interpreted as "sour grapes." We must all take responsibility for the current medical establishment, and only we, simply or collectively, can navigate through it to our best advantage—and perhaps change it to better suit our needs, if we so desire.

The carrot on the stick is good health into old age. Instead of experiencing a tortuous ordeal, you should anticipate the flowering of your life. Just as the fruit off the tree is the highest expression of development and intelligence in the plant world, so old age should be the same in the human world. Your work is done. You have paid your dues. Now, the opportunity exists for the kind of growth that Eastern traditions refer to as going into the forest; a time of contemplation, relaxation, exponential spiritual growth. Anticipation of one's own death as it approaches can generate a feeling of release rather than dread. Write about your experiences and expect that it will be read. You have the combination of experience and knowledge. Combined with the perspective just mentioned, you have a great deal to teach. Simple lessons or complex.

ACKNOWLEDGMENTS

As mentioned early in the text, even in pre-civilization, human activity quickly became too complex for an individual to thrive alone. This fact is even more obviously apparent 5000 years later. I have a niece who recently published a book on language in which she cited forty-seven people who contributed to her effort. I recently read a book about doctoring, in which the author of a two hundred page treatise cited thirty-seven people who assisted him.

Somewhat intimidated, fearful at times that I would not have more than five or six people willing to attend my funeral, I began to tear into my memory bank to see if I could dredge up some names to cite for this undertaking. Sadly, I could only find a few people. Perhaps this is consistent with the fact that I have spent almost my entire career in solo practice.

First, I wish to thank someone whom I have never even met. That would be Woody Allen, the most frequently quoted person in the book. He has taught me a great deal, most importantly the value of self-deprecatory humor, which is closely linked with not always knowing the right way, and humility.

I greatly acknowledge the help of my eighteen year office manager, Suzanne Lee. At a time when the average medical office employee stays for one year, ten months, sixteen days, five hours, and nine seconds, she re-wrote the book on commitment and loyalty. Not only did she keep me financially solvent and out of jail, she managed to nurse my hand-written manuscript through the appropriate electronic devices to get it into a manuscript form that would allow countless agents and publishers to reject it.

Suzie would never have had a chance to work her magic were it not for the phenomenal accomplishments of one of my long-standing patients. When Cheryl Anderson heard about my plight of having a manuscript of hundreds of handwritten pages, with countless cross outs, arrows pointing up-down-left-right, marred by coffee stains and the remnants of sneezes, with limited options regarding salvage, she said, "I'll do it for you". I said "no! I wouldn't wish that on my worst enemy." She said "please!" and the deal was done. She and Suzie went to work, and the rest of his history.

Thirdly, I thank my publisher John Paul Owles. At first, I wondered if his motto "We believe in authors" was just a clever gimmick. I became even more suspicious when the only reason he gave to me for handing me a contract was the realization that he and I grew up in the same city (Chicago), and graduated from the same University (of Illinois). (What the Sam Hill does that have to do with publishing a book?) Actually, I recently visited the museum of railroad magnate and philanthropist Sam Hill in South Central Washington, overlooking the Columbia River. It is very much worth a visit. However, I am acknowledging John Paul in this paragraph, not Sam Hill, as he did nothing to help me with this book.

The book would not have been written were it not for the undying support of my wife, Dianne. For years, she kept telling me "you are a great writer. You need to write something." Years of psychiatric services and antidepressants would not get her to cease and desist. Most importantly, she is the only person who reliably laughs at my jokes.

Donna Jensen is a remarkable person. For many years she has been my lay teacher and advisor, guiding me with her deep wisdom, encouraging me through difficult times, and assuring me that my stars are aligned to give me a chance for good results. Sometimes, if we are lucky, the more mothers the better.

The picture on the cover of this book was taken by Drenda Morey. She and her husband Mike are very long-standing patients of mine. She states that she loves me, and I definitely love her. She and Mike are pure and fine. The picture was taken on my last day in my Bellevue office, after 37 years. I met Drenda when she was a young woman, when I was taking care of her sick mother. She is representative of all of my patients past and present to whom I am eternally grateful for their trust and for their willingness to be intimate with me. They have been my great teachers, more than all of the eminent professors, by far.

Lastly, I acknowledge another person and family whom I have never met, Christian Cameron Wright, and his parents Cameron and Tiana. They shared their grief over the loss of their six-month old child by placing a picture of his beautiful face in the newspaper. I keep this picture above my desk to remind me of the fragility of life, the beauty and innocence of children everywhere, and of the child within everyone, and of all sentient creatures.

PROLOGUE

The Paradoxes of Biologic Systems

L ife is full of paradoxes. As one begins to break out of the illusion of certainty and of seeing the world in terms of black and white, what we truly think we know to be bedrock truth is culturally defined—and the more the paradoxes of life emerge.

Living stuff itself, that is things endowed with life forces, are fundamentally paradoxical. It is abundant, pleomorphic, and enduring in one form or another. Paradoxically, it is exceedingly fragile. The paleontological record attests to numerous previous mass extinctions. In our times, we are seeing a massive die-off of species to rival other mass extinctions but now studied in great detail. Often, it appears to be that relatively slight perturbations in the environment of a given species can lead to the Armageddon of that unfortunate group of creatures. Are we destined to be one of them?

Modern day humans are not immune to these same environmental occurrences. Our bodies have truly amazing self-healing capabilities. Take a very straight forward example: A gash, through the skin and into the deeper tissues, left alone under most circumstances will restore itself to normality in a short period of time. What is not often appreciated is the extremely complex cascade of processes that work in precise coordination to bring this about naturally, without even the need for conscious thought. Alternatively, our experiences in life repeatedly demonstrate to us in glaring fashion that either by accident or illness, life can be snuffed out in an instant.

The Illusion of Invulnerability

Unfortunately, the march of remarkable advances in medical science has created an illusion of invulnerability. It tends to lull us into a state of thinking that such advances will always save us, pulling us back from the brink of the abyss. Please consider an overlooked fact, simple but of great importance: It is much easier to stay alive than it is to stay healthy. Stop and think about this for just a moment. To stay healthy requires a conscious effort, a plan, a conscious application of the plan, and luck. Recall the pundit, whose identity is lost in the mists of history, who told us "It's better to be lucky than smart."

To stay healthy, we need a plan, and we need commitment. It's never too early, or too late to start. The journey is difficult. The rewards are worth the effort, many times over.

The Illusion of Certainty and the Bell-Shaped Curve—Homo Sapiens Sapiens—Seekers of Knowledge:

It has been stated many times that knowledge is power. Of course, knowledge is relative and subject to interpretation. Yet some knowledge, any knowledge, enables a person to have a deeper understanding, and at least the ability to ask the right questions. It is hoped that the "knowledge" presented in these pages can act as a catalyst for you to examine what you want, what you need, and how to get it.

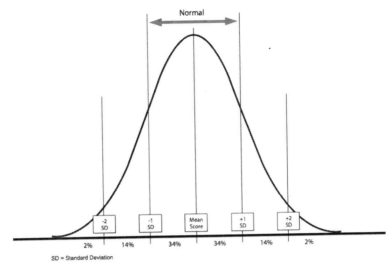

Bell-Shaped Curve.
1 standard deviation =67%; 2 standard deviations =97%

We humans are desperate seekers of knowledge. It is so declared in our name. It is built into us, just as sniffing the fire hydrant is built into our canine companions. We want to know. We are driven to categorize, to organize, to box concepts, all of which is an attempt to endow us with at least the appearance, if not the fact, that we understand something better.

We all have a team of individuals whom we consult at various times and ask advice. Certainly, we do this with doctors. I doubt that many doctors would ever present this next concept to you, or even think about it. But it is a very important concept, simple yet complex, elegant and profound. At one time or another, most of us have seen a rendition of this. It is the concept of the bell-shaped curve.

Medical data, just as biological and sociological data, can be described in terms of probability. One standard deviation on each side of the median is considered to be medically "normal." The second standard deviation away from the median merges into "abnormal," whether describing something as simple as body height, or more complicated such as the potential for a positive response of a certain type to a certain form of treatment. Please note that 4.2% of the population, although technically "abnormal," may be functioning in a satisfactory manner. Lastly, the far reaches of both sides of the curve, comprising 0.3% of the population, clearly boxed into the "abnormal" designation, may respond in remarkable and unpredictable ways to the certain type of treatment mentioned above. Such a response could appear to be "miraculous," or simply the normal biologic response for that small group of people. When doctors describe the likelihood or unlikelihood of something happening or not happening, patients can take or leave that advice. It is simply based on statistical likelihood and other unknown factors influencing the possibility of a good outcome "against the odds."

The Illusion of Cause and Effect

Medicine and doctors have always been embedded in the prevailing culture. Acquisition of medical knowledge is subject to the same endemic biases associated with the generation of any other type of "knowing."

Another example of our inherent drive to know is our heavy reliance on the observation of two events linked in time or space. The immediate inclination is to declare that one caused the other. In the recent past, for example, the appearance of the witch in the community caused the crop failure. Light the fire! Such linkages occur numerous times every day in our lives. However, even our distant predecessors realized that *cum hoc ergo propter hoc*; two events occurring together are not necessarily representative of a cause-and-effect phenomenon. That is, correlation does not imply causation. This concept has become an important part of our legal justice system. Yet patients, and yes, even doctors make these potential mistakes frequently. Hopefully, the doctor has enough knowledge to filter through this, but that is not always the case. It never hurts to remove the blinders and take a second or third look. In medicine this is called creating a "differential diagnosis," that is, a list of possible explanations for the problem.

The Illusion of Separation: Ego and Greed

The concept of me, me-first and only-me, will be discussed later in detail. This sense of absolute separation is perhaps the root of all of our problems. It comes from the so-called ego, in turn a function of the so-called reptilian brain. This plays out in a multitude of ways, many of which could be defined as variations of greed. Patients and doctors both enter into the relationship with these partially or totally subconscious forces at work. For instance, the patient's one-sided need for an approbation or legitimization may require him or her to demand a series of expensive tests. These are usually paid for by someone else. The doctor sees the patient as a potential annuity, capable of providing steady income for years to come. Sadly, this occurs every day in the patient-doctor relationship. We need to do much better in this respect. Until universal greed is controlled, the need to watch your pocketbook will remain a sad fact of human interaction.

The Ultimate Finish Line—Death— and How to Get There Gracefully

"Certainty? In the world nothing is certain but death and taxes." (*Benjamin Franklin*).

As is true for any ingenious quip, there are numerous ways that this can be interpreted. The element of sarcasm is difficult to miss. Sarcasm, although frequently humorous on the surface, carries an element of bitterness, frustration, or resentment. Perhaps our relationship with taxes hasn't changed much in the last two hundred and forty years. I suspect that as soon as we had representation (for the taxes) that we fought for, we likely did our best to avoid paying them. Even a superficial examination of the historical record tends to verify how remarkably similar were the issues and problems hotly debated and dealt with centuries ago, with those present right now. First presented in *Ecclesiastes*, "nothing new under the sun" seems to ring true.

I suspect that concerns about death were much more on the surface in the late eighteenth century than they are now. Death then was visible everywhere. People's lives were lived in close proximity to animals whose short life spans, rough treatment, and slaughter in full view of the many was an aspect largely not encountered in modern times. Infant and maternal mortality was an everyday experience. Epidemics and plagues wiped out large populations quickly.

Death is now largely hidden from us. The carnage of wars such as our Civil War was a great boon for the mortuary business, as thousands of unclaimed bodies littered the battlefields. Animals are now slaughtered in factory farms, their abject misery and suffering carefully hidden from us. Our loved ones, both human and animal, are dealt with by professionals. As Woody Allen expressed it, "I'm not afraid of dying. I just don't want to be there when it happens." Closed casket ceremonies are the norm. In addition, life expectancy has risen dramatically, giving us nearly forty more years than that available in Franklin's time.

Lastly, consider a trick that the mind plays on us. Isn't there a glimmer of a notion deep in the recesses of our thinking that death is somehow something that happens to somebody other than us? Isn't there a very private, albeit absurd, notion that through some minuscule crack in the fabric of reality that we will escape this fate? My own experience has reinforced this observation countless times. As I cautiously begin to broach the topic now termed "end of life issues" with patients who are clearly pre-terminally ill, with a list of serious diagnoses twice the length of an average grocery list, I am often presented with a look of dumb-founded surprise. If I could read that person's mind, the response would be, "You're not talking about me, are you?"

This recently occurred to me during the last hospitalization of a 94-year-old woman, who angrily looked at me and shouted, "I am not going to die!" Unfortunately for her, she died at home two weeks later. I say unfortunately because in my opinion, she is representative of the majority of people who die an unconscious death. In other words, she missed the main purpose of life, which is to become conscious; to awaken. Their tenacious hanging on "for dear life" acts as an impediment towards openness and potential for a very high level of connectedness. What could be construed as a brave fight against all odds can deteriorate into a cowardly act of blind stubbornness, leaving all those left behind wishing for something richer. We desperately need to learn how to die better.

Every day presents us with countless choices. Health care is no different. We make choices about health-related issues minute-by-minute. Some of these appear to be overtly "good" and some overtly "bad." Each person maintains a high level of autonomy in making these decisions, right up until the moment of crossing the finish line. It appears to me that it is less important that the decisions appear to be right or wrong, than that they be made consciously, with awareness of potential consequences and ramifications involving the individual and other people. No blaming; especially not of oneself. Perhaps with forethought and luck, crossing the line can be an anticipated release with no regrets. Read on and familiarize yourself with choices and consequences.

Are Doctors Really Different from Used-Car Salesmen?

Historically, with a few dips in popularity, for the most part doctors have been held in high esteem by their contemporaries. Historians are haunted by the notion that history is written by the victors, or the literate, or the wealthy, or the exceptional. The point is that even sophisticated approaches looking at the philosophy of history, or the history of history, have been unable to dispel the concern that the vast majority of common people have been voiceless (of course, this is referring to the pre-texting, pre-e-mailing, pre-blogging, pre-twittering era, etc., where anyone can say anything to vast masses of people). For instance, as is well known, the Romans excelled in many areas of human achievement. For those who might be interested, it is relatively easy to find details regarding commerce, governmental functioning, warfare and other activities in astonishingly great detail. However, what did people do on a daily basis? What did they eat? How many hours did they work? What did they say to each other? Did they take vacations? This type of daily routine of the masses is much more difficult to delineate. In some way, the archeological findings of the Vesuvian catastrophe can give us more information than any written document. Obviously, most people were illiterate, thus leaving the documentation to the educated and wealthy elite.

So, for most eras we don't know how people went about doctoring, or how they felt about doctors on a personal basis. Over the last five hundred years, this information has come to light, and doctors have generally fared well. Once again, recall the obvious fact that doctors are embedded in society. Questions regarding doctors' ethics, motivations, goals, ambitions and other subjective qualities have not, and likely cannot, be studied scientifically. Everyone is entitled to their own opinion, in such matters that are not provable.

In my opinion, as an "insider," doctors are not much different than the mass of their contemporaries. I think that they score slightly above average in terms of empathy, compassion, self-sacrifice, and honesty. This should give one the confidence to allow themselves to be vulnerable, as patients. However, I also see two major limitations. First, the difference between doctors and others is relatively small. Recall that in a wide variety of human contests, the difference between the winner and the losers is usually a very few percentage points, or a few milliseconds or millimeters. Secondly, the doctor-to-doctor difference can be huge; that is, Doctor A, a great humanitarian, and Doctor B next door, a selfish con-artist.

For the record, don't be afraid to buy a used car. In my professional and personal experience, I have met used-car salespeople worthy of your trust. The same can be said for doctors.

SECTION I

BARRIERS TO GOOD HEALTH

FEAR (OF BAD NEWS)

Bodily abuse and enormous concern about the state of the body is another one of those paradoxes. Few people look forward to reprimands. Many people anticipate reprimands when going to see the doctor. Behavior of doctors and patients is as diverse as any other biologic parameter. Should a doctor reprimand (take a parental approach)? Commiserate (take a partnership approach)? Plead (take a childlike approach)? All three of those approaches are right or wrong for the individual patient. Perhaps the best answer is that the doctor's skill-set should include an instantaneous assessment as to which approach is most likely to be successful for which patient personality profile. Although possible, and utilized with great panache by some doctors, most are lacking in such psychological prowess.

The end result is that doctors are fearful and tentative in many encounters, just as are patients. The Tower Cancer Research Foundation has stated that 13% of cancer patients postponed seeing the doctor because of fear of being told they had cancer. "Hope, fear, procrastination, and lack of medical insurance" were all deemed to be important impediments.

In recent years, the phenomenon of "White Coat Hypertension" has attracted much attention. Although a great deal has been learned about this phenomenon, the full spectrum understanding and application of it is still not clear. It refers most strictly to the appearance of high blood pressure, when taken by a medical person in a white coat. Of course, it also applies to high blood pressure in the doctor's office, taken by any medical person even without a white coat. It can also occur outside of the doctor's office. Finally, it can even occur when the patient takes their own blood pressure. Obviously, the common denominator is that application of a blood pressure cuff to the arm of a susceptible individual can cause blood pressure to rise. As common as this is, its exact incidence has not been easy to assess. In one large study done in 1999 and published in the *American Journal of Hypertension*, in a general medical clinic, it was deemed to have an incidence of 39%. The underlying factor provoking this fascinating response is thought to be anxiety.

The conclusion is that fear or anxiety can have a large impact upon the willingness of an individual to subject themselves to medical scrutiny. Despite open discussions in the media about medical topics, as well as advertising by cancer clinics, heart clinics, and others about how compassionate and gentle their approach is purported to be, this will likely continue to be a barrier. Lurking behind this fear, whether generated by the doctor or projected on to him or her by the patient's own psyche, lies a sad fact. The patient apparently detects a basic disinterest of the doctor or a distrust that the doctor can be comforting and supportive. Too often as children, we have been dealt with harshly and have been left feeling absolutely shattered and abandoned. These traumas become indelibly stamped into our psyche and may return to haunt us at crucial times. For the doctor, they must strive to always do their best to provide the ambiance of a safe haven.

COMPLEXITY OF MODERN LIFE/ MULTITASKING

The age in which we live has taken on any number of names, referring to different aspects of the astounding access to information available to us. The gigantic leaps in the availability of information with previous technological advances (such as the printing press) in some ways appear to be a dwarfed by the sheer numbers of people with whom we can communicate. The Age of Communication and the Age of Information appear to be two sides of the same coin. We are flooded with information to the extent that it becomes even more difficult to sort out the valuable from the useless.

Multitasking has for many people become a means of survival. We have so many tasks, some old and some new, now mixed into any number of combinations. Doing two, or three, or more (?) things in a simultaneous time span has become commonplace. The implication, although often implicit, is that multitasking is a positive attribute, symbolic of achieving competence in everyday life.

The question as to whether this is true or not may be raised here but will not be debated at this juncture. All that can be stated is that multi-tasking is a reflection of competence in the modern world. I don't think many people would debate that. What can be debated is whether proficiency in this arena results in an underdevelopment of some other attribute of modern life, such that the loss exceeds the gain. Here is a sad example. Once or twice per day, an encounter with a patient is interrupted not by me, but by their cell phone. Even more incredibly, most of the time, the call is apologetically answered. Those awkward moments have a high potential to scuttle any degree of intimacy between patient and doctor.

Besides interrupting a patient after fifteen seconds, some doctors are repeatedly interrupted by their staff. If so, I suggest you find another doctor. It is true that we sleep less now, work longer hours, and frequently feel time constraints. This sets up a barrier to good health by a number of avenues. Many of us are getting less sleep than we need for optimal health. This itself can be the generator of a list of health issues including propensity for accidents, hypertension, diabetes, poor performance at work or school, and many others, to be discussed later. We are called upon to operate under conditions which are far too stressful to be considered optimal. Stress is documented to be a major factor in suboptimal functioning of, or even breakdown of the immune system.

Try to simplify your life. This may require courageous changes, including those which may reduce income. Set aside a time to "detoxify" in whatever way seems right. Great armies in history have fallen because of over extending their supply lines. Take time to replenish, to re-supply yourself, in any way that feels good. Program this into your schedule. You must do this, or you may not be able to carry on your mission.

PATIENT-GENERATED APATHY/ DYSTHYMIA

As stated by Thoreau so poignantly, "The mass of men lead lives of quiet desperation." It has been stated that law enforcement personnel and medical workers see the worst traits of people. The former obviously see the results of absolute selfishness, me at all cost, and unbridled violence against others. The latter see a more subdued type of recklessness or inattention, partially directed at self, and often self-destructive, but clearly observable nonetheless. So once again, I admit sampling bias is generated.

However, in my daily dealings with people, I agree with Thoreau. People in the presence of a doctor may allow themselves a certain level of openness, that may not occur elsewhere. The frequency with which deep dissatisfaction is presented is very high. The causes of such are as many and varied as are the natures of the people manifesting them. The point is that feelings of unhappiness, dissatisfaction, and even desperation are ubiquitous. I personally feel most saddened when I perceive the situation clearly by their own description, perceive the solution, but also perceive that the unhappy person is so fixed in a state of rightness and intransigence that nothing is likely to change the dynamics. There are also many ways to indicate to the listener (me) that my advice is not being solicited. I am serving the purpose of hearing the cause for their misery and allowing them to decompress before going ballistic. Sometimes the space left for a response allows for no more than the generic "relationships are often very difficult."

Perhaps all is not lost. There is likely some slight therapeutic benefit in simply codifying and voicing the displeasure. At least it does nakedly identify it. This type of interaction is built-in regarding discussions of "depression" and the role of antidepressants. Of course the antidepressant will not bring back the loved one or the retirement income, but just talking about it may help, a little. The doctor may feel intensely uncomfortable without a clear solution, and the patient may sense this. A solution need not be outlined right then. Arbitrary advice given on a few tidbits of information is unlikely to hit the mark. A sympathetic ear from the doctor or anyone else is helpful.

At best, this is very tough going for both the patient and the doctor. Most of us think we have an idea of what depression is and feels like, and this will be discussed later. Dysthymia is different than depression and is much more common. It is a deep dissatisfaction, usually spanning a number of areas of a person's life. The person knows that the doctor cannot fix this. Perhaps they are concerned that the doctor will see it, even if it isn't openly discussed. All of the variety of symptoms which can accompany dysthymia, some of which may be unrelated and independently important may thus not come to medical attention. Finally, the dysthymia may be so severe as to give the patient the notion that, "Frankly, my Dear, I don't give a damn." In other words, the appointment to see the doctor is never made. Going to see the doctor is a little like going to your twenty-fifth high school reunion, in that you don't want to be perceived as a failure. Being dysthymic is perceived as a failure. Why do we greet someone with, "Good morning! How are you?" The response is always "Fine!" when a more honest answer would be "Miserable, lonely, irritable, angry, and I wish you hadn't asked." Let's train ourselves to refrain from the "How are you?" It is reflexive and inauthentic, and it increases the sense of alienation in the person saying, "Fine." Most of us are not "fine," much of the time.

Please note the obvious. The barriers to good health overlap substantially. They are different aspects of a problem which in its broadest sense has to do with trust, and to a lesser extent, intimacy. Our basic sense of distrust, stemming from early childhood dealings with family and others, drives us in the direction of perfecting social skills of glibness and superficiality, the killers of intimacy. These attributes unfortunately and invariably lead to further disappointment.

Is there an antidote for glibness and superficiality? The answer is, "yes, of course," involving an approach of a different kind. Our disappointments result in a reflexive response of pulling inward, based on the assumption that we are not loveable or desirable. The antidote is hidden in the depth of ourselves. Awakening to our lovability via the path of humble lovingness of ourselves, despite our warts, is the crucial first step. All but a very few of us have something which is loveable (Hitler was a vegetarian and loved animals), or cute, desirable, or beneficial to others. If you cannot think of anything loveable about yourself, look at a picture of you as a baby, or small child, in all of your beautiful innocence. That is it! Self love leads to self esteem, which leads to the ability to receive and transmit lovingness. Study a picture of you in your bell-bottom plaid slacks, trying to conform because you needed to fit in and feel accepted. If nothing has worked, try to identify one living creature in your life who unquestionably loves you. That can kick-start the process. Extension of that love outwards is the antidote. Lovingness, love given, and received is always the antidote. Alternately, start from scratch. A commitment to do anything for the betterment of any sentient being, or any worthwhile cause, immediately enriches the world. Starting is the most difficult task. Starting with lovingness in your heart for yourself is your ticket to success.

DOCTOR-GENERATED APATHY/ DYSTHYMIA

Many of the limitations of patients, summarized as being involved with aspects of trust and intimacy, apply to doctors as well. Apathy and dysthymia, as noted, are exceedingly common in medical practice, in one study clearly identifiable in twenty-two percent of people seen in a primary care clinic. There is no reason to expect that doctors are any better off than the general population. In fact, a number of surveys have shown that amongst the "professional" contingent of our population, physician job satisfaction is generally lower than most. Other studies have indicated that doctor's perception of job stress has increased dramatically over the last 20 years. All of this has to do with long hours, decreasing pay, and threats of even deeper cuts to specialists, reduced autonomy, increased scrutiny, increased frequency of medical malpractice claims, and many others. In some surveys, up to forty percent of doctors would not again choose medicine as a career. Suicide rates for male physicians are forty percent higher than the general public, and the rates for female physicians are remarkably twice as high (two hundred percent) as the general population!

Need more be said? The person that you meet in the doctor's office, with all of the factors listed above, may be a person who feels under siege. Meeting such a person is a huge barrier to good health. You may only be scheduled for a ten or fifteen minute visit, another huge barrier. Even if he or she is still passionate about medicine, any combination of sleep deprivation, patient overload, running late, and other factors can act as barriers to effective care. Long hours need to be cut back. On the other hand, decreasing pay to specialists is a good thing and will eventually pay dividends. Reduced autonomy is somewhat of an illusion, but needs to be accepted, whether illusory or not. Patient overload is particularly prevalent in large clinics with very high overhead. Doctors can be proactive in these types of situations, by creating situations with intrinsically lower overhead. Return of the empowered PCP, with much higher pay scale and much reduced workload is essential to the mental health of all doctors.

MALPRACTICE CRISIS

So what can you do about the beleaguered doctor? As just mentioned, many of the barriers overlap, and several will be discussed later. Each of the listed problems can be dealt with individually. Some will demand complicated solutions. Others are relatively easy to deal with. The one that comes to mind immediately is one often talked about--and usually just as quickly shelved. This has to do with what can be called the malpractice crisis. You the patient (consumer) need to get on board with this. This is a win-win situation for you and your doctor. Accurate data regarding medical malpractice is very difficult to obtain, as the bias factor is high. A few published figures can be quoted. Seven percent of psychiatrists are sued each year. Eighty-nine percent of OB/GYN doctors have been sued during their careers. We also know that only about 10% of jury trials are won by the plaintiff. The average doctor is sued every eight years.

I fully concede that my bias, from the inside looking out, is that medical malpractice reform is desperately needed for several reasons. The ease with which a doctor can be sued is a barrier to medical care. Doctors are aware of their vulnerability in this regard, and it cannot help but heighten the barrier to trust and intimacy, already mentioned, which obviously must be mutual to be most effective. It drives many doctors into early retirement at a time when they are needed to pitch in and be part of a solution. Part of the solution is getting the load of patient visits down, and time of the actual visits up. This is very difficult to accomplish in the current climate, and every early retirement based on malpractice concern is a loss for patients and doctors.

As noted, for the most part, doctors work long hours and want to be helpful. First of all, "the patient" represents a biological system. Such systems are enormously complex and unpredictable. I have been called upon to review many cases of impending litigation, as an expert witness for both plaintiff and defense attorneys. I have testified for plaintiffs on a few occasions, but much less often than for defendants. However, my involvement with all of these cases has convinced me that although there was a bad outcome, it almost invariably occurred in a very complex setting. It usually appears to me that the doctor did not make a clear-cut "mistake," but that a decision made turned out to be incorrect. I see a clear-cut difference between an act of ignorance or negligence versus a freely-made decision based on good reason, good conscience, and good intention. Please note that I review medical malpractice issues related to pulmonary medicine, and that my experience is in that area alone. What I see is a wide gap between patient-family expectations and medical realpolitik. In other words, in the cases I have reviewed, far too much is expected medically from patients and families most of the time.

Secondly, fear of medical malpractice has a huge effect on driving up the cost of medical care. This topic falls under the category of "defensive medicine." As I work in the trenches every day, I can attest unequivocally that a substantial portion of the tests that I order are to limit my legal exposure. How much? I can only guess, but perhaps thirty to fifty percent. In the emergency room setting, the figure is likely much higher. Please note also that every test ordered, including simple blood tests let alone "invasive" studies which are intrinsically much more dangerous, can reveal findings which are irrelevant, but which in and of themselves may require investigation. These investigations can even lead to biopsies and surgeries! So what starts out as the need to be "thorough" ends up being a self-perpetuating chase, that drastically expands the cost of medical care and also places the patient at risk of serious iatrogenic (doctor induced) complications. This is an uncompromisingly nasty situation, which is rarely helpful and can end in a lose-lose result.

The alternative to defensive medicine has already been alluded to. It starts with a detailed history and a careful examination. It may not need to go further than that. The risk for the patient from a history and exam is nil. The doctor needs time to accomplish this most basic tool of medical practice. The less time available for a thorough history and physical, the more testing that will follow. Certainly a blood panel might be expected, as a large amount of information can be obtained from a simple needle stick at a moderately low cost. After the results are available to doctor and patient, they may wish to reconvene to go over results and discuss whether further testing is urgently needed, or whether a period of observation can be undertaken (weeks to months). Alternatively a "clinical trial" may be recommended, whereby the patient undergoes some kind of trial with medication, or auxiliary treatment, again awaiting the response over weeks to months.

All of this is contingent upon the doctor having enough time to do the proper history and physical, review all of the findings, and create a plan. It is contingent upon the patient having a deep sense that this thoughtful process is being carried out with his or her best interest at the very center of the whole process. If these basic criteria are not met, then the process can gradually spiral out of control with referrals to other doctors (who will likely do further tests, performed by them), rapid escalation of costs, increasing frustration on the part of all concerned, and possible emergence of incidental information (a "spot" on the x-ray or scan far removed from the area of concern) mandating further workup and more specialists. This is the modus operandi of the medical system in the midst of a "malpractice crisis". It is a lose (doctor loses credibility), lose (patient loses confidence in the leadership of the medical team and becomes susceptible to iatrogenic problems), lose (society "loses" larger amounts of money) situation. It happens every day, multiple times. It needs to be stopped.

As long as doctors and patients interact, every once in a while a mistake of great magnitude will be made, and a patient will be harmed. The doctor will likely be mortified and suffer a great deal of angst for his or her oversight. The best term to describe a true malpractice event, in my opinion, is negligence. This comes from the word neglect. This term implies a carelessness. So, when carelessness enters into the doctor-patient relationship, the doctor becomes appropriately vulnerable to sanction. To me, there is a huge difference between the doctor proceeding carefully, but making a wrong decision, and the doctor having been careless, meaning "I don't care" enough to be careful.

Effective malpractice reform would go a long way toward relieving the dysthymia in the medical profession and would represent a gift from patients to their doctors to improve working conditions for this beleaguered group of professionals. The only real losers would be trial attorneys, advertising openly on television and other media. You would still be able to sue a doctor who demonstrates negligence, i.e., neglect, i.e., carelessness, i.e., "I don't care enough to be careful."

As of January 2012, this topic, which would cost the taxpayer nothing, was once again omitted from the largest health care reform bill in the last 40 years.

CORPORATE TAKEOVER

There is a well-developed culture within the medical community that poses, "Doctors make terrible businessmen." It is so pervasive that it is likely true. Granted, any given medical community may have its relatively short list of doctors who functioned in practice, just like everyone else for perhaps 10 years, and then drifted off into the business world, sometimes maintaining a small practice and more often abandoning it completely. These individuals tend to be financially very successful, and may, through their expertise, help some of their colleagues improve their financial pictures. Some of these people lose, or give up, the "doctor aura" which can leave their ex-colleagues wondering why they made a career detour through medical school in the first place. Some of them take positions as administrators or even CEOs of large medically-oriented corporations so that for this subset, the "MD" after their name is likely a career-enhancing emblem.

Given that doctors consider themselves to be poor business people, the origins of this likely rest in the notion that at least historically, doctors as a whole do have an element, or degree of altruism above and beyond that shared by other professionals. In other words, at least early in their careers, they are driven by altruistic ideals to help patients, sacrifice, and believe that financial rewards are a much lesser consideration. Unfortunately, as the demands of paying very high overhead bills, family and personal needs, pressure to keep up with the extravagant Dr. Jones, difficulties paying off medical school debt, and the daily grind of trying to manage a small army of employees mount, the landscape changes drastically and quickly. Use of an "office manager" may temporarily help. However, with constant turnover of personnel, deteriorating esprit de corps, and even threatened law suits from former employees, the doctor desperately looks for an alternative.

Once again, in the era of Dr. Goldstein (not exactly prehistoric times), the vast majority of doctors practiced solo or in small groups of two or three. When I began practice in 1974, this was still true but beginning to change. Within the last fifteen to twenty years, the change has been revolutionary. The solo practitioner or small group is now the distinct minority. Groups have become progressively larger and more diverse, and groups have merged with other groups, and more and more mergers. Presently, it is not at all unusual in metropolitan areas to find groups with hundreds, if not a thousand doctors, scattered over a wide geographic area.

The attraction is the notion that the bigger the army, the more powerful the force. Big groups can bargain with insurance companies. They can advertise widely; they can pay for vacations and continuing medical education events. And of course, they completely relieve the doctor of administrative hassles, which are now dealt with by people with masters or doctorate degrees in business administration or health administration.

If it sounds too good to be true, it may be so. Despite attempts to get a clear picture about which system works best, that is solo versus larger group practice, there are too many variables, differences in structure from group to group, reporting biases, and local peculiarities to arrive at convincing data in this regard. It is not clear whether medical practice overhead of 60 to 70% is inherent in all practice settings, or more common in some rather than others. It is even less clear because of the subjective nature of the question as to whether or not doctors are happier, or function better in one environment or another. Doctors are competitive, this being another internal conclusion about self, or "We couldn't have gotten through medical school." They want to be treated fairly and rewarded just like anyone else. All it takes for doctor-A to become bitter and unhappy is to learn that colleague-B in mega group-C is only working half-time, or only seeing half the patients that he or she is seeing while making the same income!

Sorry! Corporate sets the financial policies and negotiates with individual members. Corporate tells you how many patients you must see in an hour or a day. Corporate may dictate almost every aspect of the way the doctor practices. It is not unusual, in some practices, to have return patients booked for 10 minutes (on-the-dot) appointments. The dictum "One appointment—One issue" becomes a necessity. This is a big barrier to good health.

Should we, as a society, go backwards? Would that be better? We must all take responsibility for what has evolved. If doctors and patients are unhappy with these trends, it is up to them to change it. Recall that you, the public, are now termed consumers. Corporate policies arise out of perceived consumer needs. Perhaps consumers, i.e., patients' needs, are really no different than they were in 1940, and the rise of corporate medicine is strictly a doctor-generated phenomenon. If this is true, these patients still hold the hammer, although it may be somewhat of a small and flimsy one. If you are dissatisfied with corporate medicine and the 10-minute visit, you can explore alternatives. Although it may be difficult to envision the clinic of two hundred doctors dissolving into two hundred solo practices. Such a drastic change may not be needed to meet your needs. Societal constraints have a quality of aliveness, implying responsiveness to environmental factors and pressures. It can be difficult to argue with the premise that ultimately, in a democracy, for better or worse, we get what we want. The question then becomes, "is what we want what we need?" That concept will be dredged up again, as you move along through this tour.

DESYCHRONIZATION OF SUPPLY AND DEMAND: THE COMPARTMENTALIZATION OF MEDICAL CARE

Recall that in my introduction of Dr. Goldstein, I pointed out that he was a "GP," that is, general practitioner. He was trained and licensed to do almost everything medical. Often, these people identified themselves as "Physicians and Surgeons." That just about covered it, save for brain surgery.

DOCTOR: "What can I help you with, Mr. Magoo?"

PATIENT: "Doctor, I have this stabbing pain in my penis. And it sometimes causes my testicle to swell."

DOCTOR: "I beg your pardon, Mr. Magoo. What did you say? I am a little hard of hearing."

PATIENT: "I'm embarrassed. It's my penis and my testicle."

DOCTOR: "Mr. Magoo, I think you have come to the wrong place. I am a neurologist, not a urologist!"

PATIENT: "I'm very sorry doctor. I didn't mean to insult you."

Perhaps medical practice and medical knowledge has become too complex for the likes of Dr. Goldstein. The county medical society to which I belong lists 142 specialty areas. It is easy to see why patients might have difficulty choosing the correct doctor, particularly if their "PCP" (primary care provider), which is the contemporary offspring of the GP, does not have a new patient opening for eight weeks.

Basically, in the broadest sense, and perhaps the silliest sense, practitioners are divided into those that are "cognitive" versus those that are "interventional" or "surgical". The implication is that the cognitive disciplines, such as family practice, pediatrics, internal medicine, and psychiatry just sit around and think about your problem, while the interventionalist will have you prepped, draped, and fixed, as soon as you can produce your insurance card. If you are really astute, you might note that the cognitive group includes the major component of the PCP contingent, while the interventional group includes all of the surgeons and surgical subspecialists, as well as radiology, anesthesiology, many medical subspecialties, and interventional pain management groups.

What you probably would not intuit is that the PCP group is on the lowest end of the physician pay scale, and the highest end of the paperwork scale (non-remunerative work). The surgical contingent, as well as internal medicine subspecialties like cardiology and gastroenterology, is on the highest end of the physician pay scale and lowest end of the paperwork scale. So, if you were a medical student, running up a debt of $120,000 over four years in medical school, what specialties might attract you the most? As can be surmised, we see a strong, steady trend away from primary care specialties. Previously, positions in internal medicine training programs were highly contested, with most programs filling their slots quickly. Now, even some of the most prestigious programs do not fill, at least not with US-trained personnel. The reverse is true for the high-paying, "prestigious" interventional specialties and subspecialties, filling their quotas quickly and consistently.

Both research data, and simple observations of practice patterns, strongly indicate that in most circumstances, contact with and evaluation by the PCP is statistically most likely to improve care and save health care dollars. The bottleneck, of course is access and time. Fewer PCPs are available. Those who haven't burned out yet are booked up, seeing 30 patients per day. Does the patient have a PCP? Can the PCP see the patient on short notice? Will the PCP see the patient based on their schedule and anticipated remuneration? Is the PCP already experiencing burnout? Is the PCP available per telephone during times when the office is not open? If these criteria are not met, the worried patient will likely proceed to the emergency room. This scenario plays itself out repeatedly in almost every community. The results on fragmentation of care, and cost of care, are staggering. Emergency room medicine will be discussed in some detail later. Once in the ER, the physician in charge may or may not call the PCP. Perhaps the PCP is simply not available. Reports may or may not filter back to the PCP in the days and weeks ahead. The patient may or may not be kept in the hospital, and may or may not be seen by one or several specialists. These consultations may or may not get back to the PCP. After hospitalization, the patient may have to have an interim stay at a "Rehab Unit" (previously called nursing home). Another new doctor is called in for that. That confinement may or may not be transmitted to the PCP. If the patient eventually makes an elective appointment with the PCP several weeks to months later, after seeing the ER doctor, being admitted to the hospitalist team and seeing several of them, discharged and follow-up with one or several of the newly assigned specialists, a Rehab Unit doctor, and finally a trip to the PCP, it cannot be difficult to imagine that this patient has been victimized by compartmentalization of medical care.

Is this scenario a problem? Is this what we want? If we truly care to "fix" the system, is this an arena that we can restructure or reinforce? As stated repeatedly under the topic of barriers to care, this is our system! We, as doctors and patients can change it, if we so desire. As one might presume, since this topic is listed under "barriers," it is likely that my own opinion (biased) is apparent. So, why don't I just say it? Okay. This system, involving serpentine fragmentation of medical care, is a big problem. In other words, the system is broken.

If this were acknowledged, the solution could be relatively easily ignited, setting off a forest fire of change. We need a great increase in primary care physicians, remunerated at the top of the physician pay scale, with the necessary paper work cut dramatically, or reimbursable. A PCP worth his or her responsibility should likely not see more than 10 to 15 patients per day (instead of 20 to 40). To make up for this increased payout to PCPs, salaries to all the others, including surgery and its subspecialties (ophthalmology, ENT, urology, vascular, orthopedics, and many others), anesthesiology, and most of the medical subspecialties (cardiology, gastroenterology, pulmonary, oncology, and others) should be substantially cut sequentially, to ensure a steady supply.

Would this type of change resurrect Dr. Goldstein? The answer is no. As I stated, he died years ago. He would never do your prostate removal, major cancer surgery, cataract removal, coronary bypass and many, many other interventions. However, the careful, thoughtful, meticulous coordination and direction of care provided by him or her would help bring the pendulum back towards its normal place of rest. It would go a very long way towards making you feel connected and cared for. It would likely resurrect feelings of affection between patient and doctor. So, although Dr. Goldstein could not return to the climate he left, he could return to take the reins as the true head of the medical team, respected by his colleagues, well remunerated, more relaxed, enjoying his or her work, and doing everything possible to ensure your good health. This dreamlike configuration of the medical landscape is not only possible, it is not really that difficult. Do we really want it? How badly do we want it? Achieving it will certainly require rattling of a few cages that should have been rattled long ago.

FINANCIAL STRESSORS

Commerce is the life-blood of civilization. It is likely that trading of goods and services commenced long before true civilization arose. Life for early humans became so rapidly complex that few individuals had the skill or inclination to be totally independent. By the time formal civilization made its appearance 5,000 years ago, such people felt secure or insecure partially based on establishment of, or lack of, trade agreements with neighboring people. The same pattern is strikingly evident at the present time.

Medical services are not very different than any other service. People value it, or devalue it to whatever level their experiences and personal finances dictate. Modern-day medical insurance companies are well aware of this, as reflected in the universal application of deductable expenses and co-pays. Obviously, their perspective is that the less it costs the consumer, the more that medical service will be used. By manipulating costs to the consumer, they expect to inhibit usage of the service, thus improving their bottom line.

Generally speaking, medical services have been thought to be relatively recession-proof. This is somewhat true. No matter how hard we may try, there are too many variables to keep us away from doctors all of the time. However, there is always some leeway, and in fact, likely often. Should I see the doctor or not? All the considerations buzz around the brain, and the answer pops out. What is obvious is that the answer that pops out will likely be affected by the specifics of the deductible arrangement and the level of co-pay. The trend has been to see an increasing level of deductible expenses, designed to inhibit medical expenditures by shifting the burden of payment to the patient. The reward is a variably lower cost of the policy. Deductible policies into the thousands of dollars are now commonplace.

The same general concept is true for co-pays. Just a few years ago, co-pays of five dollars or ten dollars were the norm. Now, it is much more common to see co-pays of twenty-five dollars to thirty dollars. Recall that since many people only see their doctor for ten minutes, that figure becomes an onerous one.

What about the reports of many millions of people in this country who are uninsured or underinsured? Although the number varies according to different "experts" doing different head counts, all agree that it is substantial. The current health care bill just passed may come close to eliminating the ranks of the uninsured. Although neither I nor most of the members of congress have read the 20,000-page bill, the "need" for 20,000 pages attests to the enormous complexity and likely yet to be determined results. As far as we can tell, there are markedly insufficient funds projected to pay for it. Once again, it is likely to be those already insured who will foot the bill, with greatly increased insurance payments.

A very small number of these people have come up with a remarkable solution, which amounts to a self-imposed medical expense account. If one could discipline themselves enough at age 30, to place a given amount of money, monthly into an interest-bearing account, over the course of the next 20 to 30 years, when medical expenses are usually relatively low, a large sum of money does accrue for times of medical need. If and when insurance coverage appears, that money would then amount to a gift to oneself. Obviously, this process requires considerable discipline and commitment.

I just mentioned that medical services are not much different than others, but there are some differences. The financially-stressed patient can and perhaps should ask the doctor for a discount. A positive response may or may not be possible, based on the size and complexity of the medical practice arrangements (the corporate factor). Also, a naysayer could make a case that it is inappropriate to "reward" a person for "irresponsible" behavior; irresponsible because should that person find themselves with a huge bill for emergency hospitalization, it is likely that the trickle-down effect will result in increased rates for people carrying medical insurance. Each doctor will act according to their own dictates. But it doesn't hurt to ask.

Please note somewhat as a sidelight, a situation which for the most part may be unappreciated. This has to do with the broad topic of governmental intervention into our private lives. In this case specifically, the contrast is between fees in medicine and fees in dentistry. As another sidelight, please note that many medical schools and dental schools share a common campus. In medical school, the joke was that the difference between the two types of students was that the medical students were obviously smart enough to get into medical school, and the dental students were not that smart. Medical costs are a government regulated fact. Medicare sets the bar, so to speak. Medicare pays the doctor approximately 50 cents for every one dollar billed. All other insurance carriers set their reimbursements based on that, with "welfare" approximately 25 cents on the dollar, and private insurance between 60 and 80%. In other words, all medical insurance payments are discounted (another good reason why the uninsured person should ask for a discount). Most doctors nevertheless make a very good living, perhaps at the price of very long hours.

The joke regarding medical and dental students has now shifted from the point of view of the cynic. Dental students are the smart ones! They choose dental school. With unregulated dental charges, many people cannot afford dental care. Period! Those who can make huge contributions to the retirement funds of their dentists. The financial rewards for dentists, who by medical standards work abbreviated hours, is enormous. One of my patients, an immigrant working as a hardwood floor finisher, showed me a dental invoice and asked me to explain it to him. It was for extractions, implants, and bridges — a full mouth restoration. The invoice was for $52,000! Dental problems are painful, ubiquitous and have strongly negative consequences for general health of the body. Many people go without dental care because they cannot afford it. Where is the government when you really need it?

THE INTERNET

I t has always been fascinating to speculate how humans felt, when for the first time they sat down on a seat in a train, listened to the engine of the locomotive being stoked, and then went hurtling across the countryside at 40 miles per hour! Perhaps even more astounding might have been the first time placing ones ear against a receiver and hearing a familiar voice coming from several hundred miles away. Moments such as those, and many others have been eloquently captured in the visual and literary arts, and remain awe inspiring.

The growth of the "Internet," a genie originally devised by engineers and physicists so that they could more accurately and easily connect with each other, escaped from the bottle with the speed and explosive force of the Big Bang. It is not an exaggeration to state that since 1982, it has transformed human activity on earth. As with any other transformative breakthrough invaluable to us, we eventually must adjust and incorporate this new technology into our daily lives, hopefully without loss of our humanity. We are an intensely curious species. We are equally intensively social creatures. We want to know! Perhaps never before in history have we had the ability to witness first hand our incredible need to communicate with each other. Making such communication possible has immediately allowed us to see how important the transferring of information is to us. So important is it that it seems any information will do.

Technology breakthroughs, for the most part, with scattered notable exceptions are value-neutral. Even gunpowder is thought to have been devised accidentally by Chinese religious figures and wasn't used as part of weaponry for several centuries after that. It has never been more clear to humans, with the incredible speed of advancing technology, how it is ultimately up to us to use new technology to assist humans with their physical and spiritual struggles — or to allow such technology to be a vehicle for our own suffering or even destruction.

Looking at it from a distance, to the observer, it appears that the Internet, perhaps best thought of as a synonym for "instant, easy, communication," has thus far been highly beneficial in the field of medical science and practice. However, in my daily experiences, I see a few problematic areas. In general, the wonder of the Internet can be seductive to the point where it takes over whatever leisure time we may have. Studies have documented that we are sleeping less now than ever before. In fact, the majority of us are falling below the minimum sleep time required for good health. A point will also be made that one can make a case for generally slowing down, trying to shed excess responsibility, and allowing our nervous systems to be recharged as part of a program to maximize health.

More specifically, it is now commonplace for people to make a decision about going or not going to the doctor on information gleaned from some type of Internet exploration. Needless to say, the potential for inducing incorrect decisions is great. As mentioned previously, it is apparent with even superficial observation that we truly need each other. Aside from the simplest tinkering, I personally would never try to fix the car, remodel the house, fix the computer, make or repair clothing, and countless other everyday considerations. A skilled performer makes the difficult task look easy. The emphasis is on the look easy. It is not easy, but it can be made to look easy.

There is nothing gained by chuckling to oneself, as a patient rambles through the information they obtained from looking at Web MD or some other medically-oriented internet website. The individual pieces of information gleaned are likely factual. However, the integration of information into a cohesive, logical, testable conclusion is not possible for the vast majority of people. A skilled physician can make it look easy, but it is not easy. Perhaps after your doctor tells you that you have Tsutsugamushi fever (a real disease). Since you may only have ten minutes with the doctor, then it might be appropriate to go to the internet, and find out how the heck you can avoid those chiggers on your next trip to Southeast Asia.

I hope that there is a difference between reading on, right here and now, and Internet Medicine. This treatise may broaden your perspective about modern medicine and health, help you to fine-tune your skills at deciding to see the doctor or not; and hopefully, it may give you basic information regarding everyday ailments. Perhaps the greatest danger to internet medical exploration might be to arrive at a conclusion which is way off the mark, reassuring the person that there is no need to see the doctor. To argue that that could be a fatal mistake is not overly dramatic. It is not intended as a substitute for discussing your issues with the best health care provider you can find, even if they make it look really easy—and, in ten minutes.

Lastly, from time immemorial, medical diagnosis has rested heavily on the so-called medical history. This is basically a recitation of the symptoms by the patient, with the attentive doctor listening carefully for elements of the Rosetta stone which will allow him or her to unravel the mystery. However, another feature which has become much more common in the last twenty years or so, since the plethora of medical information has become readily available to the public, is that the patient no longer transmits symptoms. A symptom is the personal description, by the patient, of what is sensed to be a message from the body. Doctors are taught how to interpret and integrate symptoms. It is likely true that the best doctors do this best, even though it looks easy. Some do it appallingly poorly because it takes time and patience. When the patient comes in and starts listing diagnoses: *"I am here because my reflux esophagitis is beginning to cause problems with my asthma, which in turn gives me pleurisy and makes me wonder if I'm having another kidney stone, or whether my colitis is acting up again. On top of that, my mother-in-law, who is a lab technician at the hospital, tells me that she thinks my anxiety disorder is compounding my difficulties by worsening hypertension and causing me to have diastolic heart failure."* If your doctor is still awake after that recitation of diagnoses, devoid of one single symptom, he or she is likely contemplating early retirement. Symptoms are the language of diagnostic medicine! Your job as the patient is to transmit to the doctor how you feel in your body and mind. Your doctor's job is to create a list of differential diagnoses, and then to pare down that list. Anyway, by the time you finished with the recitation above and helped your doctor calm down, your ten minutes would be finished.

INABILITY TO ASSEMBLE YOUR MEDICAL TEAM

The human brain is an unfathomably complex structure. Not surprisingly, it is capable of producing a wide range of responses, behaviors, and even original thought (that is, not directly prompted by an external stimulus). It is now widely promoted by neuroscientists, with information gleaned within the last ten to fifteen years that this enormous range of responsiveness cannot mathematically be explained by the number of neurons alone, even though these brain neurons number approximately 100 billion. Neurons connect with each other, with these connections called synapses. Each neuron may synapse (connect) with 1,000 other neurons. Therefore, the adult brain has approximately, give or take a few, 100 trillion synapses. So, is this why we humans are so smart and technologically advanced? Neuroscientists preach that thinking is produced by interconnection of "neural nets," each representing focal collections of interconnected neurons. Supposedly, this is what gives us our intellectual prowess.

Admittedly, the magnitude of these numbers is difficult to work with from the standpoint of understanding how the brain works or does not work. It should certainly give us an appreciation that due to a few misfiring of neurons, or neural nets, anybody is entitled to an occasional temper tantrum or bad day.

Consider further that there is speculation among the best and the brightest neuroscientists and linguists, that much of the development of our neocortex came about during the time we were becoming facile with language. It is hotly debated whether the big brain gave us language, or vice-versa. Other species communicate with each other through a variety of different mechanisms not involving speech-language at all. The need for fast, accurate communication is likely hard-wired into most or perhaps all, and certainly all "advanced" animal species. It is easily discernable in birds, fish, insects and mammals. Our deep human need to communicate has already been noted. Other animal species communicate via electrical, electromagnetic, ultrasonic, and who knows how many other ways. Octopi have huge brains and have been studied quite extensively. They are thought to have a fairly high level of intelligence, and they communicate by changing the tint of their skin color. Scientists, struggling to communicate cross species with as little bias as possible, have been impressed at how precise this communication appears to be.

So, we humans are stuck with speech-language as our major means of communication. Overall, for straight-forward activity, it works well. However, any time that the limbic system of our brains, the so-called emotional brain, becomes involved, language begins to break down in terms of the accuracy with which it transmits information. There is a certain kind of intimacy, somewhat built-in to the patient-doctor relationship. This automatically activates the limbic system and can create problems with communication. Connecting with a health care team, consisting of the doctor, the nurse or medical assistant, the office staff, the parent organization, if there is one, the adjoining hospital, and others is not likely to be easy all of the time.

Failure can occur on many levels. If the patient is involved with an HMO, they may be assigned to a doctor arbitrarily. The health care team comes with the doctor and may or may not be interchangeable with other doctors. Different HMOs have different philosophies about referral to specialists. Outside of an HMO, although the patient may be able to select the doctor, much of the rest of the team is beyond their selection. The individual doctor may or may not have a network of fixed referral sources, sometimes based on the "you scratch my back and I'll scratch yours" principle, economically driven rather than on the basis of pure quality of care alone. Any given doctor can vary widely between being exceedingly parental to exceedingly lax. Some are very cordial, and others formal. Some are readily accessible, and some are not.

All of these features have to do with the structure of the practice, and the personalities of the patient and doctor. In some communities, especially smaller or rural, there are simply fewer choices. For instance, there may be no female doctors, or not enough specialists, or too much or not enough managed care, or too much or not enough foreign medical graduates to accommodate the community needs.

The essence of a good team is an empathetic doctor who considers a new patient to be a gift rather than a burden, and a patient who is willing to live up to the designation "patient," and be patient, at least for a while. The bulk of responsibility to make it work, in my opinion, falls on the doctor. The best doctors, having studied mental health and having had good mentors and colleagues, can "read" the patient's needs and adapt appropriately. We truly cannot, and should not, even try to change the basic nature of individual people. People are most likely to achieve contentment, a very high priority in life, when they are accepted for who they are. As has been suggested already, doctors do tend to be a notch or two above others in terms of compassion and desire to serve. These qualities, if present, need to be applied routinely.

Once again, our brains and thus our behaviors are exceedingly complicated. Speech-language, a direct product of our brains, can be eloquent or banal but in any case has built-in limitations, regarding accuracy and the desire to transmit the information we wish to transmit. Patients and doctors may "divorce" and dissolve the relationship. Most often, this is initiated by the patient, and I endorse this action as an attempt to get a better fit. The patient needs to have a good feeling about the relationship, due to the fact that it is an important one and involves intimacy.

On the other hand, we are who we are, and tend to carry our baggage with us wherever we go. We do not know how often doctors and patients search for a lifetime to find each other— and never do. We do not know whether the really good fit results in really good outcomes in terms of health. These kinds of research have not been done but can be done and might be very meaningful. In the meantime, inability to get the right fit can be a barrier to good health.

MEDIA ADVERTISING/ BRAINWASHING AND IGNORING THE OBVIOUS

The trading of goods and services, "marketing" in modern parlance, has been part of the human landscape pre civilization. The American Marketing Association describes marketing as an "… activity, set of institutions, and process for creating, communicating, delivering, and exchanging offerings that have value." This creates a mechanism through which "existing and newly created needs and wants can be satisfied by goods and services." Implicit in these straightforward comments is the remarkable confessions that some needs and services are pre-existing; others can be created.

Advertising, in this schema would likely fit into the "communicating" aspect. It is virtually impossible to conceive of a world without advertising. Undertaking a thought experiment regarding this might be fascinating—and would likely yield a world which would appear so alien to us, as to be barely recognizable as a human undertaking. Just as there is a reciprocal relationship between human evolution and human society, each affecting the other, it is likely that the humans of that human undertaking would themselves be substantially different than "us."

Thought experiments notwithstanding, the ubiquitous nature of advertising, traditionally using mass media, and most recently using the "massest" medium of them all (the Internet), are both a product of as well as a driving force for modern civilization. Advertising as a concept may be value-neutral. However, since it is a by-product of marketing, which in itself has been formative regarding modern civilization, one would make a strong case for it being a strongly positive influence. After all, it is directly or indirectly involved with the creation of countless types of job opportunities. Since everyone cannot be the Pope, or the President, or the Emperor, or the world-class icon of one type or another, helping us be worker-bees, who obviously work, would appear to be very beneficial. There is at least one burning contingency which is do we like the world we have created? All of it? Some of it? Does advertising promote *badness*, along with *goodness*?

Remember that we have these enormous brains, with unbelievable analytic capabilities. It would seem obvious that no matter what type of publicity is directed our way, we should be able to separate the wheat from the chaff and decide, using reason, whether to buy or not to buy any given goods or services. That might be true if we had only our cerebral cortex. However, we also have our ancient, reptilian, sexual, instinctual, emotional, SURVIVAL-ORIENTED brain to deal with, sitting right underneath, and connected to our cortical brain. Advertising rarely goes after our cortical brain. *You should become a member of the Neptune Society because it is dignified and cheaper and ecologically sound.* It almost always goes after our "reptilian brain," involving the attributes like, *Beer-X or Car-Y will make you younger, sexier, and more hip* so that you have a profoundly better chance of insuring perpetuity of your gene pool.

If we trick the advertising industry—and shut off our reptilian brain at the beginning of every "commercial break"—we would in fact see that a substantial proportion of what is being promoted as beneficial for us, may be in fact deleterious. From the purely medical perspective, products that might promote intoxication or obesity could be considered harmful. Although we have one hundred billion brain cells, how many people would volunteer to give up five or ten billion? Obesity is one of the main factors behind the epidemic of diabetes and hypertension worldwide, in turn behind the enormous impact of all cardiovascular diseases, including heart attacks and stroke. Promotion of meat products can have strongly negative consequences for the consumer, with increased risk of cardiovascular disease and increased risk of several common cancers—as well as the environment, by production of methane, degradation of soil, and use of water resources. Meat eaters die younger. The promotion by the American Dairy Council may look wholesome but may contribute to poor health by promoting products which have too much saturated fat, too many calories, and a few nasty amino acids.

The ancient Greek motto of "everything in moderation" is difficult to activate when the reptilian brain is being bombarded. Nevertheless, it remains, for the most part, advice to be seriously considered.

The worldwide plague of tobacco abuse is a crime against humanity. I openly and enthusiastically confess my bias in this regard, with my defense being the negative consequences from tobacco abuse that I see every day. One puff of tobacco smoke is known to negatively affect blood chemistry for one week. It causes enormous amounts of human suffering. It has permeated civilization to the extent that it now appears that even advertising is not necessary. It has such a throttle-hold on us that just one cigarette at the right age can create a lifetime slave to the habit. Perhaps not widely appreciated, we do know that environmental factors affect our genetics. From observation of my patients struggling with tobacco addiction, I truly wonder whether or not four hundred years of worldwide tobacco usage, covering approximately twenty generations of humans, has physiologically or even autonomically changed our brains and made us more susceptible to the addictive effects of tobacco.

This genie is out of the bottle. There is little that we can do now regarding the worldwide scourge, but there are some things we must do. We must frequently and repetitively speak to our children about it, beginning in kindergarten. We must elect an enlightened president and congress (is this an oxymoron?) to stop subsidizing tobacco farmers. How can any caring person justify this in 2012? There may be a fine line between reducing tobacco production and creating a tobacco black market. With that in mind, we should greatly reduce the acres of tobacco under cultivation and turn the production of it over to the government—or a tightly-regulated, non-profit, private consortium. We should price the product high enough to further discourage use but not high enough to induce black market activity. We should direct sales revenues into research involving tobacco addiction. All of this could be done quickly and effectively. The only prerequisite is a courageous president and congress, one more interested in improving people's lives rather than getting re-elected.

The United States, as a culture and a society, should be ashamed to have become likely the fattest society on earth. Alternatively, what we have done with reduction of our personal smoking habits is miraculous, being one of the lowest consuming communities on earth. We just need to take the final step to prevent mass export of tobacco from our farms to third-world countries, where cigarette smoking will take the lives of millions of people in the future. Until we do this, our personal accomplishments remain unfinished.

VIOLATIONS OF THE HIPPOCRATIC OATH

W illiam Osler of the late eighteenth and early nineteenth centuries has been called the father of modern medicine. Hippocrates, born on the Greek island of Kos in the fourth century BC, has been called the father of medicine. Through the school that he founded, contact with large numbers of students, extensive writings, and a relatively long practice of the methods and philosophy that he developed, he was the first to delineate the practice of medicine as a profession in itself. He emancipated medicine from the realms of magic and superstition. He taught that man is a product of his environment.

One very small segment of his writings successfully summarized the ethics he delineated and represented a distinct departure from previous practices. Remarkably, this so-called Hippocratic Oath, has become hallowed over many centuries as a right-of-passage for newly trained physicians. It was spoken aloud by most students at graduation ceremonies into the 1970s. It has since been modified by some schools, but is still widely in use. There are a number of tenets outlined in this brief statement. Recently, some of these tenets, such as those prohibiting abortion and suicide, have come under intense scrutiny, and thus the reason for recent modifications. However, two tenets have stood out in importance, endured the march of centuries, and are known by most physicians. These are always conducting oneself "for the good of my patients," and to "never do harm."

The passion and polarization of opinion involving the topics of abortion and death with dignity issues starkly demonstrate to us the depth to which multi-pluralism in the twenty-first century divides us. As a species, divided by chasms of such depth, we can only hope to continue to recognize our differences, but also our common humanity. After all, there has never been a shred of evidence to suggest that we

are not all *homo sapiens sapiens.*

History for the most part is written by a very small contingent of the population. We may know something about the skill set of physicians in the sixteenth or seventeenth centuries, but we know little about the personal and societal issues with which they grappled—and how those issues may have affected practice patterns. Obviously, medicine historically has not distinguished itself as a renegade or rabble-rousing profession. It likely influenced society all along through its humanitarian aspects, but it never considered the redirecting of history to be part of its credo.

Perhaps it is not clearly known how or to what extent the Hippocratic Oath may have been violated in the past. At this time, the violations are commonplace, frequent, and repetitive. A few are egregious. Most are tacit. Many have elements of both. Since there are many different forms of violation, it may be impossible to estimate what percentage of doctors do this or that. Conservatively, it is likely that a substantial minority of physicians do most of the violating, but that may be a great underestimation.

Where to begin? There are so many examples. For instance, in the previous discussion about advertising as a potential barrier to good health, nothing was said about advertising to doctors. Listen up! Doctors are daily barraged with clearly biased information coming at them from a number of sources. Traditionally, doctors have been feted by pharmaceutical companies in countless ways. A bargain is struck. You give us something, and we'll give you something. This sounds very similar to the doctor to doctor bargain, "you scratch my back and I'll scratch yours." Looking at this type of behavior from a distance, common in all walks of life, it represents a response to fear and taps into our need for tribal allegiances to feel safe. What the pharmaceutical company wants is a piece of your time. In exchange, you could in the past and can now get a variety of gifts. The gift is always wrapped in packaging which is meant to convey that you are getting educational information. On the simplest level, one or several well-dressed, well-paid representatives from the company come to your office and talk with you about a drug that they market. Besides the highly biased, one-sided "education," you then could receive pens, scratch pads, gift certificates, medical books or supplies, decorative items, and many other trinkets. Since appointments are eventually made by office staff members, they tend to favor companies who are known to offer fancy gargantuan box lunches for the whole staff, with leftovers lasting several days.

Similarly, such "educational" events may be conducted at a fancy restaurant in town, in the evening by a very well paid physician "consultant." Spouses may be included. There is first a cocktail gathering, and then a dinner during which the presentation is given. There may be additional gifts given after dinner. One colleague described to me how he and his spouse count on two or three restaurant meals per week, free of charge. (It sure beats grocery shopping, cooking, & clean up.)

Stepping up the ante, they may sponsor day long, or longer, seminars in town or out of town. Most of these are located in what would be deemed resort areas, with all expenses paid. Along those same lines, educational activities sponsored by legitimate medical associations are provided regularly. They are often located in definite resort areas with nationally well-known speakers. So far, this sounds good. However, every speaker at that meeting, at the termination of their lecture or participation, must list the medical products and pharmaceutical companies who pay their salaries. Usually, the list contains multiple companies, often competing. Incidentally, this practice is relatively new, perhaps over the last fifteen years or so. So the nationally-known expert giving the lecture about this new drug, may well be on the payroll of the company marketing the drug.

Now, for the most frightening payoff of all. In years past, research physicians and their underlings would spend weeks and months writing a "grant" which was to be submitted to a governmental authority. The grant basically represented a very detailed experimental plan, with an expense account. After perhaps hundreds of hours of preparation by numerous doctors, some of whose future in research might be hanging in the balance, the grant is submitted—and either approved or denied. Over the same length of time that doctors at conventions have had to identify their affiliations, governmental purse strings have been drawn tight. So where do the "losers" who are turned down, now go to get money? You guessed it! With relatively minor changes in protocol, a pharmaceutical company with a potential new drug in the pipeline may agree to fund the entire project! The frightening part of this is that as naïve as I may be, can I trust the research so produced? What about the notion that a slight change in a statistical analysis could give a different result? We are talking about prestigious careers in academic medicine for physician-scientists who would any day rather study the fecal matter of monkeys than see 30 patients per day in the office (I made that up). I do recall how I first heard and read about these sponsoring affiliations at a medical conference fifteen or twenty years ago I sat there in stunned disbelief.

Doctors in private practice are not immune to violations of the Hippocratic Oath. Slightly closer inspection reveals that the notions of "for the good of my patients" and "never do harm" are closely related. The only good that the doctor should aim for is to help the patient by listening attentively, making the appropriate diagnosis, prescribing the correct treatment, and generally relieving suffering. Any time the doctor begins to take into consideration his or her own needs—such as financial, or security, or prestige—the potential for violations arises. Most doctors work on a fee-for-service arrangement. In other words, they only render charges when they have a patient encounter. Does the patient need follow-up once per week or once per month? If the plan is inappropriately excessive, it puts the patient at risk in several ways. It certainly costs the patient more money. In other words, it likely harms the patient. Does the patient need the surgery or procedure, or is it completely *elective*? An overly zealous approach could put the patient at great risk. I met a patient who previously had been hospitalized for one month by a beleaguered doctor, whereas most such illnesses would have required only two or three days. It was only when hospital administration insisted that he release her that he did.

There is supposedly a ruling that prohibits doctors from referring patients to facilities in which they have a financial interest. However, there are many ways to see a patient and request a large number of in-office tests which are not indicated (called "fishing") at very high cost to the patient. Data obtained incidentally in this fashion can be very difficult to interpret and could result in further inappropriate intervention with attendant risk, as well as causing the patient needlessly to worry. I see this every day.

There are many other examples. It saddens me to see this type of activity. I know that an explanation can be created under the veil of being thorough, but most of the time the veil is far too thin to be convincing. All that I can do, is distance myself from these physicians and not refer my patients into their clutches. Otherwise, patients need to be just curious enough to protect themselves. It is relatively easy to get a second opinion when in doubt.

Whatever may be wrong with the delivery of health care in the industrialized West in general, and the United States specifically, misbehavior by physicians stands in stark contrast to what is expected of us. Since the society and physician are intimately connected, all of the blame cannot be placed at the feet of physicians. In order to get physicians back on the right track, they will have to come under pressure from some authoritative source. In other words, it is unlikely to come from the ranks of physicians themselves. The reason for this has to do with the progressive compartmentalization of medicine, each compartment seeing themselves as having competing interests. When we dredge up pictures of "competition" and "interests," it frequently boils down to the force that makes the world go around—money. Within the course of my career, I have seen a number of trends involving specialty societies, which I was supposed to belong to at one time or another. The American Medical Association lost its ability to influence doctors and in turn to speak for them with the swing away from the general practitioner ("GP") to the specialist. Dr. Goldstein was of course a GP, which was the dominant group in medicine up until 1965 or thereabouts. Since then the specialty societies have taken over, and membership in the AMA, founded in 1847, has dropped to approximately 20% of all physicians.

The American College of Physicians, representing internists, very influential in 1967 when I entered internal medicine, has lost membership due to the emergence of powerful organizations representing all of the major medical subspecialties. Internal medicine, once looked upon as the Queen or King of medical science, has lost a great deal of prestige. In recent years, internal medicine training programs, even at prestigious universities, have not filled their quotas, at least not with US-trained medical graduates. The latest to leave the ranks are the hospitalist group, now numbering more than thirty thousand and mostly internists. The American College of Chest Physicians (ACCP) and the American Thoracic Society (ATS) have looked after the interests of this relatively small group of physicians reasonably well. Once again, all these various medical societies have charters which are very broad in scope, including care given to people who are financially underprivileged. Members pay dues. Members, like all other unions, want good working conditions including fewer hours, abundant vacations, and professional independence. The main thing they want is high salaries, especially the most dollars per hour possible.

Obviously, don't look to the professional societies to correct the violations of the Hippocratic Oath. The whole thrust of these organizations is pointed in the other direction. Unfortunately, the only organization big enough and strong enough to enforce change is ... The Government. The good news is that at least on paper, you are the government. There could be a grass-roots movement to impress upon congress that the structure of doctoring in the United States is broken.

We want health care costs to fall, or so we say. If we truly do want to see a major drop in health care costs, you, the consumer, will have to participate. You will need to abandon your ability to sue doctors for minor issues or errors of judgment ("Tort reform"). You can and should continue to sue doctors for clear-cut mistakes, which are easy to document and reprehensible. Unfortunately for you, however, those egregious mistakes represent only a small percentage of all malpractice suits lodged at this time. You will also need to stop demanding expensive services that you are not paying for, such as imaging studies like MRI, physical therapy services, and laboratory studies done repeatedly. All of those should truly be initiated at the discretion of your doctors.

On the positive side, your irritation with doctors is justified. You have lost your basic trusted advisor (Dr. Goldstein) and are now seeing a variety of specialists, who are ordering extensive tests that give them additional profit. They don't see you or know you as a complete person.

Getting back to the place where you have a doctor who takes you on—and wants to know you and act in your best interest—won't be easy, but it is doable. You may have to become an activist to get that. If enough of you do this, the big, bad GOVERNMENT which represents you will make it happen. Right now, those doctors who fall under the category of "PCP" work the hardest and make the least dollars per hour. If I told you that they make approximately $55.00 per hour, you might think that is too high. Recall, however, that before the fall of General Motors Corporation, some of their workers had paychecks that brought them up to $70.00 per hour. People in the construction industries make anywhere from $20.00 to $100.00 per hour, depending on what they do. When looked at that way, the doctor's salary of $55.00 per hour looks like a bargain.

However, very few doctors work a forty-hour week, which would give them approximately $100,000 per year. What they do is a 60-hour work week bringing their salary up to about $150,000 to $175,000 per year, somewhat typical for family practice, pediatrics, and internal medicine. What has happened is that instead of seeing twelve to fifteen patients per day, and doing a really good job with a really good financial reward for sixty hours per week, they have to increase their patient load up to twenty-five to thirty patients per day. This guaranties that they cannot do a good enough job commensurate with your expectations. Office visits are reduced to ten to fifteen minutes, and nobody wins. The doctor is pushed hard by the clinic to see more and more patients. The doctor knows that they are not being nearly so thorough as they need to be, and "burnout" sets in. You feel neglected and angered by the abrupt visit. No one is happy, and rightly so. On the other hand, when you see the specialist, they routinely order a plethora of tests, which you may see as their attempt to be thorough. Perhaps this is true. Or perhaps the tests are ordered under the guise of being thorough, thus allowing the specialist to see a much lower volume of patients and receive a much higher paycheck, because the tests, supposedly necessary, are reimbursed at a very high level. People who are involved with surgery, including anesthesiologists, are in a class all their own. Surgeons and anesthesiologists are reimbursed at exceptionally high levels, allowing these doctors to see five to ten patients per day and still make very large incomes.

The situation is clear. We need to reverse the trend of the vanishing PCP, vanishing because medical students quickly learn where the money is doled out. They may have student loans to pay off, or at least that is the excuse given. What we desperately need in this country is a cadre of PCPs, who are very well compensated for the very difficult work they do. Hopefully, these are the people who choose medicine as a profession because they are compassionate, wish to help people, and are willing to work hard to make that happen. An army of Dr. Goldsteins. So we need a complete revamping of the salary structure for doctors. Only the government can pull this off. Instead of full-time doctors working forty to sixty hours per week with yearly salaries varying from $120,000 to $500,000 or more, everyone, including surgeons, anesthesiologists, pathologists, and medical specialists should be brought to a relatively narrow range of perhaps $150,000 to $200,000 per year. We need to stop young people from selecting medicine as a career to make huge sums of money. I know that this is possible to do, but I doubt full implementation without a government takeover. Perhaps I am underestimating the cadre of PCPs who will reign in unnecessary expenditures. Given proper training and authority and particularly relief from the crushing fear of malpractice when clashing with specialists, this would bring back the best of medical practice, which is a partnership between doctor and patient, with welfare of the patient always placed first. The new cadre of PCPs, seeing twelve to fifteen patients per day (mostly thirty-minute visits) will give you a feeling of security as their concern for your welfare will be obvious. They will still be working fifty to sixty hours per week, but all of the negative elements that lead to burnout will have been removed. Despite whatever the naysayers might scoff at, I know that the transformation can occur, if we so desire.

ELECTRONIC MEDICAL RECORD (EMR)

Hold your horses, Pardner! Is this a typo? How can a new technology, lauded and financially supported by the government, supported by numerous major health care organizations, and promised to be the vehicle for greatly reducing mistakes in medical practice be listed under "Barriers to Care?"

"Health Care System." This is a term that we hear frequently. What is it, and what is it supposed to do? The term "system" implies some type of a network, or grid, perhaps with interlocking parts, the function of which is to perform some type of task. The issue of "care" and "caring" was discussed regarding the issues of what might justify that a suit be brought against a doctor. Briefly, the conclusion, suggested by me, implies that the key should not center on the making of a well-conceived course of action, which turned out to be wrong, but a lack of caring, or not caring enough to be careful. Care and carefulness are attributes, which are easily seen scattered throughout the animal kingdom, but perhaps most ubiquitous and deeply ensconced in humans. "Health" is well being of the mind and body. So given this breakdown of the term, the health care system of this, or any country, represents a network of people and tools, working together through the medium of caring and careful attention, to help members of society to achieve and maintain well-being of body and mind.

In this definition of a health care system (biased, as are virtually all opinions and conclusions), there is nothing stated regarding computers. Despite the unbelievable penetration of computers into the daily lives of people over the last twenty-five years, there are still realms of experience where they are not necessary — and possibly disadvantageous. Hopefully, they are not utilized as we enter a facility for religious worship, meditation, or prayer. They are intrusive in virtually all activities whereby we intend to experience the natural world. They do not accompany us in our attempts to achieve ecstatic moments, whether — in the concert hall or the bedroom.

Having said that, I do not believe that computers should be an integral part of the patient-doctor interchange. Perhaps the following statement has not been precisely made thus far. The key element in the establishment of an effective health care system is a concerned, careful, sympathetic doctor, performing with balanced brain function for the betterment of you, the patient. Absent this, we are left with an elegant, state-of-the-art, beautifully constructed car, with no wheels. Recall my contention that as the science of medicine is exploding logarithmically, the art of medicine is collapsing. Doctors have forgotten what their mission is. They feel overwhelmed. They are pushed to go faster and to rely on technology to bail them out. Most see too many patients to perform excellently. Unable to be excellent, they change the focus to winning, by trying to get enough money to retire ASAP. (The crucially important difference between excellence rather than winning will be discussed later).

Lastly, to pull all of this meandering together, recall the basic pathway towards establishing a diagnosis—the medical history, obtained face-to-face between the patient and doctor. Recall Dr. Osler's observation that "the patient is telling you the diagnosis." The meticulous history, obtained through skilful questioning, becomes the first element of the medical record under discussion.

One could have imagined, if not predicted, that as the age of computers rushed into our lives, at some point the electronic medical record would emerge on the scene. This expectation in some way could be likened to the appearance of an epiphenomenon. Epiphenomena are seen commonly if looked for in the workings of the world. They represent the appearance of a certain property of a system, whose individual elements would not be associated with that property, but which in the setting of a degree of complexity of the system, arise naturally. In essence, they are a by-product of complexity.

So once again acting as the gadfly and setting myself up as an antiquated reactionary, here is my take on this.

1. Once again, change is intrinsically value-neutral.

2. Computerization of the modern world has obviously been enormously helpful in countless ways. However, the technology has already fallen into the hands of those who are misusing it, with the aim to take something from you, including even your life.

3. Computers in medicine have allowed us to accelerate the process of acquisition, and dissemination of knowledge.

4. The love affair with and fascination with computers in members of our society reached a critical mass, whereby well-meaning members of the medical profession had a vision of improved medical care mediated through improved medical record keeping via the electronic medical record (EMR).

This last tenet is a completely false notion. Thus far the data does not support improved outcomes using the EMR in the vast majority of situations in which that has been investigated. Medical care remains an intensely personal undertaking. It does not lend itself to computerization. The human organism, with its vast complexity, includes huge domains of sensitivity and nuance generated by mega structures such as the limbic system of the brain, and microstructures, such as the individual cell, neither one of which in the foreseeable future can be computerized.

The ability to improve the medical record has advanced greatly in the last twenty years, long before the emergence of the EMR was conceived. Simple steps such as using the SOAP (subjective-objective-assessment-plan), technique for organizing thoughts, and eliminating cursive writing by emphasizing transcription which have helped enormously. There are many other easily installed changes in record keeping, including the commonly adopted "problem" list which made the medical record of 1960 look like the Model T. All of this is free of charge.

Installation of the EMR is extremely costly. Complete installation of such a record for an average-sized hospital could cost ten million dollars to twenty million dollars. Who do you suppose pays for that? Installation in the clinics of doctors can cost up to $32,000 per doctor. Your government is so committed to the EMR, that it is largely subsidizing this conversion by sharing the financial burden with doctors, one of the highest paid professional groups in society.

What do we get for this huge expense? The EMR drones on in repetition. There are many, many different templates, varying greatly in cost, quality, practicality, and especially readability. Many of them are misleading. The three-page document is meant to look as if the doctor spent forty-five minutes with the patient. However, that is the result of a fifteen-minute office visit. It consists largely of a review of old data accumulated in previous visits, mostly obtained by patients filling out questionnaires—but not interviewed by doctors. One is hard-pressed to find the two or three sentences, which apply to the current visit. Inaccuracy, which may be present in any medical record, when repeated over and over, can increasingly take on the aura of TRUTH.

What about the miracle of having your entire medial history embedded in a credit card size device, which you can take anywhere in the world and present to the medical professionals in whatever remote area you find yourself? This notion is generated by naked fear. The instances whereby this scenario would be critically important are extremely rare. I have spoken to physicians per telephone, caring for my patients in many parts of the world, and have afterwards felt that the communication just completed was largely unnecessary, as they already knew everything I told them. My suspicion is that the patient, or concerned family member, requested that the call be made. Reversing this, I personally cannot recall a single incidence whereby my call (prompted by a request) to some far flung backwater was truly helpful at that moment.

In conclusion, I suspect that most of this sounds like, and looks like "blowing in the wind." I have no pretensions that the EMR industry is destined to dry up after these statements are read. However, the single clearest statement is that the health care system does not lend itself to the same level of computerization that one might see in a car company, or in the space program. Tinkering with it beyond a basic level can result in a huge barrier to proper functioning of the system, whereby a patient and a doctor enter into a sacred relationship. Focusing on the keyboard and the computer screen can sabotage this most critical aspect of information gathering.

"Whooh! That was a rough ride."

Section II

DOCTORING CIRCA 2012

HOW DID THE DOCTOR
GET INTO THAT WHITE COAT?

And now, the moment of truth. The sun bears down on the arena. The heat is palpable. The gate clangs shut with a definitive resonance. Silence momentarily engulfs the world, further intensifying the moment and sharpening the definition of the two naked figures. No place to hide. Life and death at stake. Who will live and who will die? How much suffering along the way? Generations of breeding and inbreeding have created a genetic knowingness, and a deep respect, and even reverence. But the outcome of this intensely personal drama is always unforeseen. A few moments of strutting and posturing, seeming to go on forever. And then, "Hi! I'm Doctor Burnsout."

So, who is that person wearing the white coat? Perhaps one-tenth of one percent of them are complete imposters, having just printed their diplomas at Kinko's down the street. But don't worry about them, because the following profile will emphasize the composite of the 99.9% of "real doctors" who are their competition. Incidentally, before we leave the imposters, it is interesting to note that many of these people carry on their ruse for many years and receive high marks of approval from their "patients."

HOW DOCTORS LEARN

Becoming a real doctor takes a huge commitment over an extended period of time. It is akin to running the gauntlet, with both predictable and extemporaneous snake pits placed along the way. It is both a marathon, and a rite-of-passage, with the award being entry into an exclusive club. Incidentally, "real doctors" or "RD" is what medical students call each other.

The easy part is college. Traditionally, a college degree has not been a pre-requisite for entry into medical school. Please note that of the approximately one hundred thirty medical schools in the US, there are substantial differences in every imaginable feature, including numbers of students, types of students, curriculum, teaching techniques, requirements etc. For most, a college degree is required or expected, and a "B+" or higher grade-point average is expected. This alone speaks to the fact that medical students are smart or diligent or both. An interview is required, as is the need to pass, and hopefully do very well on the Medical College Admission Test. Smart and diligent, in various proportions.

Medical school, for most students, is a four-year program, structurally not much different than undergraduate work, at least during the first two years. Didactic and laboratory experience in anatomy, physiology, pathology, and many other such "basics" is interspersed with very gradually increasing experience with patients. Such experience is relatively limited in time and scope, and is generally closely supervised. Exams are given, and students may or may not be appraised of the results. Perhaps most often they are "pass" or "fail," although certainly exact figures are kept and assessed by the college. Classes may extend from 8:00 am to 5:00 pm. Obviously, there is considerable study time required after hours.

The third and fourth years represent a distinct departure, as the emphasis then falls on "clinical medicine." Didactic sessions continue, but the majority of time is spent in the hospital and clinics seeing patients. Once again, such activities are very closely supervised and critiqued. There is a mixture of mandatory rotations, such as internal medicine, surgery and pediatrics, as well as a large number of elective rotations, such as neurology, pathology, psychiatry, anesthesiology, and all of the medical and surgical subspecialties, such as cardiology and orthopedic surgery. Since the knowledge base of third-year students regarding clinical medicine is nearly zero, a great deal of learning goes on. Hours vary tremendously, depending on the particular rotation, but generally mimic the hours of graduate physicians, now capped at eighty hours per week. Extensive study of books, manuscripts, and other literature is still expected. During these two years, the majority of students come to conclusions about specific career choices to be further pursued in residency and fellowship.

Following graduation, the "MD" degree is bestowed, and displaces the "RD," never to be used again. Through a complex matching system, the new doctors move on to postgraduate training. In the past, the first year, which is all that is needed for application for medical license, was called internship. For the most part, it is now considered to be the first year of residency. At the time that Dr. Goldstein was training, this is as far as he and most of his colleagues went with formal training. In other words, he then went into practice and could participate in the full spectrum of medical activity, including surgery, pediatrics, medicine and obstetrics. Given the state of affairs today, it is hard to believe that this was the norm, likely up to the 1960s.

Today, the vast majority of postgraduate physicians continue on with their training. Depending on the type of training—and whether or not they plan on a career in private practice or academic medicine—the various programs go on for another two to perhaps eight years. The latter part of the training is called "fellowship" if it involves work in a single discipline recognized by the American Board of Medical Specialties. When training is finally completed, whenever that might be, most doctors attempt to pass one or more specialty certifying exams. At the present time, board certification in three specialties is not unusual. Pass rates vary from specialty to specialty but are generally high. A physician cannot promote him or herself as "board certified" until the diploma for such is awarded.

While in medical school, students are hammered with the concept that the purpose of formal schooling and training is to provide a body of basic knowledge, representing a framework to be enhanced steadily. One professor explained it clearly enough by emphasizing that the faculty was committed to teaching us how to learn.

Once formal education, including all post graduate training ends, physicians must continue educational pursuits in order to maintain licensure. There are many avenues for this, all falling under the category of Continuing Medical Education (CME). Credits are awarded for attendance at or participation in educational activities. Such activities must be approved by various agencies to be able to award credits. Programs are arranged by hospitals, medical groups, county and state medical organizations and others, on a local basis. Specialty societies have one or several annual conventions where many thousands of physicians may attend lectures and seminars. These types of activities are a mandatory part of CME credits. Also mandatory is a certain amount of "independent study," documented by the honor system. Please note that due to the extreme bias inherent in the previously mentioned pharmaceutical company presentations, although the free dinner may be worth the effort, CME credit is rarely awarded.

In my experience, the greatest opportunity for ongoing education by far comes from interaction with patients. Not only do patients occasionally come up with rare or fascinating diseases (recall Osler's injunction to treat the patient, not the disease), but they represent a constantly present crucible in which the application of all of the physicians accrued knowledge is mixed with the absolutely unique physiology of that particular patient. For the attentive and open-minded physician, in my opinion, this represents by far the greatest opportunity for medical education. Needless to say, no CME credits are awarded for this. Once again, as Osler said, "the patient is telling you the diagnosis."

This personal opinion brings into focus a difficult and new issue which has arisen within the last seventeen years. For much longer than that, the very best experimental protocols for research in clinical medicine, using real patients, were deemed to be the "randomized, double-blinded, placebo-controlled" studies. Allow me to break that down. "Randomized" refers to the selection of and placement of patients into different experimental groups to be compared, according to arbitrary assignment based on "first come, first served." That is, patients are assigned temporally, as they enter, regardless of any personal characteristics. "Double-blinded" means that neither the patients nor the researchers know what grouping any individual patient is in; that is, not knowing what treatment, if any treatment, they are receiving. "Placebo-controlled" refers to the need to have a group which receives no treatment, thus representing the natural course of the condition. Such studies must be "powered" sufficiently, by having large numbers of patients, and perhaps be continued for a sufficiently long time, to pass statistical muster. All of this is designed to reduce bias as much as possible. Recall that many of these very expensive studies are funded by pharmaceutical companies.

The "problem" arises when contemporary medical education leaders emphasize to doctors that their everyday clinical decisions should rest on "evidence-based medicine" principles. This means that they "apply evidence gained from the scientific method…conscientious, explicit, and judicious use of the current best evidence in making decisions." Some are even suggesting that such evidence and application is becoming the "gold standard." Although proponents of the evidence-based medicine model all acknowledge the potential usefulness of personal clinical experience, the emphasis is definitely on medical research and the contemporary medical cannon. Notwithstanding all of the pitfalls of clinical research, de-emphasis of physician experience may be misguided. It can certainly create insecurity in physicians, already insecure about their malpractice exposure.

In the "real world" of clinical medicine, for many doctors, the apex of book knowledge occurs as they leave academia and enter private practice. On the other hand, their experiential knowledge is likely at its lowest level. As the doctor moves through the years of patient-centered experience, the latter expands dramatically. The key is to keep the former from eroding. Actually, with all the CME activities available, this is easy to do. In summary, one might surmise that the doctor may be at his or her peak somewhere around mid career; that is between ten and twenty years after completion of formal training (generally, approximately ages forty to fifty, depending on which specialty is in question). Perhaps this could act as a reasonable starting point for those selecting a doctor.

HOW DOCTORS PRACTICE AND HOW TO SELECT ONE

Despite the fact that you are now astonishingly versed about the training of a modern-day physician, knowing more than you ever cared to know, the sun gets hotter, the intensity builds, and who will make the first move? There are still two crucial features lacking before you formally engage with the doctor. First and foremost, you don't know anything about the character of the doctor, or even whether he or she has a character or is a character. Secondly, you still haven't selected THE doctor.

Unfortunately, character is a feature which may remain obscure until after the actual partnership begins. After all, neither the bull nor the matador choose each other. Doctors are smart. Doctors are diligent. They likely score above average in compulsiveness and determination. But what about character? As mentioned earlier, I think that they overall have a somewhat higher level of compassion than most, although that represents a fragile attribute, subject to the vicissitudes of an ongoing career. For the most part, they behave professionally, are able to exert emotional control over themselves, and work well under difficult and stressful conditions. On the other hand, at any given time, thirty to fifty percent of physicians would like to change their practice venue, to improve the relationship between work and family life.

Obviously, doctors are products of their environment and upbringing. Medical educators need to keep in mind that the intensity of the medical school and post-graduate training programs is often offered with little or no emotional support and encouragement. What thus emerges and grows is extreme competitiveness. We will later learn how this brain state emanates from the preemptive (reptilian) brain and runs counter to compassion, a product of the new brain, so essential for dealing with all of the people he or she meets with every day in the normal functioning in the role of the doctor. To the extent that competitiveness persists, it does not leave adequate space for compassion to emerge.

When all is said and done, however, doctors are not radically different than a cross-section of people in general. They have the same wants that any composite of people do. They can be just as petty, insecure, petulant, and self-absorbed as anyone. These statements are likely disappointing, as we tend to expect so much of them.

A few tell-tale signs may be helpful in the selection process. Keep in mind that empathy and compassion may be predictive of their overall quality and efficacy. Perhaps most indicative might be doctors who give their time away, perhaps to a local "free clinic" or via medical trips to a poor country. Those who have served in a government agency which administers care to the indigent, before beginning private practice stand out. In my opinion, all doctors should participate in seeing "welfare" patients. As noted before, the remuneration is so low that it might be impossible to stay in business seeing mostly welfare patients. However, incorporating ten to twenty percent welfare patients is doable for almost all doctors and enlivens and animates the practice. Unfortunately, many doctors see none of these patients, even upon referral from another doctor. Discounting fees for uninsured patients likely speaks well for the doctor, even though it may not translate into matters of empathy and compassion. Lastly, before resorting to the ultimate arbiter, the children's counting rhyme dating back to 1850, and known by all ("eeny, meenie, miny, moe…"), referral from a trusted acquaintance may be very helpful and more likely to succeed.

Needless to say, the above considerations, and perhaps others equally representative of good character, may not be easy to access. The doctors with the best character, in my experience, tend to be understated and may not be boastful or self-aggrandizing. Perhaps, such information may be listed on a website. Perhaps a yellow pages ad may hint at something. If nothing else, it might be advantageous when first calling the office to ask the receptionist "What is the single best thing about your doctor?" You might be amazed at the positive (or negative) responses that you might receive!

As far as selecting THE doctor is concerned, there are a series of obvious objective criteria which should be considered. Let us simply surrender to the likelihood that the character issue may not be discernable until after the relationship begins. The rest of the process is more clearly definable, and might please those dedicated to the evidence-based philosophy. Please note that each choice will be highlighted by a few notable pros and cons.

SOLO

A single doctor practice was the norm for many years. Don't forget Dr. Goldstein. It is now distinctly less popular than before, although still fairly common in smaller communities. It did not fail because of any particular intrinsic defect, but because doctors felt that they had better options from the personal standpoint when joined with other doctors. These likely included hopes of reducing overhead, having a reliable on-call arrangement and vacation schedule, having a larger presence in the community with perhaps access to more patients, and greater ability to quickly interact with colleagues in terms of "curb-side" consulting (this refers to getting a snapshot second opinion, without actually having the colleague see the patient).

As a sidelight, I am of the belief that human interaction and communication is somewhat predictable and repetitious. In other words, the way that an individual reacts with family and friends is not fundamentally different than the way groups act with bigger and bigger groups, regions act with regions, and countries act with countries. The behaviors are similar, but the stakes get progressively bigger. On the personal level, the decision of a couple to divorce may possibly be the first step in an attempt to destroy each other. This becomes a cessation of diplomatic interaction on the international level, just before the intercontinental ballistic missiles are sent on their mission to save the world from whatever. Both of these sides of the discord spectrum are reflections of the fact that although we are genetically almost identical, we are culturally very different.

So, it is unclear whether the lofty aims of the doctor joining hands in partnership have met their expectations or not. Some yes, some no. Certainly, no "slam dunk."

Again, there is nothing intrinsically wrong with the solo system. In fact, there are some distinct advantages. Most importantly, from the standpoint of both patient and doctor, the concept of "the buck stops here" can be rigidly applied—the "here" being at the doctor's desk. Less time is spent in endless office meetings, haggling over numerous minutiae. Vacation and on-call relationships can be worked out somewhat more flexibly. It is much easier to track finances. Most of the time, during off-hours, the patient should be able to contact their very own doctor rather than a surrogate.

What is best, small companies or big companies? What about medium-sized companies or huge companies? All have their advantages and disadvantages, and hence our ability to exercise personal choice.

SEX

This chapter is not about procreation. But fear not, as that will come later! For many patients this is an easier choice, simply because it is one or the other. Unfortunately, at the beginning of my career this topic would not have warranted a discussion. In my class of 200 first-year medical students, there were ten women. Finally, fifty years later many medical schools have announced triumphantly that they have finally enrolled approximately equal numbers of men and women.

During this long transition towards equalization of gender status, and not yet achieved, women traditionally choose fields of interest which were somewhat predictable, such as pediatrics and obstetrics-gynecology. Also, fields which could be dealt with well on a part-time basis rose in popularity, such as radiology, pathology, and psychiatry. All along, there has been a slowly increasing accretion of women in family practice and internal medicine. Lastly, over the past ten to twenty years, it is now increasingly common to see women in all of the disciplines which have been traditional male bastions, such as cardiology, pulmonology, nephrology, surgery, and all of its surgically-oriented sub-specialties such as orthopedics, neurosurgery, and even urology. Unfortunately, retention of and promotion of women in academic medicine has lagged well behind the acceptance of women in the private practice sector.

There appears to be a significant segment of the female population of patients who prefer a female physician. This appears to be perhaps most prevalent in obstetrics and gynecology. There appears to be a definitive subsegment of male patients who would not choose a female physician. Considering the dramatic changes of sheer numbers of female physicians in the last fifty years, from five to fifty percent, it is remarkable how little it appears to matter to most patients.

As of this moment, patients need consider only a few ancillary features in selecting on the basis of sex. Overall, female physicians tend to work fewer hours than their male counterparts. A higher proportion may work part time. Overall, there is a lower percentage of female physicians in rural practice, and there is a tendency to spend less time on-call. Much of this likely relates to the fact that many female physicians consider themselves to be the primary caregivers of their families. As mentioned before, tragically, although the suicide rate of physicians is higher than any other professional group, the suicide rate of female physicians may be as much as twice as high as their male counterparts. The reasons for this are obviously very complex and will likely never be definitely known.

AGE

This consideration involves several obvious observations. Throughout the years of medical school and post-graduate training, doctors are constantly enmeshed in a highly academic environment and surrounded by truly brilliant physician-scientists. For the most part, and to varying degrees across different programs and universities, the missions of these individuals has been described as tripartite in nature, namely teaching, research, and patient care. The environment is electric! The trainee is continually pushed and prodded to do better. The end result is that upon completion of training, one has a huge reservoir of factual knowledge.

This apex of raw knowledge is usually manifest between the ages of twenty-eight and thirty-five, at which time the physician enters practice. Obviously, for some patients this information may be the single strongest attraction. On the other hand, I have already commented upon the phenomenal opportunity for continual improvement in knowledge-base by careful assessment of one's own personal activities over the years. Therefore, a strong case can be made for combining the attributes of book knowledge and experience by seeking a doctor in mid-career, perhaps around the ages of forty to fifty. Although a few misguided patients may select a doctor like me, well beyond the fifty-year cutoff point for "mid-career," there have been doctors in my community who appeared to be fully competent and functional up until age eighty. Once again, this is a decision which sometimes is very personal. I think that aiming for age forty to fifty is the best compromise, overall.

SINGLE-SPECIALTY GROUP

This is a rather simple concept to grasp. This is a collection of doctors who basically do the same thing and have some type of partnership arrangement. The group could be anywhere from two to twenty, or even more. This type of arrangement is created for basically the same as those listed in the first paragraph of the discussion regarding perceived deficiencies of solo practice. The larger groups might be twenty or more internists, or pediatricians, or family practice doctors, encompassing the "primary care" model. The smaller groups of two or three could be the same but would more likely represent surgeons, urologists, neurologists, nephrologists, and others. The mid-range groups of five to ten or so, might be orthopedists, cardiologists, ob-gynecologists, and many others. Perhaps the pertinent features of these larger groups, from the standpoint of patients, is that in general, the larger the group, the less likely you will see your doctor, particularly during off-hours when the office is closed, or if you have an urgent problem. Also, the larger the group, the more likely are the corporate-like policies and procedures to be commonplace. This can be a significant barrier between you and your doctor, or between you and a responsible, caring person who will listen to your medical or administrative issue—and act on it. Obviously, all of this depends on the efficiency of the clinic. The bigger the institution, however, the harder it is to find where the buck stops.

MULTI-SPECIALTY CLINICS

By definition, multi-specialty clinics have an assorted array of different medical specialties represented. The most simple might be only two or three, possibly medically related or not. Many of them have a large number of specialists, with one or many individuals in each specialty. The corporate model is most pervasive in this arrangement. The goal is clearly to provide a setting for one-stop-medical shopping, whereby everything you will ever need is available within this institution. This does not mandate that you see doctors only in this clinic, but you will be strongly encouraged to do so.

These clinics can become enormous, with fifty to hundreds of physicians being commonplace. All of the potential problematic issues noted in the larger single-specialty groups can be seen here as well. This is by necessity the apex of corporate medicine. The larger of these groups may be located on campuses with numerous buildings, research activities, doctors in training, in addition to staff doctors, and even their own hospital. If this description sounds imposing or intimidating in any way, please note that some of the best known of these multi-specialty group practices include some of the most famous and prestigious medical institutions in the United States, including the Oschner Clinic, Cleveland Clinic, and the Mayo Clinic. Many of these clinics, with a midrange numbers of physicians, establish satellite clinics in different parts of the community including suburbs and outlying areas, providing name recognition, and acting as a conduit to funnel patients into the main clinic or hospital.

So, we have essentially made a tour from one end of the medical cosmos to the other, the office of the solo-practitioner, to the office of a similar doctor in a huge multi-specialty clinic. Which is best? Certainly, the trend has been towards progressively larger clinics. At least in the early stages of this metamorphosis, the trend was initiated by physicians. The original intent, no matter what might have been pronounced, was to better the life of the doctor, not the patient. We don't even know if that basic need has been realized. It seems as if this is like a snowball set rolling down the hill, picking up momentum and getting bigger and bigger. We don't really know where the major stimulus for continuing this trend is coming from, whether it be doctors or patients or even the corporation itself. It is almost certainly not the doctor. I think it may be the bureaucracy of the corporate body, akin to the way government can grow exponentially, unless we have checks and balances to limit this. If the stimulus is coming from the patient, and it may be, then so be it. As stated before, doctors are generally not rabble rousers. Most seem much more comfortable following than leading. Bureaucrats know how to lead. Patients can lead by voting grass-roots initiatives or by personal selection. Medicine remains embedded deeply in society. If bigger and bigger looks better and better to patients, that is what will happen. Perhaps there will be some type of correctional trend backwards, in the future. We are the patients. Ultimately, this is a facet of society where we can, and will, get what we want.

BOUTIQUE MEDICINE

We often forget that citizens of the United States live in the richest country in the world. Much of Europe, parts of Asia, and scattered other countries share a standard of living far above that of the vast majority of people on earth. We forget it because many of us bemoan our financial status and definitely don't feel rich. Nevertheless, except for the very lower-most portion of our population, perhaps restricted to homeless individuals, we are the richest.

Those of us, who place healthcare at a very high priority, can now elect to partially step out of the conventional system and try to get very personalized service. The specifics of each boutique practice vary, but the common denominators are as follows. The patient pays an annual fee out-of-pocket. This could be as little as $1,000 per year, up to $20,000. Most are likely in the range of $5,000 per year, usually paid monthly or quarterly. For this entrance fee, the patient gets a "package" which could include an annual physical, easy access to the doctor "24-7" usually via cell phone and/or e-mail, guarantees as to limitations of the size of the doctor's practice, electronic medical record, and an office space and equipment of top quality and décor.

In my opinion, although there is nothing illegal or even unethical about this business model, there is really only one possible advantage to this type of practice. That is, you should get much more time with your doctor, and he or she should therefore be much more likely to know your case so well as to minimize oversights or erroneous conclusions.

Originally, physician groupings were conceived and dedicated by physicians for the benefit of physicians. This model is one hundred percent devised by doctors, mostly for their benefit. In a properly balanced boutique practice, the doctor will make much more money for a significantly lower workload. Patients may benefit as a sidelight. Please note that the services provided by boutique physicians can still be found in the conventional medical model. As outlined, if we can successfully train and financially reward primary care physicians in sufficient numbers, the "guarantees" of the boutique practice will be available to all.

In summary, the arrival of boutique medicine represents a symptom of a serious disease. The disease is the marked imbalance between numbers of and respect for primary care physicians coming through the pipeline, versus specialists coming through. It represents a response of physicians to enormous stressors and of patients to deep dissatisfaction with the existing system. It is not an evil empire. However, it is tainted by having been born from a gridlocked system gone astray and not being accessible to the majority of the population. A boutique type practice is the ideal. It should be available to all. To make it happen, there needs to be a dramatic restructuring of medical pay scales and the availability of and enthusiasm for primary care. It can happen. Until then, if you can afford a boutique practice, go for it!

ARNP—PA

Within the past twenty-five years or so, the "Advanced Registered Nurse Practitioner" and the "Physician Assistant" have appeared on the medical landscape and somewhat surprisingly proliferated by carving out a solid niche in the medical practice schema. This may be because these medical personnel provide elements of what Dr. Goldstein provided, and which people miss dearly. Briefly, there are similarities and differences between the two. This summary is not intended to be in-depth. However, this population of caregivers needs to be mentioned, as they are likely now a permanent fixture of the medical community.

Although formally designated "mid-level providers/practitioners," both ARNPs and PAs function in a very broad array of work, basically tracing the same types of career choices that MDs make. Nurse practitioners begin with an RN (Registered Nurse) degree and go on to advanced training at universities from there. PAs begin with undergraduate degrees and then go on to a formal school for PAs, with attendance there usually for three years. Either group then may go on to specialty training and eventually to licensure. Opportunities and responsibilities vary somewhat from state to state. PAs differ in that they are directly responsible to a given physician, although the degree of oversight may be minimal. ARNPs can work independently from physicians.

From the standpoint of clinical medicine, they can function in the same capacity as an MD. Were they to appear in the hospital or clinic, as a substitute for the MD, the patient would likely not detect the difference. Perhaps the majority of either group work in clinics, including solo to multispecialty. Some of these may work in the hospital as well. They too are required to do continuing medical education and pass periodic licensing exams.

Even into the late 1800s, in some states and countries, the MD degree could be awarded to a person who basically did an apprenticeship with an MD, even with a minimum of formal education. So, in the real world, what are the differences between the MD, and ARNPs or PAs? The actual practice differences are blurred. In my experience with them, there appears to be no glaring differences. Perhaps one could speculate that ARNP, and/or PAs, might even be better at some of the basics such as history taking than MDs. Perhaps, overall, they spend more time with individual patients. On the other hand, there is no question that their formal training is less rigorous and considerably shorter. As to whether you, the patient, should select one in preference to an MD, I cannot state confidently. Having said that, ARNPs and PAs would appear to be viable alternatives for many types of routine, or so-called "mid-level" medical issues.

COMPLIMENTARY AND ALTERNATIVE PRACTITIONERS

C omplementary and alternative medical (CAM) practitioners are the esthetically correct designation of a wide variety of practitioners, previously called "Alternative Medicine." Perusal of a textbook of CAM listed over 100 separate disciplines. The most widely used would include chiropractic, naturopathic, Ayurveda, homeopathy, and others, with these also having the extensive philosophies to compensate for possible lack of proof of efficacy, when scrutinized by modern scientific and statistical approaches.

Scientific and personal knowledge does not allow me to expound on these disciplines individually. They are, no doubt, very popular and for what appears to be several reasons. In general, one would say that they fulfill needs not met by conventional medicine. For instance, many of them emphasize strongly the mind-body interaction, emphasizing spiritual and other-worldly issues. Should this seem bogus, what about the scientifically-accepted notion that a body is composed of largely empty space! Many of them have very old, and even ancient, philosophies which are eloquent and speak to the issues of nature, and being in harmony with nature. Conventional medicine barely mentions these considerations. The beautiful dissertations in Ayurveda about food substances, food preparation, and the actual process of eating are breathtaking, as are the attempts to weave the life force into the fabric of the universe. The intensely-done history taking, essential in the search for the homeopathic remedy, is a skill which was acknowledged by Osler, and which could benefit all physicians. Chiropractic is very useful for spinal issues and other musculoskeletal problems. Homeopathy can provide very safe therapies for everyday ailments. Unfortunately, the skill and training of CAM practitioners may be lacking and difficult to document. One potential application might be to seek help from a CAM practitioner if your conventional medical regimen is failing. Be cautious about credentials. This is where a strong recommendation from a personal acquaintance would be helpful.

WHEN TO SEE OR NOT TO SEE THE DOCTOR—THAT IS THE QUESTION

After one or several promises of the impending arrival of the moments of truth, with several abortive stuttering steps in that direction, I will now "bring home the bacon" and provide some solid medical advice. The first topic might as well be bacon. The reference above in quotation marks extends back to twelfth century England and refers to a reward of a side of pig to a man who could swear in church that he had not argued with his wife for one year and one day. It was unknown then, but widely acknowledged now, to be one of the most dangerous foods available—to be ingested with great trepidation, lest one plug-up the last remaining artery standing between apparent "health" and a step off the cliff.

THE NATURE OF SYMPTOMS: LOCAL, SYSTEMIC, SEVERITY AND DURATION

With the exception of a dire emergency, such as when a person is suddenly rendered unconscious, the vast majority of patient-doctor encounters occur when the patient initiates a visit. Most often this occurs in response to an observation by the patient that the body is alerting them to a potential threat to its solvency. In other words, the bringing to consciousness of a new and unexplained phenomenon, whether it be subtle or intense represents the appearance of a symptom.

In order to be a reasonably informed patient, it is helpful to know some basic information about symptoms. For the most part, we would like our bodies to hum like a brand new sewing machine, allowing us to do whatever we want, whenever we want. For most children and young people, this is the case most of the time. With normal aging, despite the body's remarkable ability to fix itself, in contrast to the sewing machine, our genetic makeup and constant interaction with the environment induces the appearance of problems, which cannot be fully or immediately repaired. These problems manifest as symptoms, the language of nature, to assert that a problem has arisen.

Obviously, the nature of the symptom will be dependent on the structure or function involved. Symptoms can be local or systemic. Local refers to a relatively restricted area of the body. Systemic refers to effects felt in one way or another over much or all of the body. Many local symptoms are brought to our attention by the appearance of pain which is by far the most common symptom. Pain is an unpleasant feeling, yet one which is essential to life. Rare individuals who cannot feel pain are doomed to a life of disfigurement and premature death. So, acute pain is our friend. Chronic pain may have some life-preserving properties, but more often, the margins between beneficial and harmful become blurred. As a general rule of thumb, note this concept. A pain felt anywhere in the body, including chest, head, and abdomen, no matter how severe, lasting five (or perhaps ten) seconds or less, rarely connotes an important process. Thus, if not frequently repeated, it can generally be ignored.

Some symptoms are observed but not felt. These would include many things on the body surface, such as bumps, lumps, rashes, and changes in color. Symptoms from some organs such as changes in hearing, vision, smell, or touch may signal the appearance of trivial to serious issues. Also included would be things such as an itch without a rash. Anything which even slightly alters consciousness, such as dizziness, memory issues and lightheadedness gets our attention quickly. The same is true for the unexpected appearance of blood almost anywhere, from the whites of the eyes, to urinary, vaginal, skin, or rectal bleeding.

Lastly, most of the so-called systemic symptoms are relatively painless, that is perceived but without pain. Prominent in this group is fever. Often, with fever there may be chills. Other notable systemic symptoms include nausea, sweating, and weakness.

There are three crucial aspects of most symptoms, all having a strong influence as to whether or not you need to see the doctor—and the urgency involved in making an appointment. These three are location of symptom, severity of symptom, and how long it has been present. Regarding this last consideration of "how long," there is the associated consideration as to whether it is continuous or intermittent, and if intermittent, what is the periodicity or pattern of timing. The following example will illustrate the importance of these. In reference to location, a pain in the central part of the chest, even if mild and experienced many times before, is much more worthy of a visit to the doctor than a similar pain in the big toe. Granted, the toe pain may signal the onset of a gout attack, which could be very painful and limit mobility for a while. However, it is also likely to resolve on its own and is non life-threatening. The chest pain, however, could signal the presence of a severe blockage of a major coronary artery which could result in a fatal outcome. One lesson to be learned here, is that with the exception of the five (or ten) second guideline just mentioned, chest pain, new or different than before, is a symptom which almost always requires you to see the doctor.

Regarding severity of symptoms, for instance in the case of rectal bleeding, the appearance of blood staining on the tissue, in a person with known hemorrhoids may be a symptom which could be relatively ignored. On the other hands, passage of bright red liquid or clotted blood per rectum, although perhaps not truly serious and still representing external or internal hemorrhoidal bleeding, should never be ignored.

Regarding length of time the symptom has been present, there is a general rule-of-thumb to keep in mind: The longer a symptom has been present, the less likely it represents a serious disorder, and perhaps the less likely an explanation will be found, even if looked for. The corollary of this is that new symptoms should get your attention quicker than something which, for instance has occurred once a year for the last ten years. Consider a symptom "new" if it has been present for less than two years. As far as the periodicity of a symptom is concerned, even very small amounts of rectal bleeding noted with most bowel movements over the past few months should be much more alarming than a very infrequent appearance over the past ten years. So, in this case, frequency, or persistence, takes precedence over severity.

To summarize regarding these three key events about symptoms, location of a pain is very important. Coronary blockages are common and potentially life threatening. With the exception of the five to ten second rule, chest pains should not be ignored. Abdominal pains, if not severe, are common and usually not life-threatening in nature. A variable period of "observation" is likely the best action unless the pain is severe. In that case, medical attention should be accomplished ASAP. Head pains may be severe (migraine) and are self-limited for the most part. Any type of persisting head pain or chest or abdominal pain warrants attention. Infrequent occurrences of symptoms, widely separated in time, especially if present for many years, can likely be "observed" rather than acted upon. Severity of symptoms, with few exceptions, will likely force the patient to seek attention, and appropriately so.

So, this is a protean list of problems, which in fact barely touches the surface of potential symptoms and is somewhat intimidating even to contemplate. The situation is further complicated by the fact that for better or worse, we humans communicate primarily by the use of language. Words and phrases may have remarkably different meanings and connotations for different people. This is a perfect setup for miscommunication, which in turn is a perfect setup for misdiagnosis, which in turn is a perfect setup for a poor outcome.

How can we possibly overcome these hurdles? In fact, it is difficult. Getting back to the basics, it is likely impossible in a ten-minute visit. It is even less likely if you, the patient, come in with a list of disparate issues. It is the doctor's responsibility to always acknowledge the intrinsic roadblocks and to skillfully ferret out the crucial information. The doctor needs to hear the symptoms, not a diagnosis such as "Well, it's like when you have a gall bladder attack." Symptoms are how things feel or look. (Well, it's like if someone stuck in a long needle here under my right rib cage.") The doctor needs to ask what you mean by a "cramp." Most doctors think in terms of a pain which has a ramp-up, high intensity for a variable time, and ramp-down, whereas the patient may be describing a steady continuous pain. It is always the doctor's responsibility, in every patient encounter, to think of the most serious possible problem and work backwards from there by asking the appropriate questions. This will greatly reduce the possibility of a very bad outcome. In general, pain complaints should be expressed by you or dissected by the doctor in great detail. It is this minutia of data which usually indicate whether you go home with a pat on the back or proceed to the hospital via 911. Obviously, where is the pain? "My hip" is not good enough, because that smacks of a diagnosis, rather than a symptom. "Stand up and show me where the pain is." If it extends over a broad area, "Where is the worst point of the pain?" Where does it extend? Importantly, what makes it better? Or worse? Is it worse to press on it? Better? Very importantly, "What is the duration of the pain? One second versus one minute versus one hour versus all day makes huge differences in possibilities. As a rule of thumb, a pain lasting five seconds or less, no matter how severe is unlikely to represent a serious issue. Along with this, it also is likely to be an issue which will not be diagnosable. Communicate with widely-used images, such as: *Stabbing like a needle; Sharp or cutting like a knife; Dull, like a deep pressing; Pounding like a hammer; Burning like a fire; etc.*

The severity of a symptom is not necessarily indicative of the seriousness of the problem. For instance, although the pain of a migraine headache may be intense, there are rarely serious consequences. On the other hand, a malignant brain tumor may be present with very mild, or even no headache. Doctors and patients are both "guilty" of crimes and misdemeanors in dealing with pain issues. Doctors tend to pejoratively classify patients as wimps or stoics. Patients tend to over exaggerate pain symptoms. In my experience, the commonly-used scale for reporting pain is absolutely worthless and should be abandoned. This is the well known analog scale of one to ten. Most patients with chronic pain on chronic pain medication describe their pain as "an eight." Or "a nine." A few will look at the doctor straight-faced and describe it as a "twelve." All of these numbers are based on a scale of one to ten with ten being the most severe pain imaginable. So, what is a "twelve?" Instead, it is much more useful and helpful to describe pain as mild—moderate—severe, with mild to moderate and moderate to severe also legitimately helpful. Mild does not significantly interfere with daily functioning. Moderate will allow a person to engage in most of their usual pursuits but is limiting in some ways—and may reduce efficiency. "Severe" takes over the body and renders a person non-functional. The hybrid categories are self-explanatory.

Modern neuroscience has shed a great deal of light on pain perception, such that the concept of the "stoic" versus the "wimp" should be relegated to the dust bin of history. People are born with huge variabilities built into the nervous system. It all falls back on genetics and on incredibly complex switching on or off of various genes, which subsequently alter the function of pain receptors at multiple levels of the nervous system, which ultimately affects how a patient feels. That does not mean they should report pain as a "twelve." It is not the patient's fault that their pain is severe, as long as it genuinely does severely compromise function globally.

Success or failure of a correct diagnosis and treatment begins with a recitation of symptoms. This has been known for one hundred fifty years. In sitting down with your doctor, you must convey how you feel rather than using diagnosis, like "it's another attack of diverticulitis." It is mandatory that you be as rigorously accurate and authentic as possible, avoiding exaggerations. The skilled physician can help draw the correct and necessary information from you. Review of the history may be required a second or third time to check for consistency of data. An accurately obtained history of symptoms, including the timing of events, severity, periodicity, related factors, exacerbating factors, attenuating factors and many other bits of information can either point to the diagnosis like an arrow, or zig-zag, herky-jerky through the foggy swamp. The meeting of the patient and the doctor in this matter is the Holy Grail of medical practice, the crucible for miraculous powers.

IS IT A COLD, THE FLU, OR THE START OF A SOON-TO-BE FATAL ILLNESS?

Although there is obviously a tongue-in-cheek flavor to the title of this chapter, and although this chapter alone will likely induce so much fear in you as to help to permanently establish the need for physicians no matter what the future may hold, it also does raise some important points which are worthy of special attention.

The common cold is a ubiquitous illness, experienced early and repeatedly in life, and is used as a rallying point to illustrate the failings of modern medical science ("We can go to the moon, but we can't cure the common cold."). Perhaps this is true. A "cold" is an upper respiratory infection (URI). "Upper" refers to structures above the larynx, or voice box. The vast majority of these illnesses are caused by viruses, in and of themselves fascinating little things. I hesitate to call them "creatures" for reasons which follow.

Believe it or not, it is unclear as to whether they should be considered to be living. Factually, they consist of "naked" DNA (deoxyribonucleic acid) or RNA (ribonucleic acid)—and that is all! "Mobile genetic particles." The fancy ones may have an envelope of protein around them, perhaps giving them a greater ability to enter cells. They exhibit characteristics of both living and non-living entities. They can even more convincingly be described as inert or animated based on which definition of "life" is used.

We have no issue classifying unicellular creatures as living. We have all seen these under the microscope in school, fascinated by their herky-jerky movements, but perhaps not appreciating how complex they are. It is stated that most or all of the myriad of biochemical processes that sustain the life of you and me occur in that single cell.

A cell can be likened to an old, walled city, so commonly found even up to early modern times. The wall is like the cell membrane, separating self from non-self, friend from foe. Inside the wall are a variety of activities simultaneously churning away, all of which contribute to keeping the city alive. The same is true for cells, which have numerous structures to use and transform energy, metaphorically to keep the lights on. The cell, just as the walled city, is absolutely dependant on the external environment which surrounds it, and from which it borrows or steals resources to stoke the fire of life. Given this influx of resources, the cell can live, thrive, and be about as happy as a cell can be. In fact, they are so happy that they can divide. That is, reproduce!

Viruses on their own are absolutely not metabolic. That is, they don't manufacture anything. They cannot reproduce on their own. Getting back to the walled city analogy, a virus might be like a cold fog forming and vanishing, advancing on the city. If it enters, it may bring diseases with it, as was thought to be possible in times past. Diseases could annihilate the city in a matter of weeks. If the virus enters the cell (and how it does is not always clear), the one thing it knows how to do is to commandeer the blueprints, insert itself into the driver's seat, and turn most or all of the energy production of the cell into replication of more and more copies of itself. Needless to say, as the cell-city devotes all of its energy to the invader, it dies.

Enough speculation as to whether or not viruses are alive. They "infect" everything, entering cells of plants, animals, insects, and even bacteria. What would the universe be like without them? Would planet earth be a better place or worse? If not living, are they essential to life itself? As straight forward as these simple questions may seem, I don't think they are convincingly answered, perhaps because no previous numbskull has asked such ridiculous questions.

Getting back to the common cold, symptoms could likely be predicted based on the location of the infection. Sore throat, nasal congestion and drainage, mild headache, ear fullness or stuffiness are commonly seen alone or in combination, representing the local symptoms. Systemic symptoms are often present but almost invariably mild. (This is a key point in differentiating cold from flu.) Systemic symptoms might be very low grade fever and mild "malaise." The latter term is a word borrowed from French, commonly used by doctors, and implies feeling "crummy"…mildly so. The entire process usually runs its course in three to five days. Antibiotics are not indicated during this time frame.

If symptoms persist more than seven days, and particularly if there is increasing cough or nasal congestion, drainage, and even facial pain, then this is no longer a simple cold. In fact, the virus has likely damaged the lining membranes enough to allow for the appearance of a secondary infection, producing bronchitis and/or sinusitis. Or perhaps it never was a virus, but a cross between virus and bacteria, such as mycoplasma, which can go on for much longer than three to five days. At this point, antibiotics may be helpful and are up to the discretion of your doctor. Otherwise, colds are treated "symptomatically." This means that we select the worst symptoms and recommend medication which will ameliorate the symptoms most distressing.

So, why can we go to the moon and not cure the cold? There are many reasons, including cultural, economic, biologic, and others. The key reasons likely hinge on two facts: Firstly, colds are nuisance illnesses rather than serious threats, perhaps not warranting huge expenditures to pursue a "cure." Secondly, viruses that cause colds are ubiquitous, likely numbering in the thousands of varieties and are capable of very rapid genetic mutations. All of these factors make development of an umbrella vaccine or antibiotic-type drug a huge challenge, and for all we know, impossible.

"Flu," which is short for influenza, is an illness significantly different than a cold. The similarities are that both are caused by viruses, with the many varieties of influenza virus being the most common cause of flu. The initial symptoms, seen within the first twenty-four hours may be identical. However, that is where the similarity ends. After the first day or two, influenza is dominated by systemic symptoms including fever up to 104 degrees, chills, including shivering chills, body aches, headaches, loss of appetite, and weakness. There are many other possible symptoms as well. The course is much more protracted, often lasting for seven to ten days. Once again, no antibiotics are indicated. Symptomatic treatment may be helpful. The disease can be diminished in severity or even eliminated by vaccination done at least six weeks before exposure. The very young and very old, or those debilitated by a variety of chronic diseases, appear to be the most susceptible to complications, or even death. Anti-viral antibiotics, especially used within the first twenty-four to forty-eight hours may ameliorate the severity and truncate the length of the illness. The influenza pandemic of 1918, obviously in the pre-antibiotic era, is estimated to have been a major causative factor in the deaths of more than twenty, and perhaps as many as fifty, million people.

Within the recent past, people have become aware of a condition called sepsis. Physicians frequently call it sepsis syndrome. Syndrome refers to a certain constellation of symptoms, somewhat predictable for whatever syndrome is in question. Sepsis is what used to be called "blood poisoning." It refers to the entry of bacteria into the bloodstream, with the potential of widely disseminating what was previously a focal infection. The three most common causes of sepsis are pneumonia, urinary tract infection (in particular, kidney infection), and cellulitis. Cellulitis is a skin, or "soft tissue" infection, which is usually painful and visible. Sepsis may be much more common than we think. In otherwise healthy people, it may be cleared spontaneously by the immune system. Alternatively, it has the potential to overwhelm the immune system. If this occurs, then the sepsis syndrome comes into play with "multiple organ system failure." Patients are quickly rendered severely ill. Even with aggressive treatment in the hospital, sepsis syndrome carries a substantial risk of death. The most common symptoms of sepsis syndrome include high fever, shivering chills, profound weakness, alteration in mentation, and eventually multiple organ system failure.

Back to the opening question of when to see the doctor. Note that with the exception of alteration of mentation, the symptoms of sepsis syndrome, possibly fatal, sound remarkably similar to influenza syndrome, almost invariably self-limited. Is there a way to tell the difference, or do you just roll the dice and wait to see if you made the right (live) or wrong (die) choice?

First of all, most people are aware if there is a flu epidemic in the community. Ever since 1918, when 50,000,000 people died from an influenza pandemic, people have paid attention to this. Secondly, have you been in contact with people with a similar illness? Third, are you basically healthy? Fourth, are you able to get up and move around, and are you thinking clearly? If the answer to all of these questions is "yes," then there is a very high likelihood that you have the flu syndrome. If the answers are "no," you might begin to worry a little and to try to remember if you have completed your last will and testament.

If you have had a concomitant illness which could be pneumonia (cough, chest pain, difficulty breathing), kidney infection (back pain, discolored or bloody urine, and history of kidney stones), or cellulitis (swollen red, tender skin area, usually leg), forget concerns about your will and proceed to the emergency room. If you are a Libran and can't make up your mind after this thorough assessment of your chances, call your doctor. Likely, he or she will be able to act as the tie breaker and suggest a plan of action. Perhaps the doctor might even ask you to proceed to the office where a very simple office test could establish a diagnosis of flu in a few minutes. Don't leave Dr. Goldstein out of the equation unless he is not available.

USE AND MISUSE OF THE E.R.— THE MOST EXPENSIVE WALK-IN CLINIC IN THE UNIVERSE

Having begun training in medicine in 1962, my career has almost completely spanned the life of the emergency room. Wartime experiences and most notably the Korean War, ending in 1952, brought to the attention of military doctors the need for rapid triage of patients and quick initiation of treatment to even hope for the possibility of a good outcome. This awareness carried over as these doctors re-entered private practice. Gradually, hospitals began to set aside space for emergency services. By the 1960s, many of these nascent emergency departments were staffed by nurses. Community physicians were available, although not continuously physically present, should more advanced services be needed. Nevertheless, even by the mid-1960s, many community hospitals did not yet offer emergency services.

In 1966, the National Academy of Sciences prepared a report subtitled "The Neglected Disease of Modern Society" in which the deficiency of emergency medical services, and consequences of this, were portrayed. (If this report was written today, the title would be "Neglected No More.") This report seemed to be the spark that ignited the rapid development of the modern emergency department, as well as the ancillary services such as 911. As a consequence, the American College of Emergency Physicians was founded in 1968.

My first intimate experiences in emergency medicine occurred in 1967 during "internship" at a large inner-city hospital. At that teaching hospital, the E.R. already was a busy and fairly sophisticated department, likely atypical for the times. The police would often bring in victims of the "Saturday Night Knife and Gun Club" to be "pronounced," meaning pronounced medically dead. The strangest of all of those occurred one night as they backed their paddy wagon up to the loading ramp and asked me to come out. As they rolled a fifty-five gallon drum onto the lighted ramp, I noted a trail of fetid smoke drifting upwards from the drum. Inside the drum was a barely recognizable mass of raw and roasted flesh of a once human being, on the wrong side of the gasoline-match connection.

On another occasion during morning rush hour, a major commuter train accident nearby gave me the opportunity to see how primitive triage was even then as scores of victims—from barely scratched to dying or dead—were unceremoniously hauled in all at once. When not quite so chaotic, ER experience also showed me a glimpse of the future as large numbers of indigent, terribly ill people came in with common illnesses, seen at their worst—and desperately in need of help. Most of these people came in without the help of emergency vehicles. Very few had money or insurance.

The last forty years have shown dramatic changes in emergency medical services. "911" is a term which young children understand. Every hospital has an E.R. Emergency room physicians go through residency training programs and seek board certification. The skill set of these physicians is impressively broad, and much is demanded of them. As a group, many of them are among the best physicians that we train in terms of their overall competency. At this juncture, if you are very ill and make it to the E.R. alive, you will likely survive. All of this is good news for patients.

The bad news is now to come. The term "emergency room" rolls off our lips with such ease (except for those who call it the "E.R. room") that we fail to pay attention to the words. "Room" is not as important, as even the broom closet in the E.R. is a room. The important word is "emergency." Unfortunately, the E.R. is now overrun by non-emergency patients. Certainly, one does not need to be in a smoking barrel or victimized by a train wreck to come in. However, those who have looked at the data concede that most often, the emergency room has lost its emergency connotation, having been adulterated into a very expensive walk-in clinic.

Emergency room misuse is an almost equal blight, on one side of the ledger, while stunning accomplishments of E.R. medicine on the other side are obvious. With the tremendous expectations we have on the E.R., as one would anticipate, it is equipped with technologically advanced equipment, and with nursing and ancillary staffing of highly trained and skilled personnel. Combine this with the fact that since E.R. doctors rightly feel themselves to be the single most vulnerable group regarding malpractice issues, "defensive medicine" is practiced there to a greater extent than anywhere else in medicine. "Defensive medicine" refers to tests and procedures which may not be strictly indicated for the patient, but that are done anyway to protect the doctor should there be a future claim. All of this combines to create the "perfect storm" and to make the E.R. a very expensive place for a patient to be. It is safe to say, that depending on the medical issue and the length of time a patient stays, a cost of somewhere between five hundred to one thousand dollars per hour is usual. From another angle, for non-emergent conditions, it could be up to ten times more expensive in the E.R. compared to the doctor's office.

In summary, we as a society and a culture have allowed the E.R. to greatly overextend its mission. People are not turned away. Waiting times may be long, and triage even more crucial and difficult. Many patients appear with non-emergent issues. E.R. physicians have to be constantly vigilant as they see routine illness and severe illness side by side. Cost of care is extremely high. A substantial number of patients are uninsured or underinsured, shifting the burden of payment to those with insurance—and straining the financial stability of hospitals. Mixed in with all of the non-emergent patients, and the general chaos surrounding a busy place like the E.R., are the smaller number of truly critically ill people, who may not necessarily look that way—and who could be lost in the shuffle.

Once again, this faulty system can be changed, if we want it changed. If we do, we need a stepwise plan, and it will take time to be fully implemented. In the meantime, one immediate reprieve is to call your doctor when you think you are seriously ill. Perhaps the doctor could see you quickly and efficiently. Obviously, with advent of the E.R., doctors have substantially relinquished responsibility for sick patients. If we wish to change the system, doctors would have to be available by phone. They would need to be capable of seeing emergent or urgent patients. There would need to be changes in patients' patterns of seeking care, and perhaps even physical changes in doctors' offices and their practice patterns. It could happen, one step at a time, if we want it to. It is not really that difficult. We need more primary care physicians (PCPs), seeing fewer patients with programmed open slots in their schedule at the beginning of every day, to accommodate urgent or emergent patients.

Unless you are unconscious, or have uncontrolled bleeding, if nothing else, call your doctor before heading to the E.R.

Perhaps twenty-five years ago, as the proliferation of sophisticated emergency rooms continued, and their popularity as community watering holes exponentially increased ("I'll meet you in the E.R.!"), and as most community physicians relinquished responsibility for such patients, a large chasm opened in this techtonic cataclysm. Where was the patient to go with a "quasi-emergency?" And, what is a "quasi-emergency?" First of all, it may occur when you know for a fact that your doctor is not available to you, even by telephone. This could include any after hours or weekend-holiday times. Secondly, it involves an issue which you judge should not wait until the doctor is conveniently available. On the other hand, you also know with a reasonable degree of certainty that this condition is not inherently dangerous or life threatening.

This chasm, in fact, was largely filled rather quickly by the appearance of medical establishments which have been variously termed, but perhaps most commonly something like "Urgent Care." Essentially, these are walk-in clinics, which means that no appointments are needed. As best I can tell, these facilities are usually staffed twelve to eighteen hours per day by competent people. They are set up to do a wide range of services, such as screening for truly serious illness, suturing, removing foreign bodies from skin, and treating most acute illnesses and injuries, with the exception of major fractures. Once again, as best I can tell, waiting times and costs of care are reasonable by today's standards.

The major question, or concern, then is why do these facilities appear to be less "popular" than might be expected. Do they give inferior care, or is this just patient choice? I suspect the latter. So, the next time the need for quasi-emergent care is needed, this may be a good alternative for both you, and the emergency room staff.

As a sidelight, many hospitals have established extensions of their facilities to outlying areas, calling some such facilities "clinics" and some even "Urgent Care." Do not suspect this trend is done in the tone of the Good Samaritan, or for your convenience. It is done as a result of intense inter-hospital competition for patients—and also to compete with the free-standing Urgent Care clinics just mentioned. These hospital-run facilities function much more closely to the mold of the E.R., including cost, than Urgent Care.

ROUTINE EXAMS: GOOD FOR THE PATIENT? GOOD FOR THE DOCTOR? OR, GOOD FOR NOTHING?

At the time that I began my career in medicine in 1962, it was still a widely prevalent pattern to admit patients to the hospital for an indefinite period of time, basically for the convenience of the patient and/or doctor. Since it was "standard of care" to admit a patient with a documented heart attack for six weeks (no misprint!), it was common to admit someone for two to three weeks with nondescript, undiagnosed chest pain. It was also common to admit patients for perhaps a week for a "check up." Lastly, the same offer could be extended to a person suffering from stress, to be basically admitted for "R & R" (rest and relaxation). As archaic as these practice standards of care may seem now, since daily hospital charges were so relatively low, "payers" did not seem to object.

Obviously, no physician can currently legitimately expect to admit a patient to the hospital for a routine exam. In fact, after 1966 as the government became more involved as a payer, and as technology and costs began to skyrocket, research was done involving one of the longstanding bastions of medical practice, that being the "annual physical."

Once again, the most common event leading to a patient-doctor encounter is the appearance of a symptom or symptom complex (a variety of symptoms representative of a single disease). In fact, this is appropriate. As a result, it becomes imperative for a patient to be attentive to the messages emanating from the body, and to assess such messages ideally from a stance midway the hypochondriac and the ostrich (with its head in the sand). It is so important to warrant restatement. It is as equally inappropriate to come to the doctor with every brand new symptom, as it is to ignore a loud, banging symptom going on for a long time. Obviously, the severity of a symptom, very severe to barely detectable, should have some bearing on the decision. All of the other issues, such as location of symptom, length of time present, pattern of appearance—disappearance, all need to be considered. With the typical "non-descript" symptom, if there is doubt or if you are worried, see the doctor.

So, what if there are NO persistently disturbing symptoms? Does that mean that you NEVER see the doctor? Note that the following comments and recommendations are excluding children and adolescents. Also, it represents what I think is an amalgam of evidence-based medicine and personal experience. Also note that an individual who exercises at a high level of physical activity has a built-in, back-up mechanism which is tuned in to producing symptoms earlier in the time course of a disease, than someone who never exercises strenuously. STRENUOUS EXERCISE, in my personal opinion (no evidence-basing here), is the single-most important factor in getting a leg up on deep health. The only possible exception might be a negative one, i.e., NOT SMOKING. What is not always appreciated is that strenuous exercise, of a hundred different varieties, is a total-organism experience. It involves a strong element of mental toughness as well as body toughness. The mental toughness is an important element, as this often fades or diminishes in the face of physical illness. In a way, the mental aspect acts like a double check. If the exercise can be done with a minimum of ego investment, that is for your benefit

---

**Reduction/Elimination of
Most Chronic Diseases**

1.) Eat a good diet
    Low in animal fat
    High in fiber
    Fruits, vegetable, nuts

2.) Stay thin:
    High School graduation
    weight or less

3.) Never smoke or use any
    nicotine products.

4.) Regular strenuous exercise

---

and for the benefit that you can bring into the world as a healthy, vibrant person, rather than to subjugate a competitor, it becomes an even more powerful tool. Recall that we are human animals and have always been predators. Our life in modern society has shown us that "hard wiring" can be re-wired in a short period of time (recall that the wolf became the dog in fifty years or less). It may appear to us now that regular, strenuous exercise is a peculiar diversion of a relatively small group of "health nuts." In fact, however, for over ninety-nine percent of the history of *homo sapiens sapiens*, the ability to move and to have stamina was literally a matter of life or death. Even in modern times, inability to keep up with the caribou migration in the Inuit culture meant that you were left behind (to die). Research involving physical activity is not easy to study because of disinterest by pharmaceutical companies, who are the major source of funding, as well as the length of time needed to produce meaningful results. Nevertheless, a growing body of evidence points to the definitively beneficial effects of regular, strenuous exercise across a wide range of diseases evaluated. So, recommendations regarding the frequency of routine physical exams will vary and may be inversely proportional to the level of physical activity of the patient in question.

In fact, a recent research article in a prestigious journal of internal medicine pointed out a dramatic reduction in the appearance of most degenerative diseases associated with aging in the setting of four variables. The factors were: (1) Eating a good diet, (2) Staying thin, (3) Never smoking, and (4) Involvement in regular, strenuous exercise.

MUSINGS REGARDING BREAST AND GENITAL CANCER IN FEMALES

It can be safely said that for the most individuals, up to the age of fifty, there are few well-documented beneficial recommendations for routine checkups. On the other hand, there are many "traditions," most involving women. It is advisable that females, at any age, should begin to have pap spears as soon as regular sexual intercourse begins. This is because of the known connection between human papillomavirus infection with cervical cancer and the likelihood of infection increasing with the number of sexual partners. For a virginal female, this would not be necessary until marriage if there are no symptoms. If marriage is delayed, first pap smear would likely be delayed until age thirty, although the traditional recommendation is twenty-one. This may sound heretical, and many young women might not be comfortable with this. Stated again, if there is worry, see the doctor!

Once married, most women see the doctor fairly regularly. What may not be widely known is that for any woman, with three consecutive "negative" pap smears, in either a monogamous relationship or sexually inactive, further pap smears can be delayed to every three years. Many women begin with mammograms in their thirties to forty. This is somewhat curious as the traditional recommendation has been to start at age fifty. To briefly summarize, the value of yearly or every-other-year mammography for women above age fifty is well documented. The data is debatable between the ages of forty and fifty. Women with a first-line relative with breast cancer (meaning mother, sister, daughter), or with multiple relatives with breast cancer, or with a male family member with such, should begin at age forty. The interval between exams is also debatable, with the advice being every one to two years.

When asked whether or not they do breast self-exams, many women reply that they don't do it because they have no idea what they are finding. Regarding this, breast self-exam is free of charge, absolutely without side effects, and proven to be helpful. Therefore, women who don't do it are demonstrating the previously noted ostrich approach. Breast self-exams are best done in the shower, with soapy breasts, monthly. The technique is simple. Many women have fibrocystic breast disease, which causes the breasts to develop a diffuse, finely lumpy texture. The texture can vary somewhat during the menstrual cycle. It is true that on first or second exam, the novice may not have any idea what they are doing, reminiscent of a medical student. However, never forget the oft-quoted medical student motto regarding exams and procedures: "See one. Do one. Teach one." The learning curve is quick! Within a short period of time, you will "know" your own breasts better than anyone else, including your doctor. So, do it!

There is something to keep in mind with cancer detection. This is definitely my opinion, and by definition, is thus not evidence-based. Nevertheless, I am convinced that it is basically true. There are a few cancers that it seems to be especially true for, including breast cancer. Specialists in breast care, including pathologists, have a large array of criteria used to predict the future activity of a cancer. Just like the weatherman or woman, statistical predictions can be made regarding such activity. Genetic analysis of tumors has added a new dimension to this, just as "Doppler radar" assists in weather prediction. The problem is that when all is said and done, we still obviously do not know what all the factors are, which are likely to be predictive in any given cancer. This seems to be especially true for breast cancer. So, when treatment for a given tumor is completed, the doctor can give you a prognosis. In breast cancer, however, the missing link is what could be described in purposefully vague terms as the "intrinsic biologic nature" of the tumor. The tumor is genetically different than you. So, even though it is "you," it is also "not you." The "not you" aspect of the tumor and you will remain at war, which could be a delicate balance of control or loss of control, which can go on for many years.

The whole point is that despite all of our attempts to find and treat cancer "early," there are unknown factors which continue to scuttle our best-laid attempts. This does not mean that we should never think of cancer, like the ostrich, or never screen for cancer. There are large numbers of evidence-based studies which indicate that these efforts can prolong life...in certain circumstances. So, cancer screening should be done the Greek way...in moderation; moderation in effort, and moderation in expected outcome. We all need to understand that despite our most meticulous efforts with screening, that is "early detection" and "early" treatment, we still have no practical ways to detect microscopic metastases, and incomplete tools to estimate the biologic nature of a given tumor.

MUSINGS REGARDING LUNG CANCER

Before we leave the topic of cancer for now, let me close with one or several fascinating features of lung cancer. This is a devastating condition with a number of aspects which have not been sufficiently appreciated. Most people know that it is related to smoking. This adds a different dimension of tragedy to the disease, in that there exists the self-imposed aspect. There are four major categories of lung cancer, each compromising roughly twenty-five percent of all lung cancer. Three of these, obviously comprising approximately seventy-five percent of the total, in numerous studies over many years have been shown to be definitely related to cigarette smoking. The fourth called "adenocarcinoma" of the lung occurs with equal frequency in smokers and non-smokers. In fact, the other three types almost never occur in non-smokers. When they do, there almost always is a confounding history of second-hand smoke exposure or "closet smoking," that is, light and/or intermittent smoking. Keep in mind that the dictum, "never say never, never say always" applies to medical issues, just as it does to all issues in life.

Now for the revelations promised above. With all of our contemporary advances in diagnosis and treatment of cancer, the cure rate for lung cancer now is roughly the same as it was seventy-five years ago: ten percent. Secondly, and perhaps even more remarkably, is the following observation. From the time a smoker stops smoking, their increased risk of lung cancer does not return to the baseline risk for a non-smoker for ten to fifteen years! This implies that a microscopic focus of cancer, or pre-cancer, in the lung at the time of quitting (the "not you") can smolder for fifteen years as the battle with "you" is waged, before one or the other claims total "victory." It is not clear whether or not other cancers share this very long embryonic period. With trillions of cells in the body, it is mathematically inevitable that cells or groups of cells mutate into malignant cells all the time. Fortunately, most of the time, our immune systems recognize this quickly and do away with the "not you." When this fails to occur, for whatever reason, clinical cancer may eventually appear.

Here are further observations regarding this fascinating disease. The first deals with "screening" or early detection. Once again, a recently detected experimental "fact" appears to defy explanation. Several lines of research have demonstrated that with modern detection devices and techniques, although we are able to diagnose lung cancer in an earlier stage now, this ability has not changed survival statistics! In other words, in comparing groups of patients who have early detection and aggressive treatment, versus those who have aggressive treatment without early detection efforts, there is no difference in survival. This definitely seems counterintuitive, but it is accepted as true at this time. If it is true, besides shaking the basic foundations of early detection, it implies that some of those small, "early" lung cancers have a biologic nature which is such that they never would have progressed to the point where they become clinically relevant! (The same kinds of observations have been made with prostate cancer). Perhaps, they may even regress?

Two final facts about lung cancer. First, survival is better for patients with lung cancer who quit smoking after the cancer is detected than for those who continue to smoke. This too seems a little odd.

Lastly, the number one cancer killer in women is not breast cancer. You guessed it! Lung cancer.

Doctors spend a great deal of time counseling patients to do this, and don't do that. It is apparent that often such advice is not followed. Habits and habitual behavior, as we all know, are very difficult to change. The addictive feature of cigarette smoking is such that the continuation of smoking after the appearance of life-threatening diseases known to be associated with smoking (such as coronary blockages, emphysema, stroke, and lung cancer) is a common, albeit tragic, phenomenon. The challenge is to continue to support and to love unconditionally those who continue to smoke. It is their journey, and it is not our right to enforce changes against their will.

THE SILENT ZONE

With the exception of the traditional recommendations given to young females, there are actually no widely recommended guidelines for males and females up to the age of fifty. So this thirty-year interval of time represents a kind of silent zone, the eye of the hurricane, with all types of childhood and adolescent issues on one side—and the emerging ravages of life's slings and arrows on the other. One could make a case that for an adult with no persisting symptoms of note, all that needs to be done is an occasional drug store or health-fair blood pressure measurement, and a cholesterol or general blood panel assessment every five years or so. This too, is often available in the community free of charge at health fairs and other venues, such as insurance exams. In summary, for an asymptomatic (no persisting symptoms) young to middle aged adult, particularly one who participates in regular, strenuous exercise, it is possible to go thirty years without seeing the doctor. Although this may sound heretical, evidence indicating that this pattern is imprudent is not available. In fact, when I occasionally see a fifty-year-old person in the office, who sheepishly confesses that they are in for a checkup, not having seen the doctor for twenty or thirty years, I congratulate them! This person has obviously been lucky (as Louis Pasteur stated, smart and luck are frequently interconnected). In addition, it is highly likely that they are skilled in listening to and interpreting body messages. They are also likely to be living a healthy life style, in all of its ramifications. So, no chastisement, but congratulations for doing so well so long.

By the age of fifty, things have begun to change. Firstly, several definite recommendations finally emerge. The major ones would include mammograms for women, prostate exams for men, colonoscopy for both, and possibly cardiac stress tests. In addition, now that the body-vehicle has fifty or sixty thousand miles rung up, it is beginning to make itself known in quiet ways. Most of the diseases of aging, including cancers and cardiovascular issues, become much more common.

BLOOD PRESSURE CONCERNS

S ince blood pressure is to be checked occasionally over this long time span, this is an important issue and deserves attention. Measurements of blood pressure began in the 1890s. It became quickly apparent that blood pressure varied widely in the population, and that elevations of blood pressure were associated with adverse events. For many years, the ideal normal blood pressure has been established at 120/80. The 120 is the "systolic," or the peak pressure seen as a result of contraction and emptying of the heart. The 80 is the "diastolic," corresponding with relaxation and filling of the heart. Interestingly, over one hundred years after these measurements were first made, we are still learning useful information about blood pressure. Certain facets of debate have gone "cold," and some have become "hot." There remain issues which are fervently debated. The following comments are once again a mixture of evidenced-based and personal opinion.

For decades it was debated whether elevations of the systolic or diastolic component of blood pressure was the crucial one. A few assumptions have emerged from this debate. Both components are important but perhaps represent different phenomena. Systolic elevation appears to be much more closely connected with the mind-body states of tension and anxiety—and is thus more variable and more likely to be part of the "white coat" syndrome. Also, when persistent, it is thought to reflect the degree of rigidity of artery walls, this being the finding in "hardening of the arteries," otherwise called arteriosclerosis.

The walls of arteries normally contain abundant amounts of muscle and elastic tissue, which are "soft" to touch and allow for expansion and contraction. This phenomenon gives rise to the palpable pulse. When artery walls become damaged from all of the noxious things that can damage them (cholesterol, diabetes, smoking, high blood pressure, etc.), the muscle and elastic components of the walls become replaced by calcium as well as cholesterol plaques and eventually fibrous tissues ("scar"), all of which "harden" the arteries.

Diastolic elevations, alternatively, more often are independent of other issues, not so frequently seen in white-coat syndrome, and likely reflect hormonal and genetic influences on the makeup and responsiveness of artery walls. For example, blood pressure of 170/80 might be a typical one for a person with arteriosclerosis. This may actually be more difficult to treat safely than a pressure of 160/105 in a young person with genetic hypertension. In trying to bring the 170 down to an "acceptable" 130, this might drop the diastolic to 60 or 65, causing the person to feel lightheaded.

With the proliferation of reliable, inexpensive, digital blood pressure machines for home use, we have learned a great deal about hypertension. The "white coat" syndrome was initially borrowed from the image of the doctor wearing a white coat. Such coats were initially embraced by medical doctors around 1900, as they tried to abandon the image of the "quack" and tried to enhance the image of the scientist. (I don't think it has been recently documented what percentage of practicing medical doctors actually wear white coats). The assumptions were that when the doctor takes the person's blood pressure, this induces an element of anxiety in some people, resulting in the term white coat syndrome or white coat hypertension. It was hoped that home blood pressure readings would help to clarify this, and sometimes they do. For instance, with a home machine, which is regularly calibrated with a mercury manometer in the doctor's office, consistently elevated pressure in the doctor's office and consistently normal levels at home connote the classical white coat syndrome.

What, in fact is considered "normal?" Remarkably, even this ridiculously simple notion is not uniformly agreed upon. Life insurance companies consider 140/90 to be mild hypertension, based on their actuarial tables. Actually, blood pressure consistently greater than 135/85 is abnormal and potentially hazardous.

There is an elegant way to obtain a huge amount of blood pressure data. I wanted to use the term "elegant" because it is so curious and cute. It is a term used by mathematicians and scientists (remember that doctors are quasi-scientists) to explain appearingly complex phenomena with simple and definitive data. Such simplified data are described as "elegant." It also gives me an excuse to mention another adorable term, Ockham's razor, extending back to the fourteenth century, again opining that in deciphering a puzzle, the simplest explanation taking the existing circumstances into account, is the best explanation. The elegant way to solve the puzzle as to whether a given patient has or does not have hypertension is to perform a "simple" 24-hour ambulatory blood pressure study. It is simple to satisfy both mathematicians and Ockham, and relatively inexpensive. It provides an enormous amount of data, that is, 48 blood pressure readings, including multiple readings during sleep. The computer can present raw data and manipulate the data in a number of interesting and informative ways to help the doctor and the patient see the issue more clearly. Ockham's razor at its best!

Most recently, the medical community has been rocked by what may be a pharmaceutical company scam. Fear not, this is neither the first nor the last such misrepresentation. It has to do with the concept of "pre-hypertension." In this format, normal blood pressure is defined as 90 to 119 over 60 to 79. Therefore "pre-hypertension" could be as low as 120/80. Obviously, this could suggest the "need" to place more people on medication. This concept should be ignored, at least for the time being.

Lastly, what to do when a definite diagnosis of hypertension is rendered? There is some good news here. Approximately 25% of the hypertensive population is salt-sensitive. This implies that for these people, a significant reduction in salt intake over at least a thirty-day period can result in a meaningful drop in blood pressure. Even more impressively, approximately twenty-five percent of the hypertensive population is alcohol sensitive. In this group, even one or two beers— or glasses of wine or "shots" of hard liquor per day—can significantly elevate blood pressure. Abstinence from such social drinking can dramatically reduce blood pressure within a few days. Both of these dietary changes are highly recommended as an "experiment." If neither is effective, weight loss and exercise can lower blood pressure by five to eight points. Calcium, magnesium, potassium, garlic and other supplements can make a similar difference. The goal is to get blood pressure below 135 systolic and 85 diastolic. If none of these methods are effective, you will likely need medication, and likely for the rest of your life. A relatively small percentage of patients, if very well-controlled for two years or more, can discontinue medication under their doctor's supervision, with continuation of normal readings for variable periods of time.

We have wandered widely from the issue of routine exams, diverted by important issues regarding cancer and blood pressure. Mammograms and prostate surveillance are both relatively easy and relatively inexpensive—and should be done. Breast cancer and prostate cancer are extremely common in this age group. Prostate screening has come under close scrutiny. Nevertheless, it still appears to be very useful for men between the ages of fifty and eighty. After eighty, it is likely no longer useful. Screening involves both the "PSA" blood test for "prostate specific antigen" and the digital rectal exam with direct palpation of the prostate with the examining finger. These studies can both be done as part of a routine physical exam. Referral to a urologist would be necessary only at the discretion of your doctor. Men with a family history of prostate cancer in a first-line relative (father, brother, son) should begin surveillance at age 40.

So-called "Family History" is often crucial in outlining a reasonable program of health maintenance and surveillance for a given individual. Family history is the course that your genetic river flows naturally. It is your personal roadmap, giving predictive information where you will go if left unattended. It is greatly to your advantage to pay close attention to this, and it will be mentioned repeatedly. Obviously in a person with a strong family history of heart or vascular issues it would be tragic to ignore this until age fifty. The very beginnings of arteriosclerosis have been shown to be noticeable in children in autopsy studies. The changes are well developed by ages twenty to thirty (first determined with autopsies of Korean War victims). Such a history demands lifetime attention to all of the risk factors of diabetes, hypertension, elevated cholesterol, and tobacco usage. Elements of weight control and exercise

Cardiovascular Risk Profile

Primary

- Smoking history
- Cholesterol levels
- Diabetes
- Blood Pressure
- Family history

Secondary

- Activity level
- Homocysteine level
- Lipoprotein A level

can make a huge difference. Children and young adults need to be made aware of these issues, with simple but explicit reasons why these issues are important. A relatively simple grading system can help you and your doctor decide if you need cardiovascular screening. Note five primary risk factors: diabetes, hypertension, high cholesterol, cigarette smoking, and family history. If each of these represents 1 point, a score of zero or 1 is low, and likely does not strongly suggest the need for surveillance. A score of 4 or 5 is high and should require regular surveillance, perhaps every 3 to 5 years. Lastly, a score of 2 or 3 is intermediate, and somewhat more difficult to decide upon. Most people at age 50 or above have 2 or 3 risk factors. Of the five, it appears to me that family history, diabetes, and cigarette smoking are the most worrisome. It is probably best to err on the side of being conservative, that is careful. The study most often done for cardiac surveillance is simple, safe, and at a reasonable cost. It is called a "stress echo" test, combining a standardized exercise protocol on a treadmill, with ultrasound of the heart pre- and post-exercise. It affords an 85% to 90% reliability of "low risk" of acute coronary events in the next two to three years." It is a "non-invasive" test, meaning nothing enters the body, giving it the highest margin of safety. For those who cannot exercise, there is a non-exercise variant which can be done, with the only drawbacks that it does involve radiation exposure, and it is more expensive. Both tests are widely used and are very helpful in the setting of a common and potentially lethal disease. This should be done.

What about the coronary calcium scoring test, which has come into vogue in the last five to ten years? It can give useful information. Perhaps the most useful would be that no coronary calcium is seen. This would be supplemental evidence against the possibility of symptomatic coronary disease. However, I have several concerns about this test.

1. It gives a "picture" but does not inform us regarding "function."

2. Interpretations of the data are controversial.

3. It utilizes CT-scanning which means radiation exposure.

4. Cardiologists, the doctors who usually recommend it, often have financial interests in the laboratories that do the tests.

I would not routinely recommend this test. If your doctor suggests the need for it, I would act as the "devil's advocate" and inquire regarding the above-mentioned hesitations.

I would also not recommend "routine" screening for other vascular areas, such as carotid arteries and vertebral arteries to the brain, or iliac and femoral arteries to the legs, and the aorta in the abdomen. These areas usually produce symptoms when they are problematic. They rarely cause sudden death. Carotid arteries should be "screened" by your doctor as part of the physical exam. The same can be said for the others.

The term "screening," comes up repeatedly. This refers to the concept of looking for a disease entity or process before it becomes symptomatic. This concept stands at the bedrock of preventative medicine. Such screening, with the perfect example being the stress

Criteria of the Best Screening Tests

1) Easy to do

2) Safe (non-invasive)

3) Inexpensive

4) Reliable

echo, is particularly relevant when the disease being screened for can be quickly fatal, like a heart attack. The very best screening studies share several common characteristics: (1) Easy to do, (2) Safe, (3) Inexpensive, (4) Reliable.

This brings us to the last of the definitely advised screening tests at age fifty, that being colonoscopy. There are a number of important points to make about this exam. First, like the "tetanus shot," this too has become a cultural icon, akin to a rite-of-passage.

Medical Cultural Icon I

Casual Acquaintance 1:

"I cut myself yesterday."

Casual Acquaintance 2:

"Have you had your tetanus shot yet?"

Given the opportunity, the check-out person at the food store, your fellow reveler at the cocktail party, your minister on Sunday morning, and many other variously informed individuals will query, "Have you had your colonoscopy yet?" On the positive side, colonoscopy is currently the best screening test to diagnose colon cancer. Unfortunately, this cultural icon drags considerable baggage along with it.

Medical Cultural Icon II

Casual Acquaintance 1:

"I turned 50 yesterday."

Casual Acquaintance 2:

"Have you had your colonoscopy yet?"

Several developments have made it obviously necessary to change the Eleventh Commandment to have your first colonoscopy at age fifty, and then every five years after that.

To begin with, there are approximately 80,000,000 people age fifty or above in this country. This implies that 16,000,000 would need to be screened each year. Obviously, this is physically impossible. Thank goodness there are not enough trained colonoscopists to accomplish this daunting task. Were there, due to the need to keep these colonoscopists fed and clothed, we would have to add an enormous

Alternative Colon Cancer Screening Tests

o Yearly fecal occult blood testing (FOBT)
o Periodic CBC and iron study blood test
o Imaging studies
    1) Double-contrast barium enema
    2) Virtual colonoscopy
o ColoSure DNA-based stool test

additional expenditure to our already enormously bloated medical budget, to the tune of about 16 billion dollars per year. In addition, colonoscopy meets none of the criteria of a good screening test. Regarding ease, suffice it to say that it is not. It entails at least 24 hours of a modified diet, followed by the drinking of a gallon (no exaggeration) of a distasteful purging agent as fast as you can, followed by a number of trips to the toilet during the night to pass the purging agent, followed by someone driving you to the facility, followed by 1 to 2 hours of preparation for the 15 to 30 minute procedure, followed by a period of recovery of your senses while the medications used are wearing off, followed by the drive home. Regarding safety, it definitely is an invasive test: that is, this large tube is advanced deeply into your body. Although the likelihood of serious complications is very low, as we say behind closed doors, "If it happens to you, it is a 100% chance." Two of my patients, during the last fifteen years have suffered major complications. Regarding expense, by the time the colonoscopist, the facility, and the pathologist who read biopsies are billed, the total cost is in the range of $3,000. How much is actually paid out is variable, primarily depending on insurance factors.

So, the time has passed for doctors to recommend this procedure to all people over the age of fifty. For those doctors (almost all) concerned about being sued for not mentioning it, it should be brought up with the patient, pros and cons mentioned, and let the patient give the final verdict. What is needed in

Colon Cancer Risk	
High	**Low**
o Colon cancer in 1st degree relative.	o Absence of such history.
o Family history heavily weighted towards cancer in general.	o Absence of such history.
o History of ulcerative colitis.	o Absence of such history.
o Previous history of adenomatous polyps.	o Absence of such history.
o Heavy consumers of meat and animal fat.	o Vegetarianism.
o Cigarette Smoking.	o Absence of such history.

the discussion is risk stratification (see chart). Patients can simply be divided into "high risk" or "low risk," taking into consideration the factors known to be involved with incidence of colon cancer. The risk issues include history of colon cancer in first degree relatives, strong family history of cancer in general, personal history of ulcerative colitis, and people with a previous history of adenomatous polyps. Obviously, the more of the risk factors involved in any individual, the more serious should be the consideration for colonoscopy. The reverse is also true, so that with none of these risk factors, the person would be considered "low risk," with colonoscopy deferred indefinitely. Vegetarianism reduces risk even further.

Obviously, there are many legitimate medical issues producing symptoms for which colonoscopy can be enormously useful. This would include problems such as constipation, diarrhea, intestinal bleeding, and abdominal pain. I do not foresee colonoscopy going the way of the dodo. It simply needs to be reigned in and utilized when it is most likely to be helpful. Concluding the topic of "screening colonoscopy," I will mention a considered opinion of mine and others. We don't even know for sure if going in and removing polyps every three to five years reduces the incidence of clinical colon cancer! So-called "hyperplastic polyps" are thought to not have malignant potential. "Adenomatous polyps" are thought to possibly have malignant potential, but we do not have good data that tells us what their true potential is. There is evidence to suggest, that similar to what was mentioned for lung cancer, the pre-clinical, pre-awareness stages of colon cancer can last for decades. And "yes," there is even evidence to suggest that some of these cancerous polyps can spontaneously involute. Just as with so many diseases, there often appears to be more we don't know about polyps and colon cancer than there is that we know. It is often stated in various syntaxes, that the only thing standing in the way of new knowledge is already entrenched beliefs.

Lastly, regarding colon cancer surveillance, for those who would be classified as "low risk," there are a number of other studies available for "screening" for colon cancer. These will not be discussed in detail, with one exception. Your doctor is familiar with these and can review them with you (see chart). Fecal testing for occult (meaning hidden, but not necessarily other-worldly) blood meets all the criteria for a good screening test. Although it can obviously miss colon cancers, it can also be effective in detection. Radiography (x-ray) studies include the time-tested, double-contrast, barium enema, and the newer virtual colonoscopy, which involves CT technique. There is a very new technique, which has the potential for eliminating colonoscopy as a screening test for colon cancer (I hope this happens soon, before a whole new generation of colonoscopists are spit out of the pipeline looking for patients). This is the first-generation stool DNA-based cancer test. It meets all of the criteria of a good screening test, and the first generation test is deemed to be diagnostic approximately 80% of the time. Colonoscopy is still better diagnostically, at about 95%.

I wish to briefly mention the statistical terms called "sensitivity" and "specificity," used in most kinds of testing. "Sensitivity" refers to the ability of the test to identify a real problem. In other words, the higher the score here, the lower will be the "false negative" rate, meaning missing cases. With the first generation DNA test, it's between 72% and 77% (between 23% and 28% of cases are missed). "Specificity" refers to the ability to not identify cases that are not real (so-called "false positive"). It seems better here, between 83% and 97%. Obviously, in assessing the value of any test, both the incidence of false-negatives and false-positives are important considerations. If further refinements of this test bring it up to a sensitivity of 90% or so, then "screening colonoscopy" may no longer be necessary, particularly for low-risk individuals.

WHAT NEXT?

A bandoning all of these theoretical or virtual patients, let's get back to you, the one paying the bill and suffering through all of these screening tests! You are now fifty years and one day old. You have dutifully seen your doctor, perhaps for the first time in thirty years, undergone an interview, submitted to a physical exam, a full lab panel, and discussed or participated in screening tests for breast or prostate cancer, colon cancer, and heart disease. Now what?

It depends on what, if anything, was found. If nothing really important was found, as might occur in perhaps (estimated) 20% of you, and if you have a healthy life style, including dietary and exercise considerations, and if you remain attentive to symptoms, evanescent or persisting, you might not need another visit to your doctor for two or three years. With perhaps 80% of you, "something" may have been found. Many of these findings may be "borderline" or "questionable" regarding all of the common concerns about cholesterol, diabetes, blood pressure, etc. There may have been any one of a host of considerations raised. These may not necessarily change the two to three year timetable.

Perhaps half of you were found to have something of definite concern. This would likely come with a set of recommendations from your doctor, including perhaps a yearly revisit, at least for a while until the situation is better clarified. Likely, a smaller percentage of you were found to have something that requires regular follow up. Regarding the above-mentioned "common concerns," it would be reasonable for your doctor to give recommendations, and possibly medications, and have you return at three-month intervals…at least for a while.

As the sands of time slip by, and as our genetic makeup continues to interact with the surrounding environment, we develop enough real or potential problems to see the doctor on a regular basis. For the lucky ones, that might only be once per year. For most of the rest of us, it is more frequent than that. The frequency and extent of re-evaluation is always negotiable between you and your doctor.

In my experience, sadly, for many patients this program may be too onerous, involving major lifestyle changes which appear to the patient to be not doable. At that point, you open yourself to the possibility that a new pejorative diagnosis is applied to you…the "non-compliant" patient. Deep down the doctor may love these patients because they get the doctor off the malpractice hook. Sometimes such non-compliance emanates from a deep belief that the doctor's suggestions are wrong or overly aggressive. More often, it relates to the various combinations of issues discussed regarding barriers to care, with the presence of a global sense of dysthymia…"What's the difference?…I'm too hassled already…Who cares?…Leave me alone and let me live my life of quiet desperation," etc., etc. In choosing this pathway, unfortunately this could be the first conscious step down the road to oblivion, to be discussed next. Remember that despite the incredible self-healing powers of the body, we all have so-called apoptosis: programmed cell-death, akin to decay, built into us. Although we shall certainly all die, as does every living thing, how fast and in what manner we die is subject to many factors under our control. The choice to ignore factors which speed up the process of decay is a tragedy which through our long history as an evolving species is most poignantly being played out now. For the first time in human history, we now have the knowledge—and we have the ability to change the apoptotic setting—to delay decay and extend healthful life to levels previously thought to be impossible.

Alternately, if this truly and consciously does represent a deep conviction, that the recommendations made are not necessary for you, tell this to your doctor. Mention that you appreciate the concern and effort. Then, as mentioned, move on with no regrets.

This ends our tour of the cosmos of doctoring, circa 2012. It is a bumpy ride, over complex issues. Doctors can provide guidance for motoring through this cosmos, and that it seems is their major purpose. They do it with varying degrees of skill and effectiveness. They are filled with the same biases that everyone else has. Very few people feel comfortable, planted in an unending field of uncertainty. So, we spout platitudes and give advice, clinging to something that feels solid…like maybe evidence-based information. But it is somewhat of a mirage. The field of uncertainty is the same field from which new information will spring, if we can tone down our biases and open up to what might be hiding behind them.

As "patients," take heart in the notion that most doctors have been innocent Pollyannaish characters at one time or another, wanting to save the world from disease and misery. I believe that that goal is still alive in most of them, although it may be hidden in their doctor-generated apathy/dysthymia. Consider their advice carefully, as you would for any other confidant. Above all, don't feel helpless. You can choose to slip into the cockpit and take over the controls, utilizing all of the preventative measures discussed, and any others which strike you as being reasonable and logical. Recall that intent very likely has a major effect on health. Deeply intending to be well, and acting on those convictions, will be helpful. Perhaps you are now beginning to get a view of one of the major paradoxes mentioned already: health and healthcare have both easy and difficult elements. For certain, succumbing to what appears to be difficult and doing nothing may seal your fate.

Section III

THE STORY OF JOHN DOE

INTRODUCTION

I nertia, generally speaking, refers to the tendency of things to stay the same. This physical and sociological concept crashes head-on with the certainty that everything is changing all of the time. So, inertia is a relative concept. During most of our biologic evolution, threats to life were so extreme and pervasive that the ability to procreate needed to be possible at a young age. The same could be said for physical prowess. At this moment in our evolution, it is generally felt that we reach our physical prime at about age twenty. For those of us hoping to live to eighty or beyond, this could cause concern, if not downright depression, facing sixty years of steady decay. Bemoaning our fate won't change it. The emphasis of all that is written in this volume is to highlight repeatedly that after the age of twenty or so, deteriorating bodily function is inevitable. Our goal should not be "old age or bust," with broken bodies and spirits. Better to slow the rate of deterioration and to hope that right-living and right-thinking will bring us to a higher level of consciousness, seeing ourselves as whole rather than fragmented. This process requires planning and determination. The rewards for those able to do this can be enormous and beneficial to all others. Inability to fulfill one's potential, alternatively, will have negative impact on all others.

The Story of John Doe – A Modern Day Descent into Oblivion

John Doe was born to young parents in 1931 in a small West Texas community, which always seemed to be hovering on the verge of disappearing into the prairie. He was the oldest of three children. Father Frank was a school teacher and coached the football team. Mother Ann was a homemaker. The authoritarian hands-on parenting of Frank stood in stark contrast to the detached, robot-like approach of Ann. John worshipped his mother, wishing to understand her better and break through her icy countenance. He sensed that something was very wrong with her but was too young and insecure to feel empowered to do anything about it. He feared his father, whom he also respected. Corporal punishment was a necessary part of growing up in the Doe family, metered out by Frank on a regular basis according to the dictates of his own inner demons.

John's outstanding characteristic was his "God-given" physicality. He was remarkably physically adept in all ways. In high school in West Texas, a boy like that would play football. And he did. And did he! In today's parlance, he would be described as a "phenom…a man amongst boys." By the time he graduated high school, he held almost every school record imaginable and was widely recruited for college. That is about the time that Ann packed her bags one day and left. John, heart cracked open, self-reproaching, never saw her again.

Although John's grades were marginal for college, he received a full athletic scholarship to the local university. His first two years in college were a continuation of his high school accomplishments on the field. All of this came to an abrupt end, when in spring practice of his junior year, he "blew out" his knee. His athletic career was over, and his scholarship was withdrawn. The local hero and celebrity status that he had been awarded for the preceding five years changed overnight. Just like the struggling community, which somehow had spawned his remarkable physicality, he joined the struggle to survive.

He applied for military service but was turned down because of his knee, which had caused him to noticeably limp. His playing weight had been 220 pounds. After several years of inactivity, his weight had risen to 240. After a number of fledgling attempts at finding a stable job, he was able to get on as an apprentice electrician in Oklahoma City. He progressed through the ranks and eventually became a journeyman electrician.

John married, and they quickly had a child. We tend to remember the bad rather than the good. This is often justified through our vulnerable formative years, as so few of us are blessed with enlightened parents, who are able to guide us through the shoals of life. John had always felt himself to be socially handicapped and could not deal with the complexities of marriage and children. The marriage failed after five years, and John's ex-wife and daughter moved to California.

John smoked lightly during high school and college; closet-type smoking. With the end of his athletic career and notoriety, he felt no reason to abstain. He began to smoke heavily and drink alcohol heavily at the time. Being a Texas football star in Oklahoma was more or less an open invitation for a contingent of testosterone-poisoned Oklahomans to challenge him physically. There were fights and assorted injuries: a broken nose, a neck injury resulting in chronic pan, and a dislocated shoulder. His work as an electrician further stressed his body. At age thirty, John married again; this time to an older woman with two children. It was time to do the responsible thing and apply for life insurance. He was turned down initially because of the finding of blood pressure elevation at 160/100. His smoking and imprudent eating habits continued with his weight up to 255 pounds. He began to feel chronically tired, attributing that to the stresses of work and family. Finances were tight, with occasional layoffs.

John's second wife was originally from the Pacific Northwest. In 1965, a joint decision was made to move there. After several years of short-term job opportunities, John was somewhat surprised to be hired by Boeing, re-igniting briefly the feeling of being feted, as he had been as a youngster playing football. He was entitled to full medical benefits. Several years later, before his fortieth birthday, he underwent his first bona-fide medical exam. The results were both important and discouraging. His weight was recorded at 275 pounds. Blood pressure was 165/105. Cholesterol level was 320. Fasting blood sugar was 140. The doctor outlined a program of diet and weight loss, as well as beginning medications. In that era, a diagnosis of diabetes with a fasting blood sugar of 140 was not yet accepted. By today's standards there would be little question.

Mixed in with all of these physical changes were mental and emotional issues. John cried frequently "for no reason." He had lost contact with his daughter in California. His father died suddenly, presumably of a heart attack. There were infrequent contacts with his siblings, who in fact were close with each other. His brother had become wealthy and lived in a ranch outside of Fort Worth. His wife was found to have breast cancer and accepted the standard treatment of the day, that being mastectomy. He felt himself growing old. He looked at pictures of himself hurtling tacklers on his way to a game-winning touchdown, unable to even connect with the figure in that picture. His one solace was a supportive relationship with his two stepchildren.

Athletics have had a special place in society, off and on back to antiquity. At times, athletes were part of the warrior class. In modern times, they are held up as our heroes, warriors going off to battle foes, sacrificing their bodies, and being paid enormous sums of money to do so. John was part of this warrior class. The events which were about to unfold would test his warrior mentality beyond anything he had imagined.

In June of 1975, while sitting at his desk at work, at age 44, John experienced a deep pain in his chest. He seemed to focus more on the profuse sweating, as that was clearly visible to his co-workers. He was not one to share intimate information. After thirty minutes, the pain left, and he thanked God. As he rose to go to the bathroom, he noted himself to be surprisingly weak and somewhat short of breath. He felt dizzy and tried to sit down. A darkening veil descended over him, and he remembered being peculiarly calm. He was found pulseless by his co-workers several minutes later. Seattle had already established itself as the citizen-initiated CPR capital of the country, and his co-workers' prompt attention saved his life. He spent almost a month in the hospital, recovering from a heart attack which left his heart severely weakened, and a stroke-like picture from a combination of the pulseless state combined with a major blockage of the circulation to his brain. At that time, he could not yet know that his physical vitality had been permanently destroyed.

He left the hospital with the usual burst of energy and enthusiasm accompanying such events. Underneath this transient sense of gratefulness was the inner knowing that there was no coming back from what had happened. His level of fatigue shuffling across the room was far more profound than anything he had experienced after hours of wind-sprints on the football field. There is healthy fatigue and unhealthy fatigue—with the mind interpreting the former as good, and the latter as bad. John knew the difference.

By January of 1976, on a list of medications totaling nine in all, including antidepressants, he had improved to the point whereby it was mandated by insurance that he try going back to work, at an agreed upon reduced work load. The first few months passed surprisingly well. Later that spring he developed leg pain, which was determined to be caused by a blockage in the artery supplying that leg and required a surgical bypass to restore the circulation. The arteries at the time of surgery were heavily calcified. He was unable to return to work for another three months.

His mental-emotional status continued to decline. He felt self-hating for his return to cigarette smoking after his heart attack. His wife was found to have a reoccurrence of breast cancer and undertook a rigorous program of chemotherapy.

He once again briefly returned to work, but it was apparent to both his supervisor and to him that he was no longer able to do the job. He was released and applied for social security disability. He found himself in a new role, acting as primary caregiver for his ailing wife. Her battle with cancer continued through several courses of treatment over the ensuing years. Remarkably during her decline and his need to be strong, he did relatively well again. He watched her wither down to 100 pounds before she died in 1980, at the age of fifty-five. John had not yet turned fifty. He felt completely depleted emotionally, as a huge vacuum opened in his life.

The ravages of his disease states continued. His long history of smoking was accompanied by increasing shortness of breath, found to be secondary to moderate emphysema. His chest pain recurred, which required the need for coronary angioplasties and stents on three different occasions through the 1980s. Despite his continued excessive weight, his diabetes did not seem to be causing any major problems. However, just before Christmas in 1994, he developed a "sore" on one of the toes of the same leg which had had a bypass. His legs and feet had become numb and painful, progressively over several years, requiring a constant supply of pain medication. Remarkably, as the "sore" gradually enlarged and became putrid from superimposed infection, it was absolutely painless.

In the midst of this, he experienced an episode of chest pain which was severe and persistent that culminated in a four-vessel coronary bypass. During the recovery from this surgery, while still in a nursing home, the foot infections progressed dramatically, as the body was unable to combat the infection because of inadequate blood supply. This resulted in amputation of half of the foot. Continued inability to heal resulted in return to the operating room for a below-the-knee amputation in August, 1996.

At that darkest point in John's life, he was greeted in the hospital by his daughter Julie. He was rewarded for a lifetime of love and support for Julie, filtering back to her in small rivulets now and then over the decades. Perhaps ever more amazing was the ease and comfort with which the reunion took place. Between hospitalizations, and during a long ordeal of learning to walk on an artificial leg, Julie returned with John's three grandchildren. The deal was sealed. Arrangements were made for John to move down to California, to live in father-in-law quarters in the home of Julie and her husband.

The transaction was consummated in June of 1998. There was not much holding John in Seattle at that time. His stepson and he were sufficiently connected to carry on their relationship. The thirty-three years in Seattle seemed like nothing more than an endless series of hospitalizations—and losses of people and body parts. Sixteen hospitalizations in all, including several for cellulitis (skin infections), one for urinary infection, one for pneumonia, two for emphysema, and one for prostate surgery.

The reconnection with Julie has transformed the lives of Julie and John. Julie has been appointed power-of-attorney over both John's financial and medical issues. John had finally completely quit smoking. He had managed to become engaged in the lives of his grandchildren and found a reason for living. He had even managed to bring his weight down. Unfortunately, "happiness" still eluded him; even more tragically, the same could be said for "contentment."

When last heard from in 2004, at the age of seventy-three, several major medical hurdles were rising higher. His kidneys were failing from vascular disease, and dialysis was looming in the background. A new ulceration on his good leg was refusing to heal and raised the threat of a second amputation. John had already conceded that he would get a wheelchair before trying to become a walking double-amputee. As of then, in 2004, he was still considered to be a "full code" patient. That means that all measure would be undertaken to keep him alive, including dialysis, amputations, respirators, feeding tubes, and intensive care. Without knowing for certain, I suspected that this aggressive approach was more Julie's desire than John's. Sometimes it is difficult to tell.

Table X is a 2004 summary of John's problem list and prescription medications.

John's story has its unique elements, as does every life. However, the overall picture of a steady downhill slide is seen every day in medical practice. It happens slowly enough, that there is infrequently an attempt to step back and get some perspective. It seems that doctors

Last Known Problem List of John Doe	List of Medications
1) Diabetes mellitus; insulin dependency with neuropathy and vasculopathy	Atorvastatin (Lipitor)
2) Hypertension	Metformin
3) Long time heavy cigarette smoking (45 pack-years)	Insulin (Lispro, Humalog)
4) Depression	Fenofibrate
	Carvedilol
5) Severe peripheral vascular disease with previous left-leg amputation and right-leg gangrene	Digoxin
	Advair
6) Emphysema	Albuterol
7) History of pneumonia	Lisinopril
	Amlodipine
8) History of cellulitis	Aspirin
9) History of GERD ("acid-reflux")	Furosemide
10) History of degenerative arthritis	Potassium
11) Chronic pain syndrome	Isosorbide
	Oxycodone ER
12) Obesity	Hydrocodone
13) Atherosclerosis heart disease with myocardial infarction, cardiomyopathy and CABG ((1995) and numerous angeoplasties/stents	Citalopram
14) Chronic renal failure (Creatinine 3.2)	
15) Stasis dermatitis	

are much better at keeping people alive, than at keeping them healthy and vibrant. John's drama began to play itself out at age forty-four with his first heart attack. He was in and out of serious trouble, hard-heartily called "circling the drain" ever since, with major hurdles still facing him at age seventy-three. Many people with similar medical tales begin a little later, perhaps in their 60s, and are still going through these ordeals into their 80s and 90s. Many people in the 80s and 90s in the hospital are officially listed as "full code." Many of them appear to be constantly struggling, if not suffering at a high level. Even more obfuscating is that in contrast to John, many of them have varying degrees of dementia and are unable to live independently. The cycle of hospitalizations, nursing home, and home goes on seemingly endlessly for these old, chronically sick people.

We have an aging population, whereby getting to age ninety is no longer considered to be unusual. We are at the cusp of a re-assessment of what really is our obligation to these people—and their obligation to us. What does it really mean to "play God?" Are we "playing God" if we allow sick patients to die, or to keep them alive at all costs? How much does society want to, or can afford to do for them? Are there exceptions to allow us to drift from the general ("patients") to the specific person ("grandpa")?

The prevailing world view is that evolution is this massive mysterious structure extending backwards to the Big Bang and forward into infinity, moving ever so slowly. Like molasses in winter. It has not yet come to widespread appreciation that cell biology has demonstrated that living things can change markedly, quickly, stimulated by environmental factors. These mutations can be beneficial or harmful, with natural selection sorting this out. Until 2004, John's life was dominated by pain and sorrow. What might not be clearly visible in the brief sketch of his life is the degree to which he suffered physically and mentally. This does not appear to be fertile ground for raising consciousness. Or is it? At what point could an environmental factor cause a genetic alteration to completely turn things around, mentally and/or physically? Is there a point when it is too late? More questions than answers. Each of us make choices multiple times every day, altering our fate and the fate of our species. We now have at least indirect confirmation of this, resting on solid evidence. Choose wisely.

RATIONING OF CARE?

John's descent into the abyss raises very difficult questions—I wish to make a statement at the beginning of this discussion which I am personally convinced is true. If we seriously do wish to significantly reduce health care costs in this country, we absolutely do need to initiate rationing of care, far above the level that we do now.

John has a very tender heart. He had a very tough childhood, as many of us do. It stained him for life, with a stain that would not wash out. When roughly knocked off the pedestal upon which we had placed him, he had nothing but poor coping-mechanisms left. He repeatedly made bad choices about health and life. In so doing, he stepwise destroyed his health and consumed enormous medical resources. He is a man for whom we can all say, "There but for the Grace of God go I."

There are millions of Johns cared for in this country at any given time. As mentioned, John made repeatedly bad choices. His plight was possibly completely avoidable. Do we want to fix our infrastructure? Do we wish to undertake the transition away from fossil fuels? Do we wish to clean up the environment and preserve diverse ecosystems for future generations? Or, do we wish to spend 16%, headed for 30%, of our GNP on desperately ill people who have been fully complicit with the appearance of their illness? It truly is our choice. It needs to be brought into the light and openly debated. Who will be on the "death panels?" Will it involve only demented people, or even the mentally intact, like John? Will setting limits stimulate people to take preventative medicine seriously? Will setting limits, akin to making laws, forewarn people of what will happen to them if they break "the law?"

There are endless numbers of questions to be asked and debated. Done properly, this could be a great healing for all those participating. If changes are initiated, likely they will be slowly installed.

Regardless, it is long overdue for the open discussion to begin.

Section IV

HEALTH OF THE BODY INCLUDING THE SOLES

INTRODUCTION

There are a few recurring themes in this text. Dr. Goldstein is not here anymore to look after you. He has been replaced by a team of highly trained specialists, each of whom feels that their specialty is the most important. Your care has become frighteningly fragmented. Although Dr. Goldstein may still be resurrected to some extent, it will never be like it was. You therefore need to take much more responsibility for yourself. We will always need skilled and compassionate doctors. Equally, we need a prevailing cultural mindset that encourages people to be as medically informed as a "layperson" can be, and that encourages and rewards good health habits.

The major textbooks of medicine, and each of the major specialty textbooks, are tomes which drone on in scientific precision for thousands of pages. What is laid out in this section is an incredibly abbreviated accounting of the most common and most important illnesses that affect people. It is written to hit the high points and to provide practical information as to how seriously to consider these—and how to deal with them.

The arrangement of topics may look strange. It is laid out roughly in the manner of the hallowed *Review of Systems*. Recall that the basis of all medical diagnosis rests with the "history," describing what the problem is, how it relates to the person as a whole—past and present—and how to pursue a diagnostic algorithm. I have already referred to the extreme importance of your own personal "Family

History," providing an unfettered overview of where you are likely to head. The *Review of Systems* is a detailed inventory of the body in which the doctor asks specific questions that can often be answered by a yes or a no. It is like going through the house after the guests have left and making sure that everything is back in order. It functions like a "daily planner" so that nothing is overlooked.

Please keep in mind a simple but key word. Whenever the word "clinical" is seen, this refers to what is seen in the real world, in the medical trenches. It is not theory, or research, but what actually occurs.

PART I
GENERAL

This topic refers to issues which were previously described as "systemic," that is, possibly affecting many different parts of the body simultaneously. It also connotes the possibility that the origin of the problem could be anywhere in the body.

Fever

This has been discussed already in the discussion of colds. For many years, it was debated whether fever was a beneficial response of the body to an insult or a nuisance to be eliminated. As can be inferred from the observation that we frequently try to reduce body temperature by various means, the nuisance idea has been preeminent recently. It is certainly possible that there are instances where elevated body temperature is helpful, but those instances are not clearly defined—and not even being explored—as best as I can tell. As always, keep an open mind.

Recall the bell-shaped curve. Body temperature is a very tightly regulated phenomenon, with a variance of one degree Fahrenheit on each side representing two standard deviations, in turn representing 95% of the population. In other words, a temperature of 97.6°F to 99.6°F could be considered in the broad range of normal for healthy people.

Remarkably, there is a phenomenon that I have witnessed that is not well explained. Frequently, patients report that, "My normal body temperature is such and such. Since I became very ill, I have taken my temperature at home, and it has been 98°. That means I'm running a fever!" On the other hand, I never hear the opposite, that is, "I have a temperature of 99°. That means I am not running a fever." For your information, being quasi scientists, doctors are forced to ignore that information. Importantly, it could foster a negative impression regarding the patient's reliability, which doesn't help either party. Using simple clinical tools, the most accurate body temperature reading is likely taken per rectum. This has fallen out of favor, with a proliferation of gadgets and devices to measure temperature elsewhere. Readings done per ear canal are reliable, depending on the accuracy of the equipment used. Oral and underarm temps are the least accurate.

As mentioned earlier with the exception of an influenza illness (chills, body aches, headache, sore throat, all seen in the appropriate context), adults with non-serious conditions generally do not show a temperature above 101°F to 102°F maximum. Fever above that level is notable and, without a flu syndrome, should trigger contact with a medical professional.

Chills

Just as with many other words or phrases, "chills" means different things to different people. From a practical standpoint, it does not carry a strong message for physicians, with one exception. For many people, "chills" simply and accurately describes a feeling of being cold, particularly inside the body. An extra sweater or blanket is sought and likely provides relief. On the other hand, shivering, especially if prolonged and/or very pronounced, can signal the presence of a disease process of greater magnitude or seriousness. Although shivering chills can be seen in the flu syndrome, they are usually relatively light and brief. Shivering chills severe enough to shake the bed, and lasting more than five minutes, are more frequently seen in sepsis syndrome, generally a much more serious condition. Conversely, the symptoms of sepsis can be very subtle, once again reflecting the possibility of huge differences in expression of biologic events in different people. In fact, sepsis may be much more common than we ordinarily appreciate and may be spontaneously corrected. Details about this are not known with certainty. However, we do know that bacteria can be found in the bloodstream frequently, but briefly after invasive procedures such as dental work or endoscopy. This is the rationale for the use of prophylactic antibiotics before such procedures in people with valvular heart disease, including mitral valve prolapse, supposedly to prevent attachment of these bacteria to the heart valves. Incidentally, this age-old ritual is undergoing close scrutiny to determine if it is really necessary. Some doctors are already recommending that it not be routinely used.

Sweating

The most common cause of sweating is elevation of body temperature, for whatever the reason. Without the presence of an identifiable illness, body temperature is closely regulated by sensors in the base of the brain and elsewhere and mediated through the autonomic nervous system (ANS). This aspect of the nervous system can also be termed "automatic," meaning it operates in response to many stimuli but is not much influenced by voluntary or conscious mechanisms. The ANS begins in the base of the brain and in the spinal cord and reaches every cell in the body, by two routes. Autonomic nerve fibers travel along the course of blood vessels, as they repeatedly divide, all the way up to the level of the capillaries, which are the smallest of the blood vessels, nourishing cells themselves. The response, which these nerves generate, occurs almost instantaneously. The second route involves autonomic stimulation of glandular tissue and, in particular, the adrenal gland, sitting on top of the kidneys causing these glands to secrete hormones such as adrenalin and cortisone, which circulate to every cell in the body. This mechanism is slightly delayed, but effects can persist for hours. Sweating is physically produced when autonomic stimuli reach the sweat glands in the skin, causing a contraction of their muscular elements which squeeze out the accumulated liquid. Once on the skin surface, as the sweat evaporates, heat is utilized in the process of evaporation, thus lowering body temperature.

Body temperature most commonly is elevated by the level of ambient temperature, and by the amount and type of clothing worn. As ambient temperature rises above the seventies, for most people, radiation of heat off the body surface may not be enough to keep body temperature at 98.6°F. At that time, messages may be sent via the ANS to cause sweating. As ambient temperature rises further, sweating may increase substantially, even to the point of being inefficient, by rolling off the skin surface, thus not taking heat with it.

Body temperature is generated through normal cellular activity, burning nutritional substrates, and generating carbon dioxide, water, and heat. The same kind of response in terms of heat production is seen with physical activity. Even mild physical activity with ambient temperature in the seventies may raise body temperature. With much higher ambient temperatures and with increasingly vigorous body activity, heat may not be dissipated quickly enough with hyperventilation (akin to a dog panting) and with sweating, and body temperature may rise precipitously. Body temperatures of 102°F to

103°F are not unusual during strenuous exertion. "Heat exhaustion" is a condition seen in this setting with temperatures up to 104°F and characterized by severe fatigue and muscle cramping. Above 104°F, and up to 106°F, people experience the onset of "heat stroke," which is a very serious problem and, in fact, potentially fatal. With appearance of this condition, sweating stops. It is not completely clear whether this is triggered by severe dehydration or whether there is "central dysautonomia," meaning a primary response of the brain stem and other autonomic centers. Perhaps both factors are operative. The end result can be a precipitous rise in body temperature, and permanent damage to the nervous system and other organs, or death.

Sweating can also occur in situations where body temperature is not significantly altered. This too is mediated through the ANS. Most of us are aware of the connection between an external stressor and sweating in particular areas of the body, such as arm pits, groin, face and head, chest, and hands. Interestingly, these areas have relatively high density of so-called apocrine sweat glands, which secrete a sweat which is higher in fat content, and thus subject to breakdown by skin bacteria to create odor. Such sweat likely has an evolutionary role as well. Its chemistry is such that it is more likely to spread over the skin as an emulsion, rather than simply dropping off as "wasted sweat." In terms of thermoregulation, this provided our physically active hunter-gatherer ancestors better thermoregulation than "normal" sweat. Interestingly, such sweat also contains pheromones, involved in the physiology of mating, which explains why our beloved pets are often strongly attracted to these areas of our bodies.

For a relatively small number of us, excessive secretion of these apocrine sweat glands can create, or contribute to a social phobia. Many approaches have been tried to quell the excessive and potentially embarrassing output. Most common are the host of "deodorants," which are variably successful in at least changing the odor and less effective in stopping production of unwanted sweat. Psychophysiologic techniques such as biofeedback have been tried but require a person to be very adept with the technique to experience success. A variety of orally taken medications have been tried, as have surgical removal of such tissue, when possible, and even use of botox. Fortunately, very few people feel the need to go to expensive and potentially disfiguring therapies for this issue.

Chronic Pain

As mentioned earlier, pain is a necessary and a life-preserving attention getter. It is the major signal produced by the body, mediated by the nervous system, providing us with information that something is wrong and needs attention. This could range all the way from the sudden realization that one's hand is on a very hot burner—and if not removed quickly, the smell of one's own cooking flesh will permeate the room—to a mild and transient low back pain experienced when first getting out of bed. Both of these are examples of acute pain, which is the potentially lifesaving information just mentioned. It occurs repeatedly throughout the day, usually transient, but sometimes lasting long enough that ingesting a medication of some kind is done—and with quick relief expected.

Chronic pain is similar in only one respect, that is, that it involves pain. In almost all other respects, it is remarkably different from acute pain. Although chronic pain has certainly been around for at least as long as written history, it has come under major consideration and concern only in the last fifty years or so. This is a curious fact and not easy to understand. One way of looking at it is to acknowledge that in past times, there was a limited ability to investigate the problem, so why worry about it? Although that might have been true, it is clearly not the full explanation. I think it to be much more likely that several factors were changing simultaneously, creating a new paradigm along the way. Factors may have included better means of investigation, a growing cadre of doctors and scientists interested in it from both the scientific and humanitarian aspects, a population with gradually increasing life expectancy, and a new societal sympathy and even compassion for those afflicted. Through more than the first half of the twentieth century, people with a large number of ailments, for which the biochemical and pathological explanations are now well established, and for which reasonably good treatments are now available, were labeled as hysterics, hypochondriacs, conversion reactions, and many other pejorative terms. Most destructive of all was that it was God's will and a punishment deserved for previous indiscretions, implying that there coexisted some types of moral and/or spiritual problem. As a society, we have come a long way in terms of open mindedness, with still a long journey ahead of us.

So, what is meant by chronic pain? Although a universally accepted precise definition is lacking, at least the basics can be outlined. It is a discomforting sensory and psychological experience, deeply personal and complex, often without well-defined cause, impairing function, present most of the time over the course of three to six months. Breaking this down one piece at a time, sensory means that it is felt by the physical body. Psychological means that it eventually spills over into the psyche, bringing in other elements, such as anxiety and depression. Deeply personal means that the only person, who can experience that sensation, is that person. Complex means that it can affect all areas of the body and mind, with many feedback loops, many of which have potential for magnifying the totality of the problem and further compromising the function. Possible lack of an obvious cause is self-explanatory and further exacerbates feelings of anxiety and depression, contributes to low self-esteem, and challenges the integrity of the patient. Impaired function is both mental and physical, disrupting ability to focus and concentrate, creating dependency needs requiring others to help, and requiring relinquishment of beloved pursuits. Present most of the time creates a sense of imprisonment from which there is a sense of no escape. Three to six months is very arbitrary but is meant to imply a certain element of permanency. In fact, there is good clinical evidence that for those who have had pain for six months or longer, which has been unsuccessfully addressed diagnostically and therapeutically, the chances of "cure" at that juncture are small. Perhaps the greatest difference between acute and chronic pain is that chronic pain is not life protective or preserving in the same way as acute pain. In fact, it has strongly aversive effects and is likely to shorten life expectancy by breaking down the immune system and triggering cellular degeneration.

It is estimated that as many as 30% of adults have some type of chronic pain syndrome. In general, the incidence tends to rise with advancing age. Nevertheless, many younger people, in the prime of life, are affected. Most of these 30% can function well enough to work and be reasonably participatory in life. However, there may be a figure as high as 10% of all adults, a staggering number given the personal and societal ramification, who by necessity experience a dramatic alteration in ability to function physically and, secondarily, mentally as well. To add to this tragedy, these people tend to be quickly marginalized. Chronic pain acts as a powerful drain on vitality. Many of these people appear listless and unmotivated. Many require medications which may dull senses. Most of them are unable to be gainfully employed. Most experience depression and anxiety. Lack of ability to be physically active often promotes weight gain. Individuals with this constellation of problems can become quickly shut off from society, friends, and even family.

There are countless varieties of chronic pain, so a detailed inventory is not possible. Table 10 lists the most common causes of chronic pain that result in the need for treatment. Any part of the body can be a source of pain. There is now a specialty board regarding the practice of chronic pain and an increasing number

Most Common Causes of Chronic Pain
• Abdominal and Pelvic
• Headache/Migraine

• Spinal Pain
  - Neck
  - Low back/sciatica

• Arthritic
• Neuromuscular   - Fibromyalgia
• Neurologic
• Cancer
• HIV

of training centers, providing broad experience and hands-on supervision for those so inclined. Most of the doctors choosing to specialize in pain treatment come from the ranks of anesthesiology, with lesser numbers from neurology and internal medicine. They are listed under "Pain Management" in the yellow pages. There are a wide variety of services which can be offered, including diagnostic evaluation. As mentioned before, often there is no definitive diagnosis established. At that juncture, it is still almost certain that some type of treatment will be offered. Some pain management specialists describe themselves as "interventionalists," meaning they do invasive procedures, usually with needles, with a variety of modalities used with the needle injection, including medications and electrical energy. Some but not all have the ability to implant wires into the spinal canal, connected to batteries or reservoirs tunneled under the skin, to provide treatment directly to the suspected troubled areas in the spinal canal. These procedures have potential for great benefit, but patients need to be carefully selected and screened so as to maximize the chances for success.

Lastly, many pain management specialists do not learn or do not practice interventional approaches, but simply diagnose and then use medication of various types. This is the area of greatest controversy, as it obviously raises the issue of use of opiate medication (a better term than "narcotics," which has always had a pejorative and even criminal ring, in my opinion) for long-term pain control. Doctors who are interested in and advocate for pain management services often state that if you are dying of cancer, you can get opiates easily and in large amounts. However, if you have an illness which is not "terminal," it may be difficult to find a doctor to prescribe for you. Many interventionalists do not prescribe pain medication. Your Primary Care Physician (PCP) probably will not prescribe opiates for you, making it possible that you will have to drive long distances to receive the medication that you need.

To further characterize the depth of the debate on this issue, there are doctors who steadfastly subscribe to the results of studies, which raise the question as to the probability that opiates can eventually increase pain when given chronically. This is thought to occur by the sensitization of pain receptors. These doctors proselytize against ever prescribing long-term opiates. On the other side of the debate is knowledge based on the now accepted fact of "neuroplasticity." It was previously thought that the brain was fully formed and polished sometime in childhood and certainly by age twenty. There is now definitive evidence that (a) in many people, the frontal lobes which are critically important in impulse control, aggression, and other critical issues are not finished developing until mid to late twenties and that (b) neuroplasticity refers to the ability of the nervous system, including the brain to change "on the fly." It is conclusively demonstrated now that neurons can and do divide and multiply. This leads to the findings using the latest imaging techniques, such as functional or metabolic magnetic resonance imaging (MRI), and the latest computed tomography (CT) scanners that show the brain and spinal cords of people with chronic pain appear to be structurally and metabolically altered in the direction of shrinkage or dysfunction or both. So, chronic pain appears to be capable of causing brain damage in susceptible people. So which group of researchers do we believe, and how do we respond? Perhaps both can be true in specific individuals. Here is how I do it, and here are my results.

In patients receiving opiates, we do not try to achieve pain-free status. This usually requires too much drug, and there would be too many side effects. We aim for a 50% reduction. Most patients are exceptionally pleased with this. After a period of stabilization, ranging usually between one to two years, I begin a very gradual reduction in the dosage of opiates. This almost invariably results in resistance from the patient. I push ahead, reducing 3% to 5% every one to two months. The hope and anticipation is that the neuronal (electrochemical) circuits set up between the painful area, spinal cord, and brain can be toned down over time. In the vast majority of cases, this can be successfully done, in a sense sidestepping the possibility that the opiates are making the pain worse. As the reduction proceeds, the pain stays the same. Some people have been able to completely discontinue opiates, while for others, the dose is substantially reduced. This procedure is simple and almost invariably works. Ideally, what is left after two to five years of treatment with opiates is a person who has chronic pain, at a tolerable level, with improved functioning compared to that noted before—and off opiate medication.

The researchers and founding fathers and mothers of the chronic pain management movement have always emphasized the need for "multidisciplinary clinics," including doctors, nurses, dieticians, physical and occupational and vocational therapists, mental health specialists, clergy, and others, all under one roof. Although this indeed may be the ideal model, it is very difficult to put together, sustain, and fund. Such models form, reform, break up, and may form again. More commonly, pain specialists work solo or in groups of two or three individuals, referring patients to other disciplines. So, in some sense, the model may still be utilized but definitely not under the same roof—and definitely with a lesser chance of close cooperation and linkage of treatments between all participants.

What happened to Dr. Goldstein?

I do not really know why doctors will not prescribe opiates for their own patients. In fact, I think it is a shameful mistake and an abrogation of their medical responsibility. We are sworn to relieve suffering. The implication is that we don't believe that the patients with chronic pain are suffering. In other words, it is a throwback to past times when such patients were felt to be hysterics or deserving of pain or punishment. It is true that there are people entering doctors' offices looking for "drugs." It is true that at least 20% of pain patients misuse medications deliberately. It is true that doctors are responsible for the prescriptions that leave their offices. It is true that they could theoretically be censored by the Drug Enforcement Agency. However, all of these facts, based on fear, are invalid in my opinion. I am afraid that doctors simply do not believe that these patients are suffering and need help. There are clearly spelled-out procedures to follow when giving a person opiate medication. Strict adherence to these principles, outlined clearly in a standardized "pain contract," (see Appendix) should minimize chances for abuse and maximize chances that patients can get what they need from their own doctors who supposedly know them best. This is another example of compartmentalization of care, resulting in needing to travel long distances because your beloved PCP will not help you.

Receptor Function

As a sidelight to chronic pain, so much of what seems to be behind dramatic biologic variation has to do with receptor functioning. "Receptors" is the term that is now being used in a global sense to explain why cells do what they do. Recall that programming begins with very, very long strands of DNA, our personal blueprint. Parts of these strands code for genes, of which there are 50,000, give or take a few.

Genes, in turn, code for proteins, which are manufactured either by DNA or RNA. Proteins are complex chains of amino acids, which bend and twist in different directions, each having a unique three-dimensional appearance. Cells are factories, making different things according to their individual instruction manuals. They make proteins internally while they use other proteins from external sources. Their surfaces are dotted with receptors of many, many different types. When a given protein comes along and fits its squiggly frame into a receptor, that may send a message to the cell to start doing something, or it may not because the receptor may be turned off. It is turned on by other proteins which also are manufactured by DNA, but not of the same strands that manufacture or replicate genes. Instead, there are vast stretches of DNA between those stretches that replicate genes, which produce proteins that turn off or turn on receptors. So genes are only part of the story of why we do what we do. A bigger part of the story is what the states of our receptors are. Do we have a large number of pain receptors or perhaps a small number? Are the receptors turned off or on? If I have an abundance of pain receptors, and they are all turned on all of the time, it suddenly is understandable how that pin prick on my arm could feel like a Spartan's spear had just penetrated into it. It has nothing to do with my previous sins, my character, my moral nature, my desire to get "high," or my desire to trick my doctor. It's all in the DNA, Baby!

Sleep and Sleeping

Sleep medicine has arrived! God save the King! Or, on second thought, maybe not. There is no doubt that the study of sleep has yielded a cornucopia of fascinating information. The physiology of sleep, just as is the physiology of many other body processes and functions, is extremely complex and, for the most part, ignored. Since one of the main findings which has emerged from studying sleeping people is disordered breathing, and since breathing has been one of the main areas of focus in pulmonary medicine, interestingly, much of the work and research regarding sleep and sleep medicine have been done in departments of pulmonary medicine. In fact, many pulmonary training programs now provide training in sleep medicine as well, usually adding another one to two years to the length of the program.

I visited a prehistoric "sleep lab" in 1972 while training at the University of Colorado. True, as I recall, it was located in the medical school. However, to get there, one had to embark on an elevator which went down for so long below ground level that it felt like it was a journey to the center of the earth. It was something that you would never do alone! Once we arrived at the lab, which was a dimly lit room with a cot and a grouping of monitors (good for sleeping, I guess), we quickly appreciated why only the most dedicated and visionary doctors would want to participate in such an

Diseases/Conditions Associated with Poor Sleeping

- Hypertension
- Stroke
- Obesity
- Diabetes
- Depression – anxiety
- Systemic inflammation
- Accidents
- Poor performance

adventure. I don't think it was until about 1985 that the lab made it out of the bowels of the earth to an above ground station. At almost that same time, I approached my local community hospital with an outlandish proposal, that is, that we would become the second or third sleep lab in the state for only a total investment of $80,000. I was turned down, thus ending my chance of becoming a sleep guru.

Well, as is usually the case, times have changed dramatically. Sleep medicine has made it to prime time. It has become the same type of cultural icon as colonoscopy, discussed widely at Tupperware gatherings and cocktail parties ("Oh really! What are your CPAP settings?"). Getting back to the serious topic of trying to stay healthy, when it seems that the odds are stacked against us, there is no question that poor sleeping has been statistically linked with a long list of common and serious problems. This includes hypertension, stroke, obesity, diabetes, sudden death, depression, anxiety, accidents, and possibly others, albeit less frequently (see chart). Whatever the cause of poor sleeping, the likely common denominator is the excessive secretion of "stress hormones" during the time when resting and regeneration is supposed to occur. In essence, the patient with sleep-disordered breathing has exchanged rest for stress. It is easy to see how this could quickly add up over the years, with "degenerative diseases" of various types emerging prematurely. Finally, some people who are identified with sleep disorders and treated appropriately show dramatic improvements in health status, feel better, and are very grateful.

So, what's the gripe? Let's recall the definition of a good screening test. It should be safe, easy, and inexpensive. The only widely accepted means of diagnosing sleep disorders at this time is a full overnight "polysomnogram," which is performed in a sleep lab. The test is safe, being "non-invasive." It is not easy requiring the person to physically travel to the sleep lab at about 7:00 p.m., undergo several hours of "hookup," and then testing which likely will last until about 5:00 a.m. Regarding expenses, this varies according to different labs. The charges will likely be $2,000 or more. Insurance rebates from $800 to $1,200, and the patient has a variable charge depending on insurance "write offs." A second study called a CPAP trial may then be requested, at a somewhat reduced rate. Follow-up studies once per year are usually requested. So, it is not really a good screening test. One of the advantages is that you will consult with a doctor who has special expertise in sleep medicine, with the possibility that some simple interventions might be helpful. The "concern" is that the doctor you see likely has a financial stake in how often and how many sleep studies are recommended to you, creating the possibility of Hippocratic Oath violations.

The most commonly identified sleep disorder of major potential concern is "obstructive sleep apnea." This is a condition whereby on repeated occasions throughout the night, the upper airway collapses, or closes, causing temporary cessation of air movement. During this time, it is possible that blood oxygen level can drop dangerously low, having a potential to cause cardiac irregularities, weakening of the heart, increased pressure in the pulmonary circulation, and even brain damage. Before getting into your car and rushing off to the nearest sleep lab, note that I said "potential." There are a variety of less dangerous events which can occur during sleep. All of these can conspire to do one or both of two things: (1) "fragmentation" of sleep, which refers to excessive brief awakening with subsequent disrupting of "sleep architecture," and (2) reduced overall sleep time. In my opinion, reduction of overall sleep time, as documented by brain wave evidence, is the most important. There is epidemiologic evidence that people who get less than six hours or more than nine hours of sleep generally have more health problems than those in between. Some experts consider a narrower range, such as 6½ to 8½ hours to be a better predictor of problems.

On the one hand, sleep studies can give us invaluable information. On the other hand, they are costly and inconvenient. In addition, a large percentage of people undergoing sleep studies leave with a recommendation to use "CPAP." CPAP stands for "continuous positive airway pressure." Since compression and collapse of the airway seems to be the major problem, the idea is to use air under pressure to help splint the airway open. Actually, it is effective and can be demonstrated to markedly reduce, or even eliminate, the resultant severe drops in oxygen content of the blood. The problem is that CPAP, or its cousin BiPAP, requires a device to deliver the air under pressure via a very tight-fitting mask strapped to the head. As cumbersome and uncomfortable as this may sound, some people tolerate it very well and even feel much better. They are not the problem. Within three months to three years, greater than half of those for whom CPAP has been recommended have abandoned it because of intolerance of the apparatus or perceived ineffectiveness. For those people, the sleep study did not fulfill its potential or promise. There has been a constant attempt to make the procedure more user friendly, and perhaps, such a system is right around the corner. But, it is not here yet.

It is possible that in our zeal to help people, we have way overshot the mark. By that, I mean since the list of associated diseases and complications is so intimidating, dare we give up attempts to deal effectively with sleep disturbances? The answer is no, and we all await a major breakthrough. In the meantime, I think that doctors who are not sleep specialists, and their patients, need to step back slightly and take a pragmatic approach. Falling back to a position of "If it ain't broke, don't fix it" would seem very appropriate to me. Here are some steps along the way.

(1) The most "dangerous" of the sleep disorders is sleep apnea. We know unequivocally that this disorder is much more common in obese people or in people who have recently gained weight. We know also that it is not necessary to become "skinny" to reverse the problem. Weight loss of approximately 10% of current body weight is very doable and much better overall than simply resorting to a machine and mask. (2) It is known that the end result of dangerous airway closure is low oxygen concentration in the blood. This can be easily measured using an oximeter placed on the finger, done free of charge or minimal charge by a company that supplies respiratory and oxygen equipment (your doctor will know). The normal reading is 96% to 98%. We do not consider a low reading to be dangerous until it slips below 88%. Perhaps for otherwise healthy people, that is too conservative, and only readings below 85% should be considered worrisome. If a simple and relatively inexpensive "fix" is needed, supplemental oxygen via nasal cannula at one or two liters per minute would suffice. (3) Avoid alcohol, a known respiratory depressant after about 6:00 p.m. (4) Trips to the sleep specialist and sleep lab are frequently triggered by concern of a bed partner. If you share a bed with another person, your kicking and snoring are more likely to be their problem rather than yours. Your stopping of breathing, if indeed a normal variant, is also their problem. If you need something to comfort you at night, use a teddy bear. They rarely complain. Kicking, twitching, and snoring are possible "markers" for a sleep disorder, but not necessarily so. Also, everyone stops breathing periodically during the night. The issue is how often, how long, and how low does the oxygen level drop. (5) Pay close attention to the following considerations: How do I feel for the first five or ten minutes after awakening? Do I have a headache?

Do I feel hangover? Answering "yes" to these simple questions means that you may not be sleeping as much as you think you are, and it suggests multiple subliminal awakenings. Note that I make no point about getting up to the bathroom two or three times, as long as you fall back to sleep promptly. (6) Do I experience excessive daytime sleepiness? (see Epworth Sleepiness Scale) Specifically and simply, do I tend to fall asleep at completely inappropriate times, such as talking on the phone or while driving a car?

Epworth Sleepiness Scale

0	1	2	3
Never	Slight	Moderate	High

Chance of Dozing

1. Sitting and reading.
2. Watching TV.
3. Sitting inactive in a public place.
4. As a car passenger for 1 hour.
5. Laying down to rest.
6. Sitting and talking to someone.
7. Sitting quietly after lunch.
8. Driving in stop-and-go traffic.

Scores greater than 12 are abnormal.

Those are very unusual behaviors and suggestive of marked reduction in effective sleep time. (7) If you, or a spouse have serious concerns about sleep or lack of such, perhaps the easiest remedy is to be kind to yourself, and simply move bedtime back thirty to sixty minutes. Chronic sleep deprivation is in fact known to be very prevalent, usually because we simply don't pay attention to the fact that most people need at least seven hours of sleep. If you have increased "sleep pressure," as it is termed, due to simply not allowing enough sleep time, this should be corrected within a month of allowing increased sleep time.

This leads to another common sleep problem, that of insomnia. Insomnia refers to the inability to initiate or sustain sleep. This is a common problem and can be difficult to solve. In light of the fact that you may only be allotted a ten-minute time slot by your PCP, it may even require a trip to the sleep specialist, but should not require a sleep study. As per other sleep disorders, this can result in daytime impairment, the severity of which will dictate how aggressively the cause and treatment needs to be pursued. Transient insomnia in response to stressors is virtually universal. Chronic insomnia, for most nights for several months is the issue of concern. In contrast to other causes of sleep deprivation, people with insomnia are often unable to nap during the day. The cause for this condition is often poorly delineated. Stress may be a trigger but does not appear to be a common ongoing issue in sustaining insomnia. An extensive history (where have we heard that before?) is needed to explore possible causes. "Sleep logs," although somewhat tedious and requiring attention, can provide important clues. As mentioned, a formal sleep study is not initially needed but may be utilized later if all treatment modalities have failed, thus increasing the possibility of a primary sleep disorder.

SLEEP HYGIENE

- All communication equipment off one hour preceding (includes radio, TV, computer, telephone).
- No stimulants for four hours preceding.
- Dim lights for one hour before.
- Reduce conversation for one hour before.
- Stay out of bed until bedtime.
- Consider warm/hot bath with Epsom salts one hour before.
- Lights off in bedroom (night light okay).
- Consider "white noise" if ambient noise is an issue.
- Consistant time of sleep initiation.
- Avoid strenuous exercise for two hours before.
- Avoid alcohol for two hours before.
- Avoid napping.

There are three major treatment modalities for chronic insomnia. The simplest is to treat medical or psychiatric symptoms that may be interfering with sleep such as pain or depression. Perhaps the best long-term treatment involves so-called cognitive behavioral therapy, supervised by a psychologist, whereby old patterns, habits, and associated thoughts are discarded and new patterns established. It is very effective but requires a skillful therapist and a diligent patient. So-called sleep hygiene is reviewed and discussed, these being behavioral factors day and night, which tend to inhibit rather than enhance sleep. Most of these issues are simple and relatively easy to invoke, although it may be unbelievably difficult to get insomniacs to turn off the TV or radio at night! Consistency for at least several weeks may be key (see chart). Lastly, sedative/hypnotic agents can be used effectively. There is debate as to whether or not these agents are safe for long-term usage. The answer to that always hinges on the "cost–benefit ratio" concept. If the "cost" of chronic insomnia is great, as it often is, these agents may improve the overall quality of life and should not be arbitrarily denied. Refusing sleep meds to chronic insomniacs harkens back to refusing pain meds for the person in pain—and has an arbitrary and dictatorial ring to it. Each situation needs to be individualized.

Sleep and sleeping is a big, complicated issue. It has been relatively ignored for most of the history of medicine. That is definitely no longer the case. Since sleep comprises up to one-third of our lives, it should be studied. As is often the case, the more we learn, the gaps in our knowledge appear to be getting larger. As has been stated before, you, the "consumer," need to have a basic understanding about health issues, to have even a fighting chance at staying healthy. We as a society need to define what appropriate care is, and what is excessive, and perhaps self-aggrandizing.

Fatigue

Back to the basics of systemic symptoms. Fatigue is an exceedingly common complaint, registered daily and repeatedly in the doctor's office. Sleep deprivation is a known and an important cause of fatigue. If you feel reasonably well, do not complain of being "tired all the time," do not obsess over sleep issues, do not wake up with a headache and a hangover, and don't fall asleep on the phone or at a stoplight, it is very unlikely that you have an attention-getting sleep disorder, no matter what your bed partner says.

Fatigue is an interesting and an important symptom, in that it obviously refers to a situation affecting the whole body, possibly arising from almost anywhere in the body. It seems to me that it almost invariably has global health implications. That is, with all of the countless processes going on simultaneously in the structure called you, what is the bottom line? Do you feel good, or bad? Do you feel energetic, or fatigued?

Chronic fatigue, lasting more than a few weeks, which may be the time span for strange viruses and other peculiar entities to pass through your body, becomes an important message that requires attention. Since it is a systemic symptom, it can arise from anywhere in the body and may be caused by hundreds or thousands of things. See your doctor, who will be obligated to do a full history, thorough physical exam and appropriate lab and imaging studies, all designed to rule out 95% of the potential problems.

What is left after this is done? Most often, nothing is found. If so, a longer period of observation is in order. In my humble opinion, the majority of people with chronic fatigue have depression, dysthymia (deep dissatisfaction), excessive stress, sleep deprivation, or combinations of such. There may be one more rarely seen cause. Because of its rarity, it gets a mention. In our era of increasing indolency, it is interesting to harken back to our Paleolithic and agrarian forbearers, who needed to use their bodies to survive. Very occasionally, particularly in older people, fatigue can be induced by an overly zealous pursuit of physical activity. This can also be seen in young athletes, usually of the type trying to maintain "world class" status.

Lastly, as is stated in modern parlance, "trust me…." Turn the TV or radio off during sleep. You may feel even better!

Alcoholism as an Example of Addiction

As has been stated previously, always slightly tongue-in-cheek, we live in a made-up world. This statement is not put forth to criticize the existing paradigm, so much as to call for a measure of tolerance and understanding regarding ways different than our own. So, what is meant by addiction? We hear about addiction to shopping, gambling, sex, eating, computer games, exercise, and other endeavors that are not always clearly separated from zealous pursuits of a hobby. Besides being another way that we tend to poke fun at each other, with "poking fun" often carrying a critical message, it is this hint of criticism that conveys our alarm over the eventual outcome of the habit/addiction. In other words, it conveys concern that the behavior could be dangerous, to you, and maybe even to me.

Actually, perhaps we are just, once again, uncomfortable as observations begin to drift toward the extremes of the bell-shaped curve. We are much more comfortable with observations that describe "normality." Normal tends to be good (comfortable). Eccentricity tends to be bad (uncomfortable). It is always most instructive to look at ourselves, in making these judgments, and then deal with the consequences. In other words, if no one is being dismembered physically, emotionally, or financially, and since we almost never have all of the facts or even most of them at our fingertips, why are we disturbed by these activities? What fears do they arouse in us? Are these fears justified, or just our stuff? Thus, here comes the made-up world again, telling us what is "normal" or "abnormal," acceptable or not, circling around to torment us.

Then, we have the hard-core addictions, such as alcohol, cigarettes, and drugs. Well, how hard core? Are they always bad? Well, at least the guidelines for addiction to alcohol and drugs are somewhat more clearly etched than those for shopaholism, or gambling, at least most of the time. And, the answer is "yes." That is, cigarette consumption is always bad (with very few exceptions; see the "Benefits of Cigarette Smoking," coming soon).

Alcoholism will be used as an example of one of the hard-core addictions. There is a great deal of overlap, such that to discuss both alcoholism and the two major forms of drug addiction may sound a little like a broken record. I may point out differences from time to time.

Alcoholism is a huge problem. Part of its immensity comes from the illusion that it is a behavioral disturbance. Thus, we tend to make judgments about the character or ethics of the alcoholic. We tend to build up a huge reservoir of anger, in terms of the inability of the alcoholic or addict to control their behavior. We may build up an equally onerous reservoir of guilt, wondering if and how we are co-creators of this disaster. Finally, as the severity of these issues worsens, the family and finances begin to crumble, and the reservoirs overflow. This would rarely occur if the problem were diabetes or cancer because those are out of our control. Right?

Back to the illusion—another of these pesky medical illusions, keeping us "asleep," or ignorant, or both. Alcoholism and drug abuse are not caused by behavioral disturbances. They often result in behavioral disturbances. As is true of many diseases, the causes of alcoholism are likely "multifactorial." In most instances, there appear to be genetic influences or predispositions, although the details of these aberrations are not yet worked out. There are certainly social or environmental stressors which are important. Mental health issues in general may involve alcoholism at points along the course. There are obviously gender influences, with alcoholism seriously impacting the lives of 15% to 30% of males and 10% to 20% of females during the course of their lives. Women, however, seem to be more susceptible to the ravages of alcoholism, with a proportionally higher incidence of both mental and physical complications than their male counterparts. Drinking of alcohol regularly before the age of fourteen highly correlates with subsequent alcohol issues. Fifteen to twenty percent of hospitalized patients have or have had alcohol issues.

Those are some of the very basic statistics involving alcoholism. However, such figures do little to describe the day-to-day disruption of life, inherent with this disease, as well as with drug addiction. Alcoholism can be defined in medical terms, using several parameters. It is debatable whether or not the definition can or should include a specific quantity of alcohol, whether it is beer, wine, or "hard liquor." Beer has approximately 4% alcohol content. Wine has 12% to 15% alcohol content. Hard liquors, which would include whisky, gin, and vodka, generally contain up to 40% alcohol. Using these rough figures, a can or bottle of beer would contain approximately 0.5 ounces of alcohol, whereby a wineglass of wine would contain roughly 0.6 ounces of alcohol. A "shot," or one and a half ounces of whiskey would contain roughly 0.6 ounces of alcohol. So, for practical purposes, one bottle of beer, one wine glass of wine, and one "shot" (1½ ounces) of hard liquor are roughly the same, regarding alcohol content.

So, in a person who never demonstrates signs of intoxication, is there an arbitrary amount of alcohol ingestion deemed excessive? The answer is "no." What can be said is as follows, and please recall that my bias comes from everyday clinical medicine. For most people not mentally affected, except perhaps "relaxed," it seems that two portions of alcohol daily would be considered to be medically safe (green light). Three to four portions daily would be considered to be of some risk for development of identifiable problems (yellow light). Five or more portions daily would place most people at high risk for the appearance of complications (red light).

Regarding "complications," there are several varieties of such. The person who just had two glasses of wine, and does this infrequently, may be at low risk for complication. However, if that person, even if feeling unimpaired mentally or physically, should choose to drive a car within four hours or so of such ingestion, and if ever stopped by a police officer for an unrelated violation such as a broken light or turn signal malfunction, an experienced police person could detect subtle signs, and a breathalyzer test could result in an elevated reading. Big complications! The point is that anytime you drink anything, and choose to drive, you may be found to be officially "intoxicated."

Most of the other complications of "social drinkers" consuming four portions or less per day, take an extended period of time, usually ten years or more, to become manifest. These complications fall generally into the realm of organ damage, including liver, pancreas, muscles, heart, and central and peripheral nervous system issues. In excess, alcohol is toxic and can affect other major organs, including bone marrow, stomach, and intestines. We tend to think that problems with the nervous system take longer to manifest than problems in other organ systems. However, this may simply be a reflection of the vast billions of cells in the nervous system acting as a de facto reservoir of function, somewhat masking loss of function. We know that isolated head injuries, causing "concussion," with minimal disturbances such as nausea, immediate confusion and/or memory issues, fatigue, and reduced motor function, can cause permanent neuronal loss or damage. Can the same neuronal loss occur every time a person drinks to the point of feeling a buzz? What about a slight buzz? The answer is that we don't know. We think that those kinds of events represent temporary neuronal dysfunction, rather than neuronal death, but we don't know for sure.

What we can see and measure is the evidence of liver damage, seen on blood studies and/or with imaging studies. The pattern of abnormality, although not absolutely diagnostic for alcohol-induced damage, is suggestive enough to offer a warning to the person. The pancreas can also be damaged, resulting in either exocrine dysfunction, with digestive issues, or endocrine dysfunction, with the appearance of diabetes. Cardiac damage can be detected in several ways, but mostly using echocardiography, with appearance of "cardiomyopathy" or reduced cardiac muscle contraction.

After many years of heavy alcohol intake, the appearance of the person may be very characteristic, such that a diagnosis can be confidently made on physical exam alone. By that time, they also likely show easily detectable evidence of neuromuscular dysfunction. Also, by that time, the effect of alcohol on the social life of the person has likely been devastating.

In summary, alcoholism takes a terrible toll on the individual and on society. It is a progressive disease, which results in progressively worsening mental and physical functioning, and premature death. People vary greatly in their susceptibility to the toxic effects of alcohol. I have seen many people in the end stages of alcoholism, who swear that they only had two to three portions per day. Perhaps, anything more than one to two portions per day places a person at risk.

The disease is treatable. The treatment is abstention. The first problem is getting to that, through withdrawal. The second problem, even greater in magnitude, is maintaining that. It can be done, but the relapse rate, and re-relapse, and re-re-relapse rates are very high. There are a variety of treatments available, and all of them work, some of the time.

The problem is not going to go away. We have known about, and used alcohol, in the form of beer and wine dating back to the appearance of agriculture and civilization 7–9,000 years ago in Mesopotamia and elsewhere. It is mentioned in the Gilgamesh epic from that civilization. We obviously have a susceptible population. We are bombarded by commentary involving alcoholic beverages, appealing to our reptilian brains. What if you are thirty-five years old, physically fit, and never go to the doctor? How would you know if you have a problem still at the curable stage? Back to basics—a little introspection combined with the acronym CAGE. Have I ever thought about the need to Cut down? Have I ever been Annoyed by questions about my drinking? Do I ever feel Guilty about my drinking? Do I ever need an Eye opener in the morning? The yes answer to any one question places you at high risk. Personally, I think the A is the most telling, representing people reaching out to help you. Isn't this what you would hope they would do?

This concludes our discussion of systemic symptoms and a few diseases/disorders that affect the entire organism.

Part II
INTEGUMENT

P lease note again that each organ system reviewed is extremely complex, represented by textbooks with thousands of pages, and monthly or quarterly periodicals of a hundred pages or so, relating the latest research findings. The attempt here is to look at each organ system in a very pragmatic manner, discussing general issues and common problems. It is hoped that it will be informative and interesting—and as always giving the reader an overview and basic understanding, resulting in the making of good choices to maintain health.

The "integument" is a term used to describe the skin and its appendages—the hair and nails. Although it does not closely resemble a typical internal organ in appearance, it functions like an organ, being metabolically active, subject to a variety of insults, capable of even causing systemic symptoms, and obviously important to the maintenance of health. It is most clearly the tissue which demarcates "us" from "not us." Alternatively, that is somewhat simplistic, in that there is a constant back and forth interchange between us and our environment, primarily through the skin and other sense organs. Obviously, the skin is a bona fide sense organ itself, through the sense of touch.

Skin, Hair, and Nails

Each organ system has a relatively limited and somewhat predictable way of notifying us about a problem. With skin, the major symptoms produced include rashes, itching, and the appearance of bumps, lumps, and a large variety of other "barnacles." Beginning with itching, the first important concept to note is that itching may be a reflection of a primary skin disease, or it may be a systemic effect of a completely separate disease emanating from another organ system. So, in considering itching, as is always the case, the "history" of the itch, culled out by your doctor, is the way to get started toward a diagnosis.

Itching

Systemic causes of itching generally, if not almost always (recall, never say never, and never say always), involves large portions of the skin surface, with perhaps a few areas of accentuation. The most common diseases to cause itching as part of their systemic expression include liver disorders and kidney disorders, generally in the setting of advanced disease of liver or kidneys. So, with no previous history of liver or kidney disease, and if you otherwise feel well, those organs are probably not causative. Blood and lymphatic disorders can cause widespread itching, and sometimes relatively early in their course. So, this possibility may require some attention, with simple blood tests and a chest X-ray substantially clarifying things and usually ruling out this organ system as the culprit.

More often than not, no systemic disease away from the skin can be identified. Then, all of the little nuances in the history, regarding length of time present, previous similar episodes, history of allergies, and possible exposures to allergens (a substance to which you are allergic), all help to determine cause and dictate how extensive a workup needs to be. Often times, no definite cause can be flushed out.

Note here that we are discussing itch without rash. In situations like this involving skin, doctors often resort to so-called empiric therapy, which means trying something because it usually works. Just like most other ailments, itching can come and go (once or repeatedly) with no cause ever determined. A trial of over-the-counter antihistamine or an "H-2 receptor blocker," like Tagamet or Zantac may help considerably. Your doctor might even try a short course of cortisone-type medications. Most often, the condition remits spontaneously. There is a peculiar condition called "non-specific dermatitis," which translates to "your guess is as good as mine." It is likely common, and it thought to possibly represent some type of dysfunction of the immune system. In fact, most of the time, when observed closely, a "rash" can be found. The rash usually consists of widespread, isolated, very small bumps, which are intensely itchy, with a wide penumbra, creating the illusion that the itch is all over. The diagram illustrates that the three tiny spots over the upper part of the chest can cause a feeling of itch over most of the area. This condition can cause marked distress and is generally controlled somewhat by topical steroids.

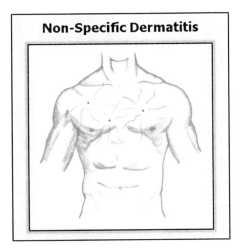

Non-Specific Dermatitis

Rash

Rash generally refers to an area of abnormal appearance of the skin surface, over an area much more extensive than a focal or an isolated lesion. "Lesion" is one of many terms used by doctors that contribute to their aura of erudition and authority. Translated, it means "thing."

It is used to describe abnormal tissues all over the body, not just skin tissue. If you spend any time around medical people, you will hear it being used. Don't be intimidated. It is just a thing. Rashes can be very chronic, even permanent, or very evanescent, lasting a minute or less. They can be itchy or not. Some have a very characteristic location and appearance and can be quickly diagnosed on that basis alone. However, rashes of common conditions such as eczema or psoriasis, and many others, can vary widely in appearance and location. At that point, the term dermatitis is most appropriate (i.e., "Your guess is as good as mine."), and referral to a dermatologist is necessary.

The vast majority of rashes do not represent truly serious or life-threatening problems. However, they can obviously have major cosmetic implications. Common conditions such as acne, if severe or undertreated, can cause significant scarring. Rashes with itching can lead to considerable morbidity (an ominous-sounding term which means "trouble"). Itching of course may lead to scratching. Scratching can lead to disruption of the skin surface, with subsequent secondary or collateral bacterial infection. This in turn can greatly complicate the possibility of accurate diagnosis and, of course, can be problematic in and of itself. Permanent changes in pigmentation and/or skin texture can occur, furthering the cosmetic insult.

Bumps

Another very common skin disturbance is the appearance of previously mentioned bumps, lumps, and "barnacles." It is likely, when first making their appearance, that these myriad types of lesions ("things") can be intimidating. There is an enormous difference from one person to another, as to when they make their appearance and to what extent that they do. Many of those on body surfaces often exposed to sunlight are secondary to damage from sunlight. Lesions developing mostly over the trunk and face, beginning in midlife, and discolored light brown or tan are so-called keratotic lesions. Other lesions are not necessarily seen but can be felt as "lumps" just under the skin surface, anywhere from the size of a grain of rice to a small lemon. A vast majority of these lesions are not serious but may require confirmation of such from your doctor, perhaps during the course of a visit for something else. I would generally not recommend surgical removal, unless they are cosmetically unacceptable, or at points on the body surface which would subject them to pressure and discomfort ("discomfort" is a term doctors use for *PAIN*). These lesions require bigger incisions than might be expected from the appearance alone. It seems to me, a non-surgeon, that over the years, surgeons are doing less and less office surgery. They tend to utilize "outpatient surgery" facilities for even minor surgery (By the way, the definition of "minor surgery" is "surgery being done on somebody else"). The facility fee alone could be from $1,000 to $2,000. If the doctor wants to knock you out because he or she doesn't like the sound of screaming, add another $500 to $1,000 for the anesthesiologist. So, the expense of removing your benign skin tumor could be worth $4,000 to $5,000. Lastly, as is true with many skin lesions, they tend to recur, and after a while, you might feel like the cat chasing its tail. The surface lesions can be removed in the office by a dermatologist or even perhaps by your PCP using liquid nitrogen. Even that is somewhat expensive. In my opinion, the only ones which truly warrant removal are the ones which are called "premalignant."

Sebaceous Cyst

There are several different types of skin lesions, which are not necessarily bumps, lumps, or barnacles, that are common and problematic. Perhaps the one of least concern might be the sebaceous cyst or abscess. This condition is similar to the hydradentis suppurativa mentioned before, except that they have a much wider distribution. Although most commonly seen on the neck or trunk, they can occur almost anywhere. They are, once again, plugged oil glands, with development and accumulation of material under the skin. They can be quite painful. They too are treated with heat and antibiotics, and they may need some type of drainage procedure done in the office (cheap). They may recur. With frequent occurrence, or if very large, they may need surgical attention (expensive).

Shingles

The second condition is so-called shingles. This is a fascinating illness which represents re-activation of the herpes zoster virus, which is (or was, as children are now vaccinated for this) the cause of childhood chicken pox. After recovery, the virus goes into hibernation in the nerve roots of the spinal cord. In most people, we never hear from it again. In perhaps 10% to 20% of such people, with advancing age, and often with some type of obvious stressor, the virus can wake up (recall that we don't even know for sure if viruses are technically "alive") and begin to migrate down the spinal nerves, all the way out to the surface of the body, where a focal rash is produced. The rash may cause no symptoms. Alternatively, it can cause itching and/or pain. The pain may be very important for two reasons. (1) It may precede the development of the rash from days to weeks. This in turn can create major diagnostic dilemmas. I recall one patient, who, after two weeks of increasing abdominal pain, with no cause found, was admitted to the hospital

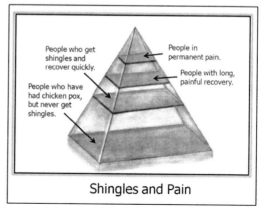

People who get shingles and recover quickly.

People in permanent pain.

People with long, painful recovery.

People who have had chicken pox, but never get shingles.

Shingles and Pain

for exploratory surgery. I visited him early in the morning on the day of the planned surgery, at which time he said that he felt the same, except for a rash which had just appeared. One look at the rash over the lower abdomen was all we needed to cancel the surgery. The rash is often laid out in such a way, no matter where it is on the body surface; that understanding of the anatomy of skin sensory innervation allows for a diagnosis with relative confidence. (2) Occasionally, the pain may be very severe and last for weeks. A very small percentage of people may experience "postherpetic neuralgia" (meaning, "I wouldn't wish this on my worst enemy") which can last for years. There are two bits of good news: (1) Only a small percentage of people, maybe 5% to 10% of the people with shingles, have severe or longstanding pain, and (2) for those who don't want to even take a chance, there is now a relatively effective vaccine available. It is relatively expensive and unlikely to be paid for by insurance. So, just like almost everything else regarding medical care, it is up to you (see diagram). Incidentally, if you have already had an episode of shingles, that should act as a "vaccination," and it is very unlikely that you will ever get it again. Lastly, the vaccine is considered to be approximately 75% effective, but does not guarantee that you will not get shingles.

Cellulitis

The third condition is called cellulitis and represents a bacterial infection, usually strep or staph, in the tissues just beneath the skin and the skin itself. It is by far most commonly seen in the lower legs, although it can occur anywhere. It is more common in elderly people and especially in those with known vascular problems, whether that is arterial or venous. As common and innocent as it is, it can produce sudden severe illness via sepsis, i.e., entry of bacteria into the blood stream. The most common presentation is that of redness and pain, almost always seen in the presence of edema or increased fluid in the legs. It is thought to occur because of tiny breaks in the skin, allowing entry of bacteria into the protein-rich fluid just under the skin, providing an ideal incubator for bacterial proliferation. If the bacteria gain entrance to the vascular system, that is called sepsis and causes a person to become very suddenly, very ill. The treatment involves elevation of the legs above heart level, and diuretics, both designed to eliminate the excess fluid/bacterial incubator. Also, most antibiotics are effective and are usually needed for seven to fourteen days. Recurrences are common because we may not know for sure if we have completely eradicated the infection or simply suppressed it, and because the factors predisposing to it often persist. If there is an intercurrent hospitalization or nursing home stay, future infection could be secondary to one of the so-called super bugs, more commonly found in hospitals and requiring certain specific antibiotics to which they are susceptible. At times, acute cellulitis gradually transforms into a low-grade chronic cellulitis which may simply be left alone.

Cancer

The last "special" skin condition is that of skin cancer. Based on the microscopic appearance of these tumors, there are three common variants, and all three are seemingly becoming more prevalent. All three appear to be partly related to intensity of sun exposure. The most common is the so-called basal cell tumor. These are also the least worrisome, in that they do not metastasize (spread widely through the blood stream) and can usually be dealt with in the office by your PCP or dermatologist. They can, on occasion, burrow deeply and do major local damage that way. On rare occasions, this could be indirectly fatal. These tumors are humbling, in the sense that they are often very innocent looking, appearing non-descript, and not always clearly different from a lesion close by which is not malignant. There can be dozens of these scattered over the body surface. So, how should we deal with these common problems? Fortunately, as mentioned, in most locations, they provide little risk of serious morbidity (trouble). They can be watched over the course of months, looking for evidence of enlargement, thickening, bleeding, or any major change in appearance. If this occurs, they can be dealt with in the office, with removal after local anesthesia.

The second type of tumor is less common but potentially much more dangerous—this being the squamous cell tumor. By the time you might notice this, it would look like a small bump or lump, protruding upward several millimeters. They are variously colored, but not very dark or black. They may be inadvertently scraped and bleed. These are not usually "watched," for very long. They can be biopsied in the office and then removed in the office if the biopsy is "positive." The potential danger of these is that they do have the ability to metastasize wildly, although this is unusual.

The third type of common skin tumor is by far the most dangerous and the one which has received the most attention in the media—this being melanoma. These tumors arise from the cells in the skin which produce pigment, and they usually identify themselves as being very dark or "classically" black. Some of these go through what appears to be a premalignant phase, but these too are dangerous and usually dark. Unfortunately, for all of us and in line with "never say always," a small percentage of these may not be very dark or black. Therefore, these are extremely dangerous, as they can be present for a much longer time before it is realized by you or your doctor what they are. Melanomas have a strong tendency to metastasize and may do so when the lesion on the skin is still very small. Treatment of melanomas is difficult because they are so aggressive. A wide surgical excision, by an experienced surgeon, is necessary. Depending on the location, there may later be a wide excision and sampling of lymph nodes, which are supposed to trap and contain migrating tumor cells. Once the tumor has extended past the lymph glands, the prognosis is "guarded," as these tumors are not very responsive to systematic therapy with drugs or even local therapy with radiation.

At this point in time, a deeply tanned patient does not impress the doctor as looking healthy. It gives about the same signal to the doctor, as the patient who would have the moxie to walk into the office smoking a cigarette. It sadly identifies you as a patient who apparently places cosmetic issues ahead of good preventative care. This may sound somewhat judgmental or arbitrary, in a world which woefully lacks unconditional love and acceptance. However, it is not as harsh as suggesting that deeply tanned or smoking individuals harbor a death wish. (Do they?) Skin cancer is a partially preventable disease. One should avoid prolonged sun exposure, or should wear heavy-duty sun block. Inspect your own visible skin once per month or so, similar to the recommendations given to women regarding breast self-exam. At first you may feel lost, but that will change quickly. At least once per year, have someone check the parts of you that you cannot see. If you are not a contortionist, and have no such person in your life, and continue to indulge in sun exposure, have your doctor do it (This is one of the few things that really can be done in ten minutes).

Causes of Temporary Hair Loss
• High Fever
• Surgery
• Anesthesia
• Childbirth
• Psychic shock
• Drugs
✓ Birth control
✓ Colchicine
✓ Chemotherapy
✓ Heparin
✓ Coumadin
✓ Others(?)

Hair and Nails

Now, to complete the issues of skin by dealing with its appendages (meaning modifications), I have little to say about hair and only slightly more about nails. There are a few pathologic (meaning abnormal) kinds of hair loss, generally rare and usually related to autoimmune conditions, which are systemic diseases. Let's skip those! Generalized hair loss is by far the most common hair condition and, with aging, affects most people, including women. Many acute and or severe conditions can cause a temporary loss of hair (see list). Many of these are most noticeable weeks to months after the insult. Generally speaking, once the underlying condition passes or is treated, hair growth returns. As noted in the list, there are a number of drugs that are commonly used and are known to be possibly related to hair loss. Most people know about the possibility of hair loss with certain types of chemotherapy. Hair loss can occur (temporarily) after birth control pills are discontinued. Colchicine is a drug occasionally used for gout. Heparin and Coumadin are both blood thinners and are very commonly used. It is likely that there are many more potential drug causative agents, but the association with others is not usually convincing. I subscribe to the notion that anything can happen. I live in an area with stands of huge fir trees, with millions or billions of fir needles in each tree. As I aimlessly wander across the floor at home, a typical pastime of mine, it always makes me happy to see a demonstration that in fact anything is possible! Out of the many millions of fir needles all around us, I see one lone needle lying there in splendid repose. The chance of this one needle out of many millions finding its way into my house is one in several millions, but it happened. Then, I usually go out and buy a lottery ticket (only kidding). If you experience hair loss weeks to months after beginning drug A or supplement B, there could be a connection. If you choose to discontinue that product, recall that it may take several months for hair growth to be restored.

Here are a few final observations about hair loss. Although thyroid disorders are often considered as possibilities, they appear to be a very unusual cause. On the other hand, substantial hair loss in aging women is exceedingly common. Since women usually begin with much more hair than men, the loss is rarely noted to be nearly so complete. As is true about everything else in biology, there are huge variations from person to person. There are genetic influences, but those too are random, afflicting some, and not others.

Unfortunately, regarding treatment of hair loss, the promise and the actuality of improvement with hair restoration products, both topical and systemic, are widely divergent. Such products do show evidence of hair growth, but it is usually of a very fine, almost spiderweb-type hair that a young child might have over their body, but that unlikely makes a noticeable difference on the top of your head. Surgical approaches to hair loss via "transplanting" have improved technically and cosmetically but are limited by the fact that such surgery is time consuming and expensive.

Recall that hair and nails are medically considered appendages of the skin. A lifetime of study, observation, and contemplation has led me to the conclusion that hair is good! On top of the head, it provides a layer of warmth and a protection against skin cancer. Eye lashes help keep unwanted debris off our corneas, reducing the potential of going blind. Eyebrows, if heavy enough, keep burning sweat out of our eyes and ensure that all of us don't have to wear those silly-looking head bands. Body hair gives us a reason to wash the sheets and clean the shower once in a while. Pubic and armpit hair are essential for…I think I'll skip this. So hair continually reminds us about the inexpressible wonders of evolution.

Nails, on the contrary, are bad! Besides allowing us to paint lovely little designs on them, they provide us with nothing but trouble. This is obviously not true for all animal species. For instance, how could cats climb up drapes or screens without nails? I'm talking about human nails. They collect dirt. Auto mechanics who have long since retired are buried with dirty nails. They crack. They break. They become ingrown and can cause abscesses and cellulitis. With advanced age, they almost uniformly become infected with fungus, which causes them to thicken, turn yellow, and crumble, usually due to a fungus. To correct this, the eleventh plague, lost to history when an angered Moses dropped the other tablet, requires us to take potentially toxic medications for up to six months, requiring frequent liver tests to make sure that this vital organ is not rotting away while we deplete our retirement funds trying to pay for this medication because our insurance company is smart enough to have figured out that it isn't necessary in the first place. However, redemption is right around the corner. After six months, our finger nails and toe nails look better than the day we traversed the birth canal. Our first several visits to the manicurist recall the exhilaration of the Allies freeing Europe during WWII. Sadly, just as the Iron Curtain descended a few years later, within a few months the telltale signs of the fungus begin to reappear in about 50% of those who had the gall to think they could get rid of it.

I must confess that nails serve one important purpose for me. As was previously mentioned in the material regarding pain, I ask patients whether their pain is mild, moderate, or severe, rather than using the analog scale of 1 to 10. Just imagine if there was a well-designed, randomized, double-blinded, placebo-controlled study showing that when patients are asked to rate their pain using the analog scale, 58.5% respond by saying, "it's a 10!" The other 41.5% say, "it's a 12!" At that point, I would ask, "So, it is like having your fingernails pulled off one at a time with no anesthesia?" So, rethinking this just-concluded diatribe, maybe nails serve a purpose after all.

PART III
HEAD, EYES, EARS, NOSE, THROAT

Note that we have just concluded a brief survey of one of the five classically described sense organs, the skin, which provides us with the sensation of touch. This is accomplished by an incredibly complex carpet of tiny nerve filaments lying within the skin. These filaments are much more densely packed in some locations than they are in others, ranging from more in the hands and feet to lesser over the back and buttocks. Just as the Colorado River, raging though the Grand Canyon begins as multiple tiny rivulets high in the Rocky Mountains, the multiple tiny nerve filaments coalesce into increasingly larger nerves heading for entry into the spinal cord. Damage to these peripheral nerves can result in a variety of disabilities, both sensory and motor (affecting muscle function), including painful and difficult-to-treat neuropathic pain. Once into the spinal cord, the sensory tracts ascend all the way up to the sensory cortex, one sensory center on each side of the brain, representing a substantial portion of the cortex, the highest level of the nervous system.

The areas to be reviewed now constitute the other four major senses: smell, taste, hearing, and vision. These too have generous displays via the cerebral cortex, again attesting to the important survival aspects that the sense organs provide.

The discussion regarding diseases of these areas in keeping with the format for discussion within the *Review of Systems* will take a very pragmatic approach, dealing with common problems. This is especially true in these areas, which have become remarkably specialized. In the 1960s, the study of ophthalmology (eyes) was still combined with the study of ears, nose, and throat. By the 1970s, the separation of ophthalmology into a separate specialty had been completed. Since then, there has been further separation regarding eye diseases, such that there are now specialists who deal with only some type of eye diseases or functions. It appears that the specialty of otolaryngology—or of ears, nose, and throat—has not yet sub-specialized to the extent that ophthalmology has.

Basically, diseases of the eye include those that might be termed supporting structures and those that are directly involved with vision per se. The lids and their lining membrane called the conjunctiva also extend over the white part of the eye known as the sclera. Injuries can occur to these structures and to the cornea, which is the clear portion covering the iris that gives the eye its color. Diseases affecting these structures are common and are usually not too difficult to deal with. The lids, being covered with normal skin, can be involved with many types of dermatitis that can occur elsewhere. With the common skin condition called seborrhea, when it affects the edge of the lid, where the lashes are, can cause a condition called blepharitis. It is common especially in older people and can be quite chronic. It may also be caused by bacterial infection. The most important part of controlling it is to keep the lid margins clean and clear of oils, using hot compresses and baby shampoo daily. A stye is a localized swelling secondary to plugging of the oil glands at the margin of the lid and is usually treated the same way—and also with gentle abrasion or rubbing. Stubborn cases will obviously require the attention of a doctor, an ophthalmologist, and possibly even a dermatologist.

Conjunctivitis is an inflammation of the lining membrane mentioned above and is usually the result of an infection. This in turn is commonly viral or bacterial and, rarely, some other type of infection. Conjunctivitis is also seen as part of an allergic flare-up. The appearance is similar, regardless of the cause, and is that of increased redness of the inside of the lids or the sclera or both. The redness occurs because of the dilation of the blood vessels in response to injury. Conjunctivitis can occur to isolated individuals, or because it may be quite contagious, it may occur in outbreaks in schools, dormitories, and other settings where people are in close contact. It may involve one or both eyes and usually comes on over the course of one to two days. In the setting of a typical upper respiratory infection, it is likely viral. In the setting of a full-blown allergic illness, that is probably the causative factor.

Hay Fever

"Hay fever" is a term given to a syndrome (constellation of symptoms) usually including runny nose, sneezing, tearing, itching or burning of the eyes, and itching inside the mouth. It is often a response to a single allergen (an allergy-producing substance), which may be present in the environment for a given period of time. This is a good example of a condition which, although clearly not serious in terms of overall health, can be very debilitating, causing both the local symptoms described above and the prominent systemic symptoms, such as fatigue and loss of appetite. It is almost always improved by being sequestered quietly in a darkened room with cool compresses over the eyes and made worse by activity, bright lights, breezes, and other stimulating factors. Obviously, based on the description, it is easy to see how it could completely interrupt or prohibit normal activities.

Fortunately, there are a variety of medications and treatments which are usually very helpful. If it characteristically is present for a relatively short period of time, usually in spring or summer, it can usually be well controlled with over-the-counter (OTC) antihistamines and/or decongestants. However, if it characteristically lasts much longer, or even year-round, or if it has not improved much with well-tolerated medication, then a visit to your doctor, who may in turn refer you to an allergist, could be very helpful. In this situation, the doctor will take a detailed history in an effort to expose what might be the most likely allergens involved. It is also likely that skin testing and possibly blood testing will be added to further try to determine if there are any meaningful allergens, either one or many to which you are being exposed. Based on the results of these tests, the allergist might prepare an injectable medication as part of a "hyposensitization" program. In medicine, "hypo" preceding a word means basically not enough or less. "Hyper" means the opposite, too much. So with the hyposensitization program, this involves an attempt to make you less sensitive to a given allergen. This is done by: (1) minimizing exposure to the allergens themselves whenever possible and (2) preparing the injectable material to be used once per week to start. This material contains increasingly larger amounts of the very same allergens to which you are responding. When given by injection, in gradually increasing concentrations, it is hoped that eventually all of the receptors for that or those allergens on your allergy-responsive cells will be filled up or blocked, so that the environmental allergens which have been the cause of the problem are no longer able to attach to the receptors on sensitive membranes and cause problems. It is a very effective form of treatment but is obviously somewhat cumbersome and expensive. In some people, it can be the difference between full functioning and nonfunctioning.

As has already been mentioned, there are a large number of OTC preparations which may be very effective. Once again, emphasizing our subtle differences standing side by side with our remarkable similarities, one type or one brand of medication may fail, whereas the next one helps greatly. If none of the OTC medications help, then you are doomed to make your ten-minute office visit with your doctor. He or she can use a number of preparations which are not available OTC and which expand the possibility of success.

Eye

After this brief tour through the land of hay fever, which can impact all of the sense organs, let us return to the part of the eye that worries us the most. Along with cancer, stroke, and dementia, most people would likely consider loss of vision to be a hurdle which they would most dread having to deal with. Light enters the eye through the cornea, which is in the clear part covering the iris. The iris is only indirectly concerned with vision, opening and closing in response to the intensity of incoming light and to other autonomic stimuli. Right

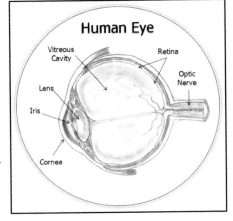

behind the iris is the lens, which is directly involved with sight, by bending the incoming light rays, which then travel through the vitreous, as they head toward the retina. The vitreous is a viscous fluid medium which fills most of the globe of the eye.

At the back of the globe, where the converging light rays are supposed to be focused lies a thin but incredibly complex membrane called the retina, which perhaps could be considered the workhouse of the visual apparatus. The retina unbelievable as it seems, changes light energy into electrical energy. This in turn is conveyed by the optic nerves along a circuitous route to the very back of the brain, where awaits the visual cortex, whose job is to interpret what the light rays entering the cornea represent. "Blind sight" is a fascinating phenomenon involving a person who has sustained a certain type of damage to the visual cortex. The person will claim to be blind, unable to see anything. Yet, they can navigate, reach out, and retrieve items, etc. They lack the integration of those stimuli by the visual cortex which makes them feel blind. All of this occurs in a tiny fraction of a second. Anything from the cornea, iris, through the lens, vitreous, onto the retina into the nervous system called the optic nerves, along the base of the brain to the visual cortex, can affect vision.

Basically, from the retina through to the visual cortex, most of the potential causes of visual loss are in turn secondary to loss of circulation and will be dealt with shortly with a discussion of the nervous system. The eye, beginning at the retina, is basically considered to be an extension of the brain. Twenty-five percent of the blood pumped out of our hearts goes up to the brain and skull, representing approximately 10% of our body weight. Doing the arithmetic, blood flow to the brain is approximately 2½ times greater than to all other body tissues. This does not represent a surplus of flow but what the brain needs to function normally. Through complex reflex mechanisms, blood flow to the brain is maintained as the number one priority, even in the face of substantial blockages in the big arteries supplying the brain.

"Stroke" is a term used to signify when a permanent loss of brain function has occurred in response to loss of circulation. In the sense of the visual apparatus, this could and does involve the retina causing partial or even complete loss of vision, usually to one eye. There is a condition called giant cell arteritis, sometimes seen in the syndrome of polymyalgia rheumatica, which is an inflammatory condition which can close off arteries. If the retinal artery is shut off, the result is sudden complete blindness in that eye. Nerves receive arterial supply as well, so that the optic nerve could be damaged by a reduced blood flow. Finally, the blood supply to the optic cortex could be cut off to impair vision. All of these would fall under the broad category of "stroke," with the example of an inflammatory cause, like giant cell arteritis, but with the vast majority occurring because of old-fashioned, run-of-the-mill hardening of the arteries.

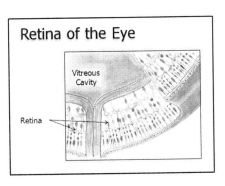

Moving forward through the eye, vision can be severely damaged by a process called macular degeneration, which affects part of the retina. It is, in fact, the most common cause of significant visual loss in people over the age of sixty. There may be genetic factors present. Cigarette smoking is known to increase the risk. Medications and supplements can slow, but usually not stop, progression of visual loss. Retinal detachment is a relatively rare condition which can cause sudden substantial visual loss. Fortunately, the situation can usually be corrected or substantially be improved using surgical or laser techniques.

The vitreous-filled globe does not actively participate in vision. However, anything that causes bleeding into the vitreous, such as diabetes, can cause severe visual impairment. Unfortunately, this can occur suddenly and unexpectedly, even in a person whose diabetes is reasonably well controlled. The best kind of diabetes to have is NONE. There are many ways whereby most "diabetics" can achieve this, by becoming "pre-diabetics," to be discussed later.

"Floaters" are common with aging. They represent the appearance of ghost-like, amorphous areas of haziness or darkness, floating across the field of vision. They are not considered to be a serious threat to vision. They are caused by precipitation of proteinaceous material in the vitreous. There is no known treatment for them.

Moving forward, we reach the lens, which is perhaps the most common source of visual loss via cataracts. Cataracts occur because of deterioration or "clouding" of the lens, negatively affecting the transmission of the light rays back to the retina. There again can be genetic factors. Eye trauma can occasionally lead to cataract formation. They are more common, and tend to occur earlier, with diabetics. Sun exposure is a risk (it seems that if the cigarettes don't get you, the sun will). In those whose vision is seriously impaired, the treatment involves surgical removal of the lens, and possibly substitution of an artificial lens. This surgery is usually very helpful in terms of restoring good vision.

Just ahead of the lens is the anterior chamber which is the location whereby a buildup of pressure from too much fluid can be transmitted all the way backwards through the eye to the optic nerve. There, the pressure can damage the optic nerve and cause complete loss of vision. This is the sequence seen in glaucoma. The most likely explanation for why fluid does not drain properly from the anterior chamber is genetic predisposition. Eye trauma can be causative in some. The iris itself can become inflamed usually as part of an autoimmune process. This can be very painful and can decrease vision temporarily, but does not usually lead to loss of vision.

At the very front of the eye is the cornea, which can be damaged by direct injury or by a variety of infections. Most often, recovery is complete; however, if corneal scarring is severe enough, surgery, or if you are unfortunate enough to have a rare type of corneal deterioration, a corneal transplant surgery is usually very effective for restoring vision.

In summary, in the absence of any significant visual problems and for a person with good general health, most people can postpone a visit to the eye doctor to somewhere between the ages of 40 and 50. At that point, if there is no evidence for cataracts, macular degeneration, or glaucoma, follow-up visits should probably be done every three to five years.

Head

Although the head is clearly of singular importance to the overall orderly functioning of the body, many of its various components are discussed under different sections. Once the skin, hair, eyes, ears, nose, mouth and throat, nervous system including the brain, and even the ephemeral mind-soul which likely resides there as well, are dispatched, what is left for conjecture?

Headache

Rather than skip the head completely, thus creating a headless survey, there is at best one universally salient topic left—headache.

Very arbitrarily, there are five major categories of headache, and each is common and presents its own challenges. Again, pragmatism prevails in the discussion, dealing with issues that are common, coming from the perspective of a witness in the frontline trenches (me), hopefully with some helpful hints.

As is true for each organ system or body part, there tends to be two types of problems seen, those being local and systemic. As you might have presumed, the same is true for headache. Obviously, headache or head pain can be seen in a wide variety of systemic illnesses. Almost any illness associated with fever can involve head pain. Perhaps the term headache is best used for one of the diseases whereby the pain itself is the focal point, whereas head pain is that which is seen as an accompaniment of numerous other systemic processes.

The three major common causes of headache are tension, sinus, and migraine, respectively. Since all are common, it is also common that more than one can be present in the same individual. In fact, this classification, which is my own, becomes somewhat fuzzy beyond the big three with the fourth being mixed, or a combination of several, and the fifth being "rebound." There is also a term which doctors use frequently, namely chronic daily headache (CDH). The relationships between these somewhat overlapping concepts will be discussed.

Tension Headache

In view of the stressful conditions in which most of us live and work, it is surprising that we all don't have tension headaches all of the time. As a sidelight, it seems likely to me that over the history of our species, there has likely been a high level of stress felt by most people most of the time. Previously, fear of famine, uncontrolled epidemics, relative helplessness in the face of accidents, maternal death at childbirth, high infant mortality, and brutality toward each other all hung like a dark cloud over our ancestors. Although some of these horrors have been ameliorated considerably, new ones have taken their place, and our sense of basic vulnerability remains prevalent. Perhaps a better term than tension headache is muscle contraction headache, which is thought to be the cause of the problem. The most common locations for this type of headache are (1) on the side of the head behind the eyes, and perhaps around the ear on the jaw joint, and (2) at the back of the head, extending down to the neck. The first is thought to represent contraction of the muscles of mastication and can result in so-called temporomandibular joint (TMJ) disease as a consequence. When this occurs at night, there can be audible grinding heard, annoying for the listener and destructive for the producer, as teeth can be permanently damaged. Tight clenching is not necessary to cause pain. If tension in these muscles is only mildly increased for extended periods of time, pain may result. The pain at the back of the head is caused by an increased tension in those muscles and the muscles extending out toward the upper back and shoulders. Alternatively, arthritic conditions of the neck are common. Pain or irritation at that area is thought to be responsible for inducing tension in neck muscles, perhaps in an attempt to restrict motion and reduce the tendency for pain. These types of headache, where the neck appears to be intricately involved, are sometimes subcategorized as "cervicogenic headache." The name is not so important, as long as it is appreciated that neck issues can cause headache.

Fortunately, these muscle contraction headaches are usually not severe. They can be chronic and very annoying. They can be treated by a variety of mechanical, medicinal, and relaxation techniques. Mouth appliances for nighttime use, contoured foam collars for daytime use, heat, ergonomic factors, changes in posture, massage, or simple awareness of the state of tension can all be helpful.

Sinus Headache

Sinus headache is much less common despite the common occurrence of nasal and sinus issues. The sinus cavities are located primarily around the nasal cavity and are connected to the nasal cavity through a series of small channels, most of which are prone to closure secondary to inflammation. Just as anyone can appreciate the discomfort felt with a badly stuffed nose, the same can occur with sinuses. At some point, the discomfort progresses to pain, which is most commonly felt in the face, forehead, and in and behind the nose. The diagnosis is usually apparent by a variety of symptoms involving the nose, ears, and eyes, such as with a cold or flu. Just as sinus disease can be acute or chronic, so can the accompanying headache. When sinus disease is low grade, the diagnosis of sinus headache can be more difficult, as the headache at times may be the most prominent symptom. Regardless, the pain is usually not severe and usually responds to OTC analgesics, antihistamines and decongestants—in oral and/or nasal form—and possibly antibiotics. Infrequently, in cases resistant to oral and topical nasal medications, an attempt at surgical treatment may be indicated.

Migraine

The last of the major forms of headache is migraine. This is a disease which continues to be fascinating and intimidating, even thousands of years after it was first described. It remains even now a "work in progress" in terms of both diagnosis and treatment.

Why the complexity regarding this entity? The answer is deceptively simple at least conceptually, in that migraine is now thought to be a brain disease, partially or completely. This represents a departure in the conceptual framework that we have held for many years, whereby the basic problem was thought to be related to overly active dilatation and contraction of the cranial blood vessels and to a so-called "neurogenic inflammation" of the blood vessels. There remain many unanswered questions regarding exactly what is the initiating mechanism, and in fact, it is likely that there are many. However, with the newest imaging techniques, it does seem conclusive that the brain itself is involved even before the symptoms begin.

And what about this so-called brain? It is the most complicated structure in the universe known to us. For that matter, even the brain of an insect is remarkably complicated, keeping its bearer alive and capable of a huge variety of complex responses. The brain of a fly has 90,000 neurons and millions of connections creating "neural nets." Futurists propose that perhaps as computer science progresses, as it is rapidly doing now, the speculation is that in the near future, as two objects approach you or interact with you on the street, one a human stranger and one a robotic facsimile, you will not be able to tell the difference! Pardon the pun, what about the biologic fact that living organisms change "on the fly," pressured by the environment as well as by internal pressures that we call evolution, operating through genetic changes and then natural selection? Will such incredibly advanced robotic facsimiles be able to do the same? In other words, will their "artificial neural nets" be as plastic as our "biological neural nets?" (neural nets are circuits between individual neurons with messages transmitted by electrical and chemical signals and with novel properties not apparent with individual neurons). There is already evidence that they have the capability of learning by themselves, rather than relying on programming alone. Given the fact that the appearance of solidity is a mirage, the brain and the trillions of neural nets contained within, with their axons and dendrites extending over vast open spaces, the "dark matter" of the brain, are likely communicating via electromagnetic and even gravitational forces. Will the same hold true for the artificial neural nets? If so, the debate could then begin as to whether or not we, as a living species, had created a new (living?) species.

Getting back to migraine, it has the major hallmarks of a neurologic event. It is a very common disorder, especially in women, and may affect up to 25% of people at some time during their lives. As is true with all biologic phenomena, there is a continuum of expression. Fortunately, only a small percentage of people have episodes which render them frequently helpless. Although there are infrequent painless varieties of migraine, the pain is usually described as severe. Recall that severe pain is defined as that which interrupts all normal functioning. In other words, the person may not be able to function and may be found lying quietly in a darkened room for up to seventy-two hours, trying to drink enough and avoid vomiting to stay hydrated, thus avoiding a trip to the emergency room (ER). A typical migraine is a one-sided, severe, pounding headache, associated with nausea, light and/or sound, sensitivity, with aggravation by movement. This is the only form of common headache which tends to be severe. Fortunately, there are a variety of medications available which are successful in quickly eliminating the pain within a period of up to four hours. Although even simple anti-inflammatories and OTC analgesics may be helpful, "triptans" which are prescription drugs, are likely to be the most successful. For individuals having on average of two or more per week, there are other types of medications which, if taken regularly, can reduce the frequency quite dramatically. Keeping a detailed log of activities, diet, and stress level may help one identify recurring triggers.

People with migraine may have a variety of triggers which may be specific for them. If found and avoided, this preventative approach can be very valuable.

The last two common forms of headache can be looked upon as hybrid or crossover forms. The first is "mixed" and can be dispensed with quickly. It represents a combination of any two or all three headache types. The problem is obvious. It may be difficult to tease out one from the other, including which one is likely to be the underlying causative one, with the others being secondary.

Lastly, the "rebound" variety may be the worst of all, in many respects. There are other names for this entity, including "transformed migraine" or "chronic daily headache." The final moniker is very descriptive. This syndrome is thought to be induced by medication used to treat other forms of headache and especially migraine. The common sequence is that with migraine which is severe and intimidating, sometimes, because of the fear factor, with the knowledge that migraine treatment is most effective when initiated early, the person will medicate for a head pain which is mild and is not necessarily representative of an emerging migraine. They may use either prescription medication or over-the-counter medication. Soon, they are medicating every two to three days, and a peculiar circumstance intervenes, whereby with waning of the medication effect, head pain resumes. Eventually, they are medicating daily, multiple times per day, each time obtaining a few hours of relief before the head pain escalates again. At this point, they have CDH and are held prisoners by it. It may be difficult to identify and may take skillful historical sleuthing by your doctor to identify. Once he or she thinks they have identified this (there is no definitive diagnostic study), the treatment of it is very difficult. In essence, the patient must be withdrawn from *all* pain medicines, including prescription and over-the-counter drugs, and go through a period of markedly increased headache, which could go on for several weeks. It takes a great deal of resolve, by both patient and doctor. It may have to be done "formally" in a drug rehabilitation facility. As is always the case, prevention is the best treatment. If you find yourself medicating for headache three or more times per week, you may be on the threshold of rebound and should consult your doctor.

Incidentally, recent evidence has linked vitamin D deficiency with migraine. Many, if not most, people in the far northern (or southern) hemispheres are seasonably low in vitamin D, which is normally made in the skin, activated by sunlight (never say never and never say always...sunlight can be good). Blood levels can be checked and, if low, supplementation should be undertaken with or without migraine. If you wish to skip the $300 blood test, almost everyone will get into the normal range with supplementation of 4,000 units per day, justifying the use of this therapeutic trial.

Magnesium deficiency and any B vitamin deficiency can predispose one to migraine. Using supplemental magnesium 750 mg per day and/or vitamin B complex may improve a migraine syndrome. Also, coenzyme Q_{10}, 50 to 100 mg per day can do the same.

Now wait a minute! Aren't doctors all about drama, like saving lives, leaping over tall buildings in a single bound, and other such jaw-dropping feats? What about things that can kill you, like brain tumors, blood clots on the brain, aneurysms, and such? (An aneurysm is a weakening of the wall of an artery, such that it thins out as a bulge develops and can rupture, causing major hemorrhage.) Aren't there aneurysms in the brain which can be quickly lethal? The truth is that all of these potentially lethal conditions do exist and can present with headache. Each one tends to have its own signature, but there is a good deal of overlap with the abovementioned common conditions. Certainly, doctors are aware of these serious problems, and in certain circumstances, with a particular clinical picture, they may require some investigation. For instance, subdural hematoma is a relatively common condition, especially in older people, especially older people who fall down, and especially in older people who fall down and whack their heads. In that setting, there can be bleeding on the inside of the skull, which accumulates and can cause symptoms days to weeks later. The condition is easily diagnosed using a CAT or CT (computed axial tomography) scan of the head and can fairly easily be treated, if needed, by draining the collection of blood. Brain tumors, benign and malignant, as well as aneurysms occur randomly and are definitely problematic. Fortunately, they are relatively rare. More about these conditions later.

Head Trauma and Headache

Consciousness, a state of self-perception and awareness, appears to be an epiphenomenon of brains. Epiphenomenon is a term meaning that once the brain (or any system) is in place and is fully operational, the epiphenomena represents a range of states or secondary features that occur naturally as by-products from the system under question, but not from the individual components of the system. Concussion is a term used to describe a loss of consciousness secondary to trauma. We tend to downplay the serious nature of this phenomenon. Recall how anxious one might feel when the lights and heat shut down in a storm. After all, there exists a complicated "grid" which is supposed to prevent this lights-out phenomenon. The next fear-generated question is, "Will it be ten seconds or ten days?" Similarly, wakeful consciousness is so intrinsic to a normally functioning brain that the light of consciousness snuffed out represents a major insult, even if it lasts for a very short time. Repetitive injuries like that are associated with the possible emergence of a variety of neurologic syndromes, even many years later. There is even a considerable amount of evidence that using the head to redirect the ball in soccer, called "heading," can result in an identifiable brain dysfunction. At question is how much of a chance does any one individual wish to take that might jeopardize the functioning of the most complex structure in the universe—the brain which is contained in your body.

Trauma, from either one event or repetitive events, can cause headache and may be a diagnostic consideration, depending on circumstances.

Ears

Somewhat simplistically, the "ear" is medically divided into three regions, namely the external ear, middle ear, and internal ear. Although separated by approximately only three to four centimeters, the transition is as great a difference in the landscape as between the Canadian–Montana border and the Arizona–Mexico border in January. In essence, the outer ear, with its signature ridge and grooves and its dangling "lobule," which has made the wearing of earrings so convenient, with its cartilaginous superstructure, covered with typical skin and ever-helpful hair covering the entrance to the canal, conveniently placed to keep out insects and other such unwanted creatures, is really not morphologically much different than other areas of the body's surface. However, the landscape changes rapidly. The external ear includes the canal leading to the ear drum, signifying the arrival at the middle ear. The drum itself is a thin membrane drawn taught across the end of the canal, as would an animal skin be drawn across a drum frame.

At this point, deep in the skull, surrounded by heavy bone, it is apparent that we have come upon something both fragile and treasured by the organism. This cave-like space is again divided—except for the tiny, round window—into two separate chambers. The smaller

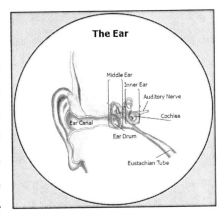

of the two is the middle ear, approximately 1.2 cm by 2.0 cm in dimension, containing interconnected bones. Toward the outside, the malleus touches the drum. Toward the inside lies the stapes, with its "foot" in the round window. In between is the incus. The drum and the three bones do what a drum is supposed to do, particularly when connected to a solid substance, which is to greatly amplify the sound waves arriving at the drum. The round window signifies the arrival at the inner ear containing two adjacent structures squeezed into dense bone, connected to each other, with markedly different functions. They are the semicircular canals, concerned with balance and orientation of the body in space, and the cochlea, concerned with hearing. Just as with the eye, where the retina is considered to be a protrusion of the brain, converting light energy into electrical energy for transport to the cortical brain, the organ of Corti, delicately placed within the cochlea converts the mechanical energy of sound waves into electrical energy to be transported into a different area of the cortical brain. The complexity and fragility of this so-called labyrinth is breathtaking. An appreciation of this both stuns us with the fact that it actually works and forewarns us of the likelihood of dysfunction ahead. So, we now switch from anatomic description to clinical function and dysfunction.

The external ear, being mostly skin and cartilage, is relatively resistant to major damage. Skin cancers are prone to occur at the very top of the ear where the sun's rays strike most directly. The skin in the external canal does produce a different type of secretion with a waxy character, designed to trap foreign objects. The canal itself varies in people from relatively straight and wide to somewhat narrow and bent. Some people produce an abundance of wax and some produce almost none. So, it is easy to understand that a buildup of wax, called cerumen, can repeatedly occur in some people. Q-tips, when used in the ear to remove wax, have been likened to the devil's handiwork. More often than not, the result of such use is to push the wax deeper, and even to pack it against the drum, creating a so-called cerumen impaction. This can also occur spontaneously. A puncture of the drum is a major calamity, requiring surgical correction and possibly resulting in permanent damage. Wax packed in against the drum effectively limits the vibration of the drum, thus hearing quickly drops off. At this point, a visit to your PCP, and possibly a referral to an ear, nose, and throat (ENT) specialist, is needed. The best way to keep the canal clear, in those who are wax producers, is to gently irrigate with body-temperature water or saline, perhaps while in the shower. There are commercial devices available to facilitate this. Your doctor can give instructions, if needed (in the office, but not in the shower). The irrigating substance should be body temperature, that is, noticeably warmer than your finger tips or checked with a thermometer, so as not to induce vertigo.

As we move back into the middle ear, there is one crucial structure which I did not mention above. This is the Eustachian tube, which is a relatively long but very narrow caliber duct connecting the middle ear with the back of the throat. This is designed to allow fluid to drain out of the middle ear and to keep it at atmospheric pressure so that the vibratory function can be best facilitated. However, because of its anatomic configuration, the Eustachian tube is prone to close off, such as with allergies and common infections, like colds. A good part of the pharmaceutical industries' production of anti-histamines and decongestants, the backbone of cold, sinus, and allergy medications, is designed to keep that little bugger and others like it open. If it stays closed, it is almost invariable that hearing will be reduced, dizziness may occur, and infection may supervene. Note that since the mouth, nose, and throat always have their complement of bacteria called "normal respiratory flora," infection in these areas with an obstructed Eustachian tube can lead to an infection in the middle ear called "otitis media," which can be very painful.

An inner ear dysfunction mostly reflects a dysfunction of the twin structures in it, constituting the cochlea and the labyrinth and accounting for our ability to both hear and balance ourselves. Hearing loss is obviously very common, seen most commonly in older people, and is termed presbycusis. There are many potential factors contributing to this, ranging from common to rare.

As has been alluded to, imbalance can be associated with inner ear problems. Sometimes this is described as "dizziness." Sometimes it is called "vertigo." You will need to try to avoid terminology when presenting this to your doctor. These types of feelings are imprecise. The worst term is to describe it as making you feel "sick" because "sick" can mean ANYTHING. If the sensation is associated with a feeling that you could vomit, the proper term would be nausea. Your doctor obviously has to be skillful enough to tease this information from you. Your role is to try to describe the feelings, unless it is a clearly identifiable one like nausea.

Most often, these ill-defined feelings of poor balance, imbalance, unsteadiness, light-headed, faintness, nausea, vertigo (sensation of spinning or movement), and who knows how many other terms, stem from ear issues. A smaller number can be much more serious involving tumors or vascular abnormalities of the ear or brain. I don't want to divulge the secrets of how to know which is which, because then you will demand your MD degree. It can be difficult, but there are often historical clues which are very suggestive of one or the other. There may or may not be physical findings characteristic or not characteristic of such. Everybody with "dizziness" or "light-headedness" does not need a CT scan or an MRI of the brain, but some do.

Regarding hearing loss, age itself, is the most common factor, this in turn possibly representing cumulative damage occurring over many years. We live in an incredibly noisy world. Most of the very noisy things to which we are frequently exposed, have come on the scene in the last fifty years. It is something that we take for granted, and therefore accept as "normal," which in turn may cause us to neglect the use of precautions against excessive noise. Loud music is everywhere. The pounding of rap music may announce the approach of a rapper in a car, a block away, despite rolled-up windows. The noise in that vehicle is intense. Since such behavior is carried on mostly by young people who still consider themselves to be indomitable and immortal, what this means is that they are setting the stage to be deaf for a very long time. Motorized garden tools are widely used and easily loud enough to cause damage to middle and inner ear structures. The same is true for household tools and even appliances like vacuum cleaners and hair dryers. Standing near (or sitting within) a diesel-powered truck can do the same. Even casually walking by a construction site makes us aware about how much noise those workers endure. Factories, flight patterns from airports, and many other exposures all contribute to hearing loss. There are also strong genetic factors, which may inordinately place some individuals at risk, even at much lesser noise levels. The solution is obviously awareness of the danger, and application of the best noise protective devices available. The latest danger to hearing loss from noise is reported to be the din, constantly heard on the Big Island in Hawaii from an invasion of Puerto Rican frogs! What next?

Other common causes of hearing loss may be much easier to deal with, such as wax impaction or middle ear infection or fluid accumulation. Some of these are amenable to home treatment with OTC medications, and some may require your doctor's help. There are many less common conditions which will definitely require professional help.

Tinnitus, or noise in the ear not generated from the environment is very common. Although it can be demonstrated in people with normal hearing, it is much more commonly seen in the setting of hearing loss. The tinnitus itself may have the same wave frequency as the wave frequency of the hearing loss (hearing loss is usually selective, rather than across the entire spectrum of wave lengths), suggesting that the brain may be involved through sensitization of those neurons involved, and involving neural feedback loops. The mechanisms of tinnitus are complex and difficult to study experimentally, and many questions regarding cause and mechanism are still not clear. For most people, it is only a minor annoyance. For a minority, it can become an overwhelming intrusion, producing a great deal of psychic distress. Once again, the best treatment is prevention of hearing loss.

There are many medications which are potentially toxic to the ears, including some very common ones like diuretics and antibiotics. Even aspirin or anti-inflammatories like ibuprofen used in excess in susceptible people can cause hearing loss and/or tinnitus. Much less frequently, there are a number of non-otologic conditions such as TMJ problems and muscle tension disorders in the head or neck which are causative.

For these people seriously distressed by tinnitus, several types of medications may be helpful, including benzodiazepines (Valium, and associated drugs) or tricyclic antidepressants. Ginkgo biloba may be helpful. For the most distressed, there are a wide variety of surgical and non-surgical therapies, with varying success rates.

Neck

Necks vary remarkably through the animal kingdom. Many species have no identifiable neck at all, with the thorax, containing the circulatory and breathing apparatus, seeming to merge directly with the head. Some species have dramatic neck expressions, and in others, the expression is intermediate. The latter appears to be true for humans. Conceptually, the neck is not much more than a conduit between the head and the rest of the body, providing an avenue for blood and nerve flow to and from the head, and for the passage of food into the intestinal tract. There are few structures tacked on, which will be discussed as well.

Many people when hearing the term "neck" think of the back of the neck first, perhaps because pain in that area is so common. Indeed neck pain is common, with three different issues contributing to this. Firstly, the neck obviously needs to support the weight of the head, which is between ten and fifteen pounds, depending on the size of the person. Although most of that weight is born by the spinal column, because of the need for rotational capabilities, the so-called "strap muscles" of the neck share considerably in supporting the head, depending on the activities involved. These muscles are vulnerable to injury, consisting of strains and tears (to be discussed later).

Secondly, the large nerves which supply the arms, emanate from the spinal cord in the neck, coalesce into the so-called "brachial plexus" in the space above the collar bone, and then divide again into the three major nerves that run into the arm. As these nerve roots exit the spinal cord to join and then separate again, there a number of tight squeezes, where they can be trapped by discs, bones, muscles, or a combination of these, such that the most common symptom would be pain. Thirdly, in addition, wear and tear of the joint spaces between the neck vertebrae can result in development of an arthritic condition in the neck, which also can be painful.

Obviously, there are numerous potential pain generators in the neck, so that neck pain is a very common clinical finding. Evaluation of neck pain, just as with any other body area can be difficult. This is especially true with the body area that involves the spine and its supporting structures. The spine is yielding its secrets to modern medicine very reluctantly. Despite the arrival of stupendous imaging modalities, we still often cannot be sure what is generating pain, in the region of the spine. Inadequate diagnosis leads to inadequate treatment, but that is the state-of-the-art regarding spinal issues in 2012.

Incidentally, we used to mention "X-rays." Although X-rays are still widely utilized, including those of the spine, there are now other major ways of obtaining anatomic pictures without breaking the skin. This includes several types of nuclear studies, ultrasound, CAT (or CT) scanning and MRI (magnetic resonance imaging... previously called nuclear magnetic resonance). Thus the term "imaging studies."

In 1969, I attended a medical convention in Denver, whereby one of the topics was "Nuclear Magnetic Resonance," described as a new concept. It sounded bizarre, if not alien. The discussants fantasized as to whether or not it would ever find a home in clinical medicine. Obviously, it has far outpaced any speculation we might have had. The physicists and engineers, the true heroes of medicine, have given us tools whereby we are now able to see things, and make diagnoses that would absolutely not be made with surgery, or even with a detailed autopsy prior to these new imaging modalities. Nevertheless, the secrets of the spine are still often hidden, even with exquisitely clear pictures.

Radiculopathy and Referred Pain

This is a good time to bring to attention an important consideration, that being the concept of "radiculopathy." As mentioned above, the nerves entering the arms originate in the spinal cord, in the neck. They terminate in the fingertips. These nerves are similar to a continuous wire, able to conduct an electrical current. Therefore, a lesion in the neck could result in a pain in the fingertip! If it causes pain in a characteristic distribution through the arm to that particular finger tip, the proper diagnosis, in this case the source of the pain would be facilitated. However, if the pain is discontinuous, such that the only pain is in the finger, that would clearly present a major diagnostic challenge. This type of pain, both potentially helpful and harmful in terms of making a diagnosis has been called "referred pain." What this ambiguous term was meant to imply, I think, is that the source of the pain is referred to an area far removed from the actual site where the pain is generated. In this example, there is nothing wrong with the fingertip. The "wrong" is in the spine in the neck.

So, radiculopathy refers to any condition involving nerves, which can travel long distances, and cause symptoms in an area far removed from the source of the pain. This has two other fascinating sidelights. First of all, there is one instance, where in fact, maybe there is something wrong with the finger. Recall shingles. The herpes zoster virus migrates out of the spinal canal and down a nerve. If the painful finger eventually displays a number of ulcerated blisters, that finger pain could have been the first symptom of shingles. Shingles, with its migrating virus can literally occur anywhere on the body surface. In the second scenario, there is nothing wrong with the finger. However, given a set of circumstances, the doctor might ask for an electrocardiograph (EKG), which then demonstrates that the person is in the midst of a heart attack. How could this be? The nerves from the finger, and the nerves from the heart muscle in that person, may enter the spinal cord and ascend toward the brain so closely together that electrical activity generated from the heart muscle nerve could "spill over" onto the adjacent finger nerve, so that the pain is felt in the finger rather than the chest. This is why people with heart problems may experience arm pain, or jaw pain, or neck pain, with or without chest pain. It all has to do with where these nerves come together in the spinal canal of this particular person. This mechanism also explains why pneumonia at the bottom of the right lung can be felt on the right side of the neck; or why many serious conditions in the abdomen, if they touch the diaphragm, can be felt in the chest or neck. Viola! You can now step up to the podium and receive your "MD" degree.

Wry Neck, Torticollis, and Cervical Dystonia

Recall that the emphasis on these pages is to discuss common issues. Cervical dystonia and torticollis are tongue-twisting medical terms, which can be "congenital" (born with it) or "acquired" (not bought, but occurring during the life of the person). There may be listed hundreds or thousands of causes, with almost as many potential treatment modalities, including the use of botox (an amalgam of botulinum toxin, the cause of a potentially fatal infection caused by a bacterium which is in the same family as the one that that can cause tetanus). Instead, I wish to mention briefly a common and interesting condition that I prefer to call wry neck. In reality, the wry necks are a species of bird, similar to woodpeckers, with the ability to turn their head almost 180 degrees, allowing them to look backwards, and intimidate potential predators trying to sneak up on them.

This remarkable neck turning ability is exactly the opposite of what happens in the setting of clinical wry neck, a blue-collar condition present in everyday life. It is characterized by a painful stiffness of the neck, which usually causes the head to be partially turned to one side or the other. Movement of the head is limited by pain, particularly severe when trying to move away from the pain. Tightness of the neck muscles can usually be felt on the side to which the heard is turned. The most typical presentation is that the victim awakens in the morning with this condition, thinking, "I must have slept on it the wrong way." After several days of marked discomfort, frustration over multiple inquiries from others as to what might be wrong, and the added difficulty of not feeling completely competent driving a car, as well as an increasing feeling of worry, you may appear at the doctor's office. The cause of the strange malady is not known with certainty. Some have felt it to be a focal muscle infection. In some people, it may be partially related to an arthritic condition in the neck. The good news is that it almost always spontaneously remits within a week. It may recur at infrequent intervals. During the misery, the pain can be alleviated by a soft neck collar bought in the pharmacy, acting to stabilize the head and limit movement, particularly at night. Heat and gentle massage may help. Hopefully, during this difficult period, you will not feel the need to turn your head 180 degrees to intimidate anything.

The Vascular Lymphatic System

The neck contains a plethora of lymph glands, which are easily accessible to palpation. "Lymph nodes," as they are medically termed, in fact are found all over the body, including those within the chest, abdominal, and pelvic cavities, all obviously inaccessible to palpation but discernable with various imaging techniques. The bulk of the lymphatic system is made up of the lymph glands and the vast array of lymphatic channels connecting them. However, the thymus gland in the chest, the spleen in the abdomen, and specialized lymphatic structures in the abdomen are also part of the system. Even the bone marrow, mostly associated with the production of red blood cells which carry oxygen, and a particular type of white blood cell which is designed to control acute infections, also produces some lymphatic white blood cells. So, this is a very expansive system, involving almost all areas of the body.

The arterial system carries nutrients and oxygen in blood away from the heart, supplying it to all body tissues. The venous system transports oxygen- and nutrient-depleted blood back to the heart. The interface at which these two meet, after the arteries divide multiple times, becoming progressively smaller, is in the capillary phase of the circulation. Capillaries are microscopic structures which permeate body tissues, coming into close contact with cellular elements. Fluid on the arterial side of the capillary is pushed out of the capillary and becomes tissue fluid. Oxygen, carried by the red blood cell and hooked to iron, also breaks away from the cell and diffuses into this tissue fluid which bathes all of the cells. The cells take up oxygen and whatever nutrients they need, and release carbon dioxide and whatever "waste" they do not need into this tissue fluid. This fluid is not static but is moving at microscopic speed, similar to how the water in the Everglades is constantly moving south. By the time this fluid reaches the venous side of the capillary network, most of it is reabsorbed, or pushed, into the venous capillaries by the ever so slightly higher pressure in that portion of the tissue fluid than what is present in the venous capillary. Thus, begins its long journey back to the heart.

Interestingly from the developmental or evolutionary standpoint, approximately 15% of the tissue fluid which leaked out on the arterial side of the capillary is not pushed back in on the venous side. This curious arrangement gives a good excuse for development of a backup system to quickly drain that last 15% of tissue fluid. To the rescue, preserving our delicately balanced extracellular milieu and preventing us from all looking like waterlogged beach balls, thus greatly complicating many of our everyday activities, comes the lymphatic system. At the tissue or cellular level, lymphatic vessels have very low pressure, and with walls, only one cell thick, they are the sump pump of the vascular system, sucking up the last of the tissue juices and heading back toward the heart. The road to the heart, or perhaps one should say the canal to the heart, is a circuitous one. As the lymph vessels head away from the tissue spaces, transporting their cargo of fluid and traces of other valuable items, they merge with each other and develop thicker walls, and even valves, like their cousins the veins. Valves in the circulatory system do the same thing that valves in your home plumbing system do—that is to regulate the flow of liquid and prevent it from going backward.

With lymph channels, however, every now and then, the pathway is partially blocked by a larger dam, which in this case is a lymph node. The lymph node is a structure with two assignments. First, it provides a home for the white blood cells called lymphocytes. These are crucial to normal immune function, by dealing with many types of somewhat more chronic or low-grade infections and also with cancer. There are three major subtypes of lymphocytes. When you hear the name of the first type, you will likely sleep soundly tonight as you recognize their assignment. As you sleep, these "natural killer cells" (NK cells) are killing viruses and cancer cells that made the mistake of entering this lymph node with the flow of lymph. They have the ability to recognize the surface proteins of these unwanted invaders and kill them. Also present in the lymph node are so-called T and B lymphocytes, responsible for a different type of warfare, using a similar recognition of non-self technique. They are so thorough that they leave a legacy of memory cells which are passed on for many generations, spanning our lifetimes. In other words, once we have had that particular infection with that particular germ and should that germ shows up again in the future, the army to dispatch it is already in place. This same kind of process is what is at the basis of whatever immunizations we might receive.

There are many such lymph nodes along the way back to the heart. The lymphatic channels empty into venous channels along the way. At that juncture, there are no further lymph nodes back to the heart. But fear not. Recall that the spleen is a relatively huge component of the lymphatic system, with the liver as a similar component. Blood pumped out by the heart (at least some of it) will have to traverse these two organs via their arterial supply, and the invaders will again have to deal with the same cellular elements that are present in the lymph nodes.

Cancer

Is anybody still awake? Since we wandered off into the lymphatic system, it must be apparent to anyone who stops to look a little more closely that our bodies exist in a continuous, somewhat precarious state of balance. The complexity and beauty of these anatomic and physiologic arrangements, with clever solutions found at every corner, are miraculous. Nowhere are these clever solutions more important than when some of the trillions of cells which constitute our physical being are wandering off course, isolating themselves, not paying any attention to the blueprint, having seceded from the union, with only their own benefit in mind. These are cancer cells. However, through the incredible complexity and beauty of evolution, and perhaps with some type of divine guiding hand, we have backup systems, and backup systems for the backup systems, to deal with these traitors. They were us. They changed their DNA, and they are no longer us, and the battle is on. If we indulge in self-destructive behavior, a list of which could fill many pages, we tip the scales in favor of the invaders. We know what destructive behaviors are, for the most part. But stress may be the worst of all. Negativity and dysthymia, and fighting with our fellow travelers, all push the advantage toward the team with the new DNA.

Back to the neck and its lymph nodes. Pain and or swelling of these glands may occur in relatively simple infections such as viral or bacterial upper respiratory infections. This is the lymphatic system doing what it is supposed to do—trapping and dispatching invaders. Those lymph nodes have a characteristic "feel" on examination. Lymph nodes from much more serious infections, or from cancer, usually have an entirely different appearance and feel. Examination of the neck lymph nodes should be a part of any routine physical exam. The two other body surfaces that allow for a direct exam of large numbers of lymph nodes are the inguinal regions (groins) and the axillary regions (arm pits). The latter are often very important during evaluation of breast cancer, as they represent the major drainage areas of the breasts.

"Glands"

The last thing to be mentioned in the neck is the thyroid, or thyroid gland. As can be surmised, the term "gland" in medicine carries an ill-defined implication. We have dealt with sweat glands, oil glands, and lymph glands. Yet to come are thyroid, pituitary, and adrenal glands. There is a pineal gland in the head. Many people consider their pancreas and ovaries or testes to be glands, but they are not by convention so-called. Then, there is the prostate gland, and meibomian glands, Cowper's gland, and other glands. In the purest sense, a gland is simply a tissue which secretes something, whether it is a hormone which has effects all over the body or a substance which lubricates one tiny area. "Endocrine glands" is an umbrella term for tissues which produce hormones. Overly simply put, hormones are chemical messengers released into the circulation which affect the functioning of cells at a distant site.

Back to the thyroid. Its neighbor, incidentally, is the parathyroid gland(s). The parathyroids lie directly under the thyroid gland and are intimately related with calcium metabolism. Calcium is in fact the most abundant mineral in the body, primarily stored in bones, with elemental calcium weighing up to three pounds. Calcium metabolism is crucial for proper nerve and muscle function all over the body, and for a large variety of other crucial issues, including bone metabolism. Alteration in calcium homeostasis in conjunction with bone disease can result in major mental changes, stomach ulcerations, kidney stones, and acidosis. Extreme deviations of calcium metabolism, either low or high, can be fatal.

Parathyroid Glands

However, in keeping with the established format, diseases of the parathyroid glands are uncommon or uncommonly demand attention. The parathyroid glands, of which there are a variable number, but usually four, can be involved with benign or malignant tumors.

Even the benign tumors can be very important, as they are usually metabolically active and can seriously disrupt calcium metabolism. The most common problem with the parathyroid, attesting to the fact that they infrequently cause clinical problems on their own, is their surgical removal, done inadvertently if and when the thyroid is removed.

Thyroid (gland)

In contrast to its shy sibling, the thyroid takes front and center stage in the neck. The thyroid, under the strong influence of the pituitary gland located at the base of the brain, which in turn is poetically referred to as the "master gland," secretes two hormones into the circulation. The first is called calcitonin and is not under the influence of the pituitary. It is part of the built-in backup systems that are so commonly found, in this case, regulating calcium metabolism. It functions as the mirror opposite of parathyroid hormone, both acting on bone. Parathyroid hormone causes a release of calcium from bone, whereas calcitonin inhibits such release. There is one fairly rare form of thyroid cancer which can produce large amounts of calcitonin. So, that is it for calcitonin.

Hypothalamic Releasing Hormones

The major hormone produced by the thyroid goes by a number of different names, but here, let 's call it simply thyroid hormone. This hormone is significantly under the effect of the pituitary, by the pituitary's release of a different hormone, whose name most of you have heard in passing but perhaps have not focused on. The pituitary hormone is logically called thyroid stimulating hormone or "TSH." TSH is the term that you may have heard, as it is the test which is considered by most thyroid specialists to be the most important in assessing the overall status of your thyroid. More about on this debate soon. Wait! It's not over yet! The pituitary in fact is not the "master gland" but just an imposter. The true master gland of the body will now stand up (drum roll)... the *brain*. So now, the situation has suddenly become much more interesting! The hypothalamus, which is definitely part of the brain and in fact of the limbic system (to be discussed later), involved with emotions and feelings and urges, sits just above the pituitary and is connected to it through a circulatory system. The hypothalamus sends and receives neural impulses from all over the brain and then decides how much of these stimulating hormones, involving thyroid, adrenal, and sex glands, will be released directly into the pituitary, in turn telling the pituitary what to do. So, as shocking as this may seem, your brain controls hormone release, which travels to every cell in your body, controlling metabolism, stress reactions, and your gonadal function. So, if anyone asks whether your brain is connected to your gonads, the answer is a resounding yes!

Hyperthyroidism and Hypothyroidism

Back to the thyroid and its hormone, whose overall influence on cellular development and function, protein synthesis, and basic metabolic activity is vast. The thyroid hormone is simplistically compared to a thermostat, affecting cellular metabolism and thus heat production. Obviously, things are much more complex, but at least, this gives a working model. The two major disease states associated with the thyroid are called hypothyroidism and hyperthyroidism. Recall that "hypo" means low or less and "hyper" means more or greater. Hyperthyroidism, or simplistically put as "over-activity" of the thyroid gland, is an unusual clinical problem.

Recall that "clinical" means "in the real world" or "practical." Likely, there are transient states of hyperthyroidism, which come and go, perhaps in conjunction with other illnesses. Regardless, sustained hyperthyroidism is uncommon. Most cases are mild and could go undetected for a long time. Rarely, the onset may be precipitous and severe, causing what is clinically termed "thyroid storm," which can be life threatening. The word "storm" is generally used to describe an image of nature which is turbulent, active, and unpredictable. That may be the picture of a person with thyroid storm, tormented, as if they had just gulped down ten cups of the strongest espresso. Fortunately, this presentation is rare. Mild hyperthyroidism clinically can be subtle and challenging and, obviously, can merge into "normal" behavior. People with this condition tend to be "hyper." They may have a tremor. They may have palpitations (pounding of the heart—fast, strong, or both). They may have insomnia. Recall the high caffeine analogy. They may have increased appetite, but lose weight. Diarrhea, menstrual irregularities, anxiety, and many other symptoms may be manifest. The challenge in diagnosis is when the person has only a very small part of this syndrome. The diagnosis can be confirmed relatively easily with simple blood tests. Once again, this is a relatively uncommon condition.

On the other hand, hypothyroidism, or underactive thyroid, is more common and may or may not be much more common. I will explain shortly. Again, in its most severe form, the diagnosis could be presumed to be present once medical history and exam are completed, to be confirmed by the blood test. Think of the opposite of hyperthyroidism. In the extreme version, the person is very lethargic. They move little. They are mentally dull. They may eat little, but gain weight. Skin is thick and dry. Speech is thick. Constipation may be severe. It is almost as if the person is heavily sedated. This extreme version is rarely seen.

Hypothyroidism—"Real" versus "Subclinical" versus?

Now for the very big topic (drum roll)… "everyday" hypothyroidism, or underactive thyroid, mild to moderate in presentation. I keep hinting that there may be more, or less, to hypothyroidism than is widely appreciated. There is also an undercurrent of what has been called "subclinical hypothyroidism." This term is felt to be bogus by many if not most experts in the field, depending on the definition. Yet, the diagnosis of hypothyroidism runs rampant. I will try to explain some of the controversies surrounding this topic. The question boils down to what constitutes diminished thyroid function and how common it is.

For many years, in my own personal experience (by definition absolutely not "evidence-based" and therefore almost automatically invalid, according to ivory tower gurus), I have noted a phenomenon which puzzled me. I very frequently do blood tests to check for hypothyroidism, and I rarely find conclusive blood tests to confirm this condition. What would those be? First, recall thyroid hormone itself, sometimes called "T4," should be low, indicating a reduced level of hormone. The range of "normal" is suspiciously too broad, running from four to twelve. Obviously twelve is three times higher than four (very few people are three times taller or three times shorter than other people). Once T4 is released from the thyroid, it is converted to "T3" which is the metabolically active form of the hormone. So, T3 should be low. To complete the diagnostic triple play, the pituitary gland should be sensing low thyroid hormone levels and should therefore be working overtime to crank out TSH to get that lazy thyroid going. So, the TSH should be high. Most thyroid experts consider the TSH to be the most sensitive test.

Here comes the rub. Because of this bias, they might be willing to call a normal T3, normal T4, and slightly elevated TSH "hypothyroidism." Some call this "subclinical hypothyroidism." So, they want me to believe that this person, with normal levels of T3 and T4, has underactive thyroid function (?). It is oxymoronic, in my opinion. Check the numbers again in three months or six months, and they will likely be the same. You still have normal thyroid hormone levels, but your thyroid specialist is telling you that you have underactive thyroid function. Despite the fact that I rarely find low T3, low T4, and high TSH, I come across many, many people on thyroid hormone supplement. I would guess that 20% of people over the age of sixty are on thyroid medication. Once on this, you will likely never get off of it. Why? Because you have been on it for thirty years, and your thyroid is now permanently asleep, so they say.

Subsequently, there have been research studies published that indicate thyroid function does, or at least the "numbers" which have been decided reflect this, vary spontaneously quite commonly. In addition, these researchers are now suggesting that it is acceptable to allow TSH to remain mildly elevated, without any definitive evidence that this is deleterious. Therefore, it seems much more appropriate to recheck thyroid blood tests two or three times over the course of six months before initiating treatment with thyroid medication.

Lastly, what about the person who comes to the doctor's office and says, "I am so tired… I wake up tired… I eat like a bird, and I'm gaining weight… and my hair is falling out… I got on the internet, and I have all of the symptoms of underactive thyroid?" This is the very patient of whom I frequently run a full thyroid panel of blood tests, which I invariably find to be normal. First of all, as already mentioned, hair loss is cyclical, with many potential causes. Secondly, most people who come to doctors' offices are tired all the time, almost always with multiple co-existing reasons for this, with stress, unhappiness, sleep deprivation, and rotten life style habits on top of the list. Thirdly, some birds, like vultures, eat a lot.

This leads us to the second group of people that are thought to have possible "subclinical hypothyroidism." Members of this group, instead of having normal T3, normal T4, and slightly elevated TSH as just discussed, accepted with open arms by thyroid specialists as being candidates for thyroid hormone treatment, have everything normal. This group of people has been of interest much more to naturopathy doctors (ND) than to medical doctors (MDs), but they have been clever enough to come up with a novel way to evaluate the concept. Measuring basal metabolic rate is possible, but very cumbersome and not practical. Since thyroid hormone is known to regulate cellular metabolism, the by-product of which is heat, they have developed an algorithm for measuring early morning underarm body temperature for five consecutive days. Readings below 97.4F are deemed to be highly suggestive of subclinical hypothyroidism and to be worthy of treatment. This diagnostic approach is not accepted by most MDs. On the other hand, it is quite safe to give the begging patient three months of medium dose thyroid hormone and see what happens to the constellation of symptoms. If there is no response, thyroid medicine can then be discontinued and other explanations be sought. As a curious and somewhat humorous sidelight, my name has been placed on a list of world-class thyroid experts and has been listed on the internet. Once or twice each year, I see a self-referred patient with supposed underactive thyroid. I think I was placed on that list because of my willingness to give them short-term thyroid replacement. There is another lab study called a radioactive iodine uptake, which is uncommonly used because of cost and radiation exposure. It appears to be more reliably helpful for overactive rather than underactive thyroid function.

To summarize, hypothyroidism is commonly diagnosed, rightly or wrongly, and huge numbers of people find themselves on thyroid replacement medication. I don't think we know the true incidence of hypo- or hyperthyroidism, and perhaps, these conditions may even have a cyclical character. Hypothyroidism is an infrequent cause of hair loss or weight gain or fatigue. In the early or mild stages of adult-onset diabetes, there may be actually an excessive amount of insulin present, with the problem having something to do with "insulin resistance" or abnormal receptor function at the cellular level. It is speculative as to whether a similar concept could be a factor with thyroid hormone, with the normal levels measured not giving a true picture of what is happening at the thyroid hormone receptor level. Now, that is an interesting concept and, perhaps, that may help clarify the concerns about thyroid hormone levels.

Goiter

There are a few other topics of importance related to thyroid, other than hormone levels per se. "Goiter" is a non-specific term which simply means thyroid enlargement. The most common cause of this is a form of inflammation, called thyroiditis, or Hashimoto's thyroiditis. This is thought to represent an autoimmune reaction. The thyroid may be smoothly and diffusely enlarged, or there may be multiple small nodules and cysts. Occasionally, a cyst or nodule can become large enough to be easily palpable, or even visible, and can raise concern about the possibility of a tumor. Iodine is necessary for the synthesis of thyroid hormone. In some parts of the world where iodine is not available through food sources or iodized salt, lack of circulating thyroid hormone can cause the hypothalamus to produce *thyrotropin*-releasing hormone, which causes the pituitary to release thyroid-stimulating hormone, which then causes the thyroid cells to proliferate endlessly, still unable to produce thyroid hormone with the results being enormous enlargement of the gland. Goiter, whatever the cause, is sometimes treated with thyroid hormone replacement despite normal blood levels, in an attempt to shut off production of TSH and stop progressive enlargement of the gland, including cysts and nodules. Thyroiditis, particularly the autoimmune variety, is very common. It tends to be chronic, but often does not cause much in the way of clinical illness and may be left untreated, as long as the gland is not progressively enlarging and hormone levels are normal.

Lastly, the thyroid can be the seat of both benign and malignant tumors. Although not very common, they are not rare. There are different varieties with divergent prognoses. The finding is that of a nodule, often first detected by the person. No matter what ancillary tests are done, a needle biopsy of the nodule is needed for confirmation. As is usually true for tumors, treatment depends on whether or not it is cancer, and on a variety of other criteria. Prognosis obviously depends on many factors but is usually good.

Our survey of common neck issues is completed.

PART IV
CARDIOVASCULAR AND RESPIRATORY

T he thorax, or thoracic cage, and chest are terms to describe the large space between the base of the neck and the diaphragm. The diaphragm cannot be clearly seen from the outside. It is a thick sheet of muscle circling left to right, and front to back, separating the chest cavity from the abdominal cavity. It lies at approximately the bottom of the breast bone in the front. As it extends sideways and backwards, it tends to drop down further toward the feet, forming a "gutter" most of the way around, with its lowermost portion extending not quite to the bottom of the rib cage.

Despite its large size, there are only two major organs within, those being the heart and the right and left lungs. There are of course many other supporting and ancillary structures, which will be mentioned. Those that can cause common problems will be discussed. There is a built-in hole at the bottom of the diaphragm, allowing blood vessels, nerves, and the esophagus to exit the chest, into the abdomen.

Although it may be difficult to believe, up until the Renaissance, the heart was thought to be the seat of the soul and to be involved with intellect, as well as its known involvement regarding circulation. To a significant degree, diseases of the heart and blood vessels, especially arteries, can be conceptualized as a unit ("cardiovascular"), as there is a good deal of commonality and interaction in terms of disease processes. Likewise, there is a great deal of interaction between the heart and the lungs. Hence the term "cardiorespiratory."

Basic Cardiorespiratory Anatomy

The heart is functionally divided into two sides, namely the right and left sides. Each side is divided into a smaller atrium, or receiving chamber, and a larger ventricle, or pumping chamber. At the exit of each chamber is a valve, making four in all. As noted before, the purpose of a valve is to control flow and, in this case, mostly to prevent backflow. From the standpoint of the circulation, the lungs are interposed between the right and left sides of the heart. Recall that by convention, arteries are defined as channels carrying blood away from the heart while veins are channels conveying blood back to the heart.

So, rather simply, here is how the table is set. Blood returning from all over the body feeds into the inferior vena cava, from below the chest, and the superior vena cava, from the chest and above. These two very large veins feed into the right atrium. The right atrium contracts, opening the tricuspid valve and pushing this blood into the right ventricle. The right ventricle then contracts as the right atrium relaxes, closing the tricuspid valve and opening the pulmonic valve. Blood then enters the pulmonary arteries, left and right, and begins to branch repeatedly, with each branch becoming progressively smaller. Eventually, these tiny and microscopic branches find themselves draped over the alveoli, which are the air sacs. It is here where oxygen diffuses from the alveoli into the blood and where carbon dioxide diffuses from the blood into the alveoli. Carbon dioxide is a product of cellular metabolism, occurring all over the body all the time. It is a potentially toxic metabolite with a tendency to cause acidification of the blood called acidosis. Recall that the other products of cellular metabolism are water and heat which are regulated by endogenous (internal) and exogenous (external) factors. Carbon dioxide absolutely must be eliminated from the body in order to avoid life-threatening acidosis. The only mechanism for release is through the lungs.

The Body's Selfless Hero(ine)

After traversing the alveoli, as capillaries, and having picked up a load of oxygen, blood courses back through progressively larger pulmonary veins until it reaches the left atrium. This chamber then contracts, opening the mitral valve and pushing the blood into the left ventricle. The left ventricle is the workhorse of the heart. One would say that it is the hardest working structure in the entire body. It is called upon to contract relentlessly, pushing blood from the top of your head to the tips of your toes approximately 4,000 times per hour, 100,000 times per day, 37,000,000 times per year, and 3,000,000,000 (three billion) times in your lifetime. Keep this in mind the next time you feel a little irregularity in the rhythm or the next time you are ready to order a cheeseburger, which is one of the most toxic foods available to us.

Basic Cardiac Electrophysiology

As is noted above, there is a sequence of contractions of the four chambers of the heart, opening and closing valves. This is obviously necessary to keep the blood flowing forward, as described, and is controlled by the so-called conduction system of the heart. This is basically a conduit for electrical impulses to carry out the sequence noted above and consists of very specialized cells found nowhere else in the body. These cells have characteristics of both muscle cells and nerve cells. The impulses generated occur spontaneously, although while in the body, the rate and size of the impulses are influenced by the autonomic nervous system and by the circulating hormones. Legendary tales report that during Aztec ceremonies involving human sacrifice, one of the objectives was to remove the still-beating heart from the chest. The Aztecs owed the success of this sacrifice to the gods to this intrinsic conduction system, which will cause the empty heart to beat briefly even when disconnected from the body.

The electrical impulse begins in the so-called sinoatrial node (node means a small protuberance) of the right atrium. The impulse spreads across the atria to the atrioventicular node, between the atria and ventricles, where it is very briefly delayed, allowing the atria to complete their contraction. It is then quickly transmitted down the two adjacent "branches," to the apex or bottom of the left and right ventricles, with smaller branches extending upwards to the top of the ventricles, so that the ventricles cleverly empty from bottom to top. As with all tissues in the body, the conduction system is dependent on a constant blood flow in order to stay viable. In fact, the conducting tissue is metabolically very active and thus is particularly susceptible to low blood flow. Because of this, abnormalities of the conducting system are common.

The conduction system works to maintain a regular cardiac rhythm and to provide a rate appropriate for physiologic needs at any point in time. Rest at night, provided there is no major sleep disturbance, is the period when heart rate is likely to be at its lowest. Rates above fifty beats per minute are unlikely to cause problems. Cardiac function, even with normal coronary circulation, muscle function, and valve function, can be seriously compromised by abnormal rates and rhythms. Abnormal rhythm is termed arrhythmia. Except in a person who is remarkably physically fit and capable of tripling or quadrupling cardiac output (the amount of blood pumped out, usually measured in liters per minute), a heart rate below forty is abnormal. In people with even mild heart disease, below fifty is abnormal. By the time heart rate gets down to thirty or less, most people will have altered consciousness because of inadequate blood flow to the brain and may begin to have shortness of breath, from lungs beginning to fill with fluid. On the other side of the spectrum, physically fit young people can generate a heart rate of 200 beats per minute or slightly more. The maximum heart rate possible drops progressively with aging, such that by age fifty, the maximum predicted would be around 160, and by age ninety, around 120. These predictions are for healthy people, meaning that such individuals could maintain those rates during strenuous activity. People with heart disease would likely develop symptoms at those rates because of intrinsic limitation of cardiac output, with whatever disease they have.

Artificial Cardiac Pacemakers

So, the expected reduction of maximum heart rate is a function of aging of the conduction system, possibly secondary to blood flow reduction and some degree of age-related scarring, both of which could slow conduction. These same processes can be prematurely advanced, causing problems with rate or rhythm which are then no longer considered physiologic (appropriate for the circumstances), but pathologic (signifying a disease process). Very slow heart rates as mentioned above, or periods of marked slowing, represent diseases of the conduction system. If severe enough, these are the circumstances when pacemaker therapy is considered. A cardiac pacemaker basically consists of an energy source, i.e., battery, usually placed under the skin of the upper chest, connected to "pacing wires" which go right to the tip of one or both ventricles. In essence, a blockage or many blockages somewhere in the conduction system has been bypassed so that the ventricles are now directly stimulated at the apex. There are many different types of pacemakers, some even including the atria, but in principle, they are similar. In some cases, it is important to try to include the atria, in that although they are not the main pumping chambers, they may contribute enough to affect cardiac output by as much as 25%. In people with a weak heart from reasons other than poor conduction system issues, this could be very important.

Concepts of Cardiac Output and Ejection Fraction

As can already be surmised, the concepts of cardiac output and ejection fraction are ultimately the final determinant of overall cardiac function. Ejection fraction is a term used often enough in clinical medicine now that a patient coming in to review test results might ask their doctor, "What's my EF now?" (EF, of course, for ejection fraction). The EF is the amount of blood remaining in the left ventricle after it completes its contraction. It is described as a percentage of the total amount of blood in a non-contracted ventricle. For instance, if the resting ventricle contains 70 cubic centimeters (cc) of blood and, at the end of the contraction, there is 30 cc left, 40 cc has been pushed out and EF would be (40 cc/ 70 cc) equal to 57%, a normal result at rest. At rest, anything below 50% is abnormal. By 30%, most people are significantly limited in terms of physical capabilities. By 20%, they would be very fragile and prone to repeated trips to the hospital. Anything below markedly limits life expectancy. In fact, EF below 30% puts people at a much increased risk of life-threatening arrhythmias (irregularities) such that they become a "candidate" for a defibrillator. The concept and technique of defibrillators is similar to pacemakers, except that defibrillators are designed to deliver a strong electrical current, i.e., "shock" to the heart muscle, in an attempt to get it back in rhythm and prevent "sudden death." Sometimes, pacemakers for slow rhythms and defibrillators for fast or ineffective rhythm can be combined into the same device.

EF can usually be estimated at the time of the non-invasive echocardiogram by using sound waves. Cardiac output is a term used less often because it requires invasive studies to get data to estimate. Regardless, cardiac output can be increased in healthy hearts by a great increase in heart rate and by a lesser but important increase in stroke volume, which is a figure based on the same principle as EF. Unfortunately, with diseased hearts, cardiac output may be much more limited and may even be "fixed," meaning not increased at all with activity. Obviously, this can greatly decrease physical capability largely because of shortness of breath and/or weakness at even low levels of physical activity.

Concepts of Cardiomyopathy

Cardiomyopathy is another term frequently used with patients. It basically means diseased or weakened heart muscle. There are many different causes of this, some occurring transiently and some permanently. For instance, a variety of different viruses can attack the heart muscle and severely weaken it. However, if our immune system can get to the viruses fast enough and disable them, the heart muscle can make a complete recovery. There are many other types of infection which can damage the heart. One of the most common causes of cardiomyopathy in South America is caused by a protozoan parasite. Other common factors involved with cardiomyopathy include nutritional, alcoholism, hypertension, and so-called hypertrophic. Uncommonly, common conditions like pregnancy or emotional or physical shock can cause it. There are many rare causes, and a group in which no cause can be found.

By far, the most common cause of cardiomyopathy is atherosclerotic disease of the coronary circulation, which results to the so-called ischemic cardiomyopathy (Ischemia means inadequate blood flow, in this case, to the heart muscle itself). Once this is known, it suddenly becomes apparent that cardiomyopathy is therefore, in most cases, a preventable disease. For the most part, we identify five major factors which are unequivocally associated with arteriosclerosis. Arteriosclerosis is an umbrella term sometimes called "hardening of the arteries," referring to damage in arterial walls. The damage can be expressed in several different way, but all of the different mechanisms funnel into the key point that vascular channels are narrowed, reducing blood flow. Arteriosclerosis implies anywhere and/or everywhere in the body. Other terms like coronary disease or coronary heart disease single out the coronary blood vessels as the site of disease. The tendency is for arteriosclerosis to be present scattered all over the body. However, it can be remarkably and peculiarly focal. The term "a chain is only as strong as its weakest link" applies remarkably well with arteriosclerosis. There can be very severe disease in one area and minimal disease elsewhere. It is not at all uncommon for there to be a "lethal" 95% obstruction of a main coronary artery and almost no blockage anywhere else in the coronary circulation.

Risk Factors for Coronary Disease and Prevention of Such

Of the five major factors negatively affecting arteries, all except for one are strongly under the influence of life style. The five are (1) cigarette smoking, (2) cholesterol levels, (3) blood pressure, (4) diabetes, and (5) genetic or hereditary factors. Perhaps, it might appear that we cannot do anything about heredity. But, even that might not be true because environmental factors are constantly dynamically affecting our genetics. In fact, hereditary factors may be a blessing in disguise, warning us of the need to pay strict attention to all of the other factors and to break the mold of our ancestors that lead them down the path of arteriosclerosis. Never has the concept of "preventive medicine" had more power than in the area of prevention of arteriosclerosis. The formula is easy. Exercise, exercise, exercise, good diet, weight control, no smoking. Those six items represent the foundation of good health. The implementation is apparently difficult, as we look around and appreciate the real world.

So, the coronary circulation, meaning the blood vessels that feed the heart itself, is preeminent regarding health of the heart by nourishing the conduction system and the heart muscle. These tissues allow the heart to function endlessly or, at least, to contract regularly three billion times during the course of your life. The job of the heart is to supply blood, with its load of oxygen and nutrients to every cell in the body. The job of the circulation is to provide open channels to the most remote tissue, and to be flexible enough to contract and dilate at appropriate times to direct decreased or increased amounts of blood to given areas depending on local needs. The circulation which reflects the least fluctuation is the cerebral circulation. Approximately 25% of cardiac output is directed to the head, constituting only 7%

or 8% of body weight and reflecting the high metabolic needs of the brain. This is maintained under a wide variety of circumstances by rapid changes in the resistance in cerebral vessels in order to keep the flow relatively constant. Other circulatory beds, as they are called, can vary enormously under specific circumstances. For instance, the digestive system receives a much increased blood flow with eating and digestion. The skin, which acts as a regulator of body temperature, can have markedly increased or decreased blood flow, depending on the need to dissipate or conserve body heat. There are many other examples of regional alterations in blood flow. All vascular beds depend on clean, open, reactive vessels to be able to function optimally. There is an unspoken or infrequently spoken concept in medicine that a person is as old as their "pipes."

"Interventional" Cardiology

The coronary circulation begins just beyond the aortic valve, in the very first part of the aorta. The aortic valve sits between the outflow tract of the left ventricle and the aorta, which is the largest artery coming directly out of the heart, supplying blood to the entire body through its many branchings. Actually, the opening of the right and left coronary arteries sit right at the juncture of the aortic valve and the aorta. There is substantial variation in people in terms of which coronary artery supplies what. In general, the right coronary artery supplies the right atrium and ventricle, and part of the conducting system. The left main coronary artery quickly divides into the left anterior descending artery, down the front of the heart, and the circumflex artery, supplying most of the back of the heart. So in most people, there are three main coronary arteries, varying considerably in size and with overlapping territories of distribution.

If obstructions are located in the larger arteries and branches and are endangering large amounts of muscle, they are amenable to so-called interventional procedures, such as angioplasty, stenting, and bypass. In smaller vessels, particularly common and problematic with diabetes, these procedures are not utilized. All cases are amenable to treatment of the underlying predisposing conditions. This is obviously especially important with small vessel occlusions, where it becomes the only means of treatment.

Angioplasty entails directing a small catheter into the area of obstruction, with access via the femoral artery in the groin. The catheter has a tiny balloon near its tip. Once placed directly into the obstruction, the balloon can then be inflated, in essence crushing the plaque and debris up against the artery wall. As primitive as this technique may sound, there is little doubt that it has been very helpful for huge numbers of people. A technique which tried to improve long-term results of angioplasty was so-called atherectomy, in which the plaque and debris are carved off the arterial wall and sucked out of the circulation. Nowadays, during the same procedure, whether it is angioplasty or atherectomy, following that part of it, a "stent" can be deployed. This is a tiny metal mesh which springs open when released and is designed to give further support to the newly opened artery. There are several different types of stents, each with its own proponents, and the field is actively changing. The stents, being foreign objects, unfortunately incite an inflammatory response, pulling in additional tissues and with the subsequent tendency to eventually close off the blood vessel again despite the fact that people with stents are given medicine for lifetime use to prevent this very vexing problem.

What does cabbage have to do with heart disease? Simple answer. When an acronym is formed using the first letters of "coronary artery bypass graft," we have CABG, pronounced "cabbage." So when the patient asks his doctor, "Is it time for my next cabbage?" This does not mean that he or she is hungry. With the interventional procedures noted above, being refined "on the run," the need to do bypass has dropped considerably. It is still done under certain circumstances and with particular types of blockages. This is obviously a surgical procedure, involving opening the chest and "harvesting" veins from the legs. It is more risky, much more expensive, and involves hospitalization for three to five days.

Here is another rub, and this is a big one. All of these procedures afford temporary improvement to a life-threatening condition. You would think that you, the patient, would get the message, recalling that coronary arteriosclerosis is a largely preventable condition, i.e., "I need to change the conditions that led to this very serious problem." Too many people view their bodies as they see their cars and other possessions. "If it breaks, we'll fix it… If the arteries plug up again, we'll do another bypass… or another stent… I have the best doctor in my town." This is a dangerous prevailing attitude, i.e., "all I have to do is take my pills," provided they are not forgotten, and all will be OK. Recall the six things that need to change… exercise, exercise, exercise, good diet, weight control, no smoking. Staying well is much more than popping pills. Failure to recognize all of these very expensive procedures as simply "buying time" leads one down the path of oblivion, just like John Doe… more and more complications, and depression, and misery, as function drops off one piece at a time.

All of the interventional procedures described above can and are frequently employed for other parts of the circulation, including kidney arteries, neck arteries, digestive arteries, and leg arteries. The principles are the same in that expensive and dangerous treatments are used to "buy time" for the area of the circulation in question. Pills are handed out. If nothing else changes, the disease likely progresses, with strokes, advancing kidney disease, dialysis, bowel operations, and amputations as consequences of the erroneous and naïve thinking that "there is nothing I can do about it" and "my doctor is the best."

I do not think it is necessary to say much about valvular heart disease. In the past years, when rheumatic fever was very common, valve damage in childhood or young adults might lead to the need for valve replacement in midlife. With the much reduced incidence of rheumatic fever over the past forty to fifty years, presumably because of adequate treatment of strep infection with appropriate antibiotics, valve destruction as a consequence is much less frequently seen. Surgery is still done for a variety of other non-rheumatic valve conditions (including ischemic) but uncommonly in most parts of the industrialized world. Unfortunately, rheumatic fever is still common in underdeveloped countries or countries with large indigent populations.

Aortic valve disease, usually aortic stenosis, is still somewhat common, particularly with elderly people, as a function of aging. Stenosis means that the valve does not open fully. Generally, this is well tolerated in otherwise healthy people, although it can limit exercise capability. However, in people with other types of heart disease as well, aortic stenosis can complicate the situation enough whereby valve replacement would need to be considered.

Mitral Valve Prolapse

Mitral prolapse is a relatively common condition occurring even in young people, being more common in women. Perhaps 5% to 7% of the population has it, although many people are unaware of its presence. The mitral valve separates the left ventricle and left atrium and closes with contraction of the ventricle. If the valve tissue is abnormal in any way, as it closes, it may billow backwards into the atrium. In more severe cases, it may bend backwards far enough to cause a separation of the valve leaflets so that some blood is pushed backwards into the atrium. Although many people have no symptoms, a variety of symptoms may occur and tend to be more prominent with increasing amounts of valve leakage. The symptoms might include "palpitations" (meaning a sensation in the chest, particularly pounding or irregularity). A particular irregularity of some consequence called atrial fibrillation is rarely seen. People with mitral prolapse can have chest pains, usually considered to be "atypical," occurring randomly, and not at all suggestive of coronary blood flow abnormalities. Shortness of breath can be experienced, usually very sporadically and even at rest. Most people do not require treatment, and they are given lots of reassurance. Those that are significantly symptomatic may need treatment to alleviate the symptoms. "Symptomatic treatment" is a term used widely in medicine. The implication is that treatment is given to make a person feel better, rather than because of concern about serious ramifications if treatment is not given. A very few people have valve leakage severe enough to require valve repair or replacement. Interestingly, mitral valve prolapse can sometimes be diagnosed with a stethoscope, right in the doctor's office by noting a particular kind of "click." Ultrasound is the normal means of documentation and assessment of severity.

The Pericardium

The heart and the origins and terminations of the great vessels running into or from it are surrounded by a membrane called the pericardium. Due to its very close anatomic connection to the heart, and the common occurrence of heart disease, the pericardium is often secondarily involved in whatever is the primary heart disease. For instance, a heart attack that involves loss of muscle all the way out to the surface of the heart can cause intense inflammation of the adjacent pericardium, which is a very vascular tissue, and with many pain sensors. Thus, the heart attack could be complicated by a pain syndrome which could make it difficult for the doctors to know if there was a problem with ongoing ischemia which might need treatment. Also, fluid could leak from this area of inflamed pericardium, which could also complicate the picture. A moderate amount of fluid could make the heart look bigger on X-ray and raise question about the adequacy of its function. A large amount of fluid could fill up the whole sac, thus restricting cardiac contractile mobility. This could be very serious, by restricting cardiac filling and pumping, and is called "cardiac tamponade". Fortunately, there are "bedside" findings on examination which can alert the doctor to this, and the fluid can be fairly easily drained with a catheter, placed with ultrasound guidance.

So, when pericardium is damaged, it responds by causing pain or by leaking fluid. The same finding can occur with other conditions such as cardiac injury (contusion) from trauma, such as from a steering wheel or a fall. Also, any time the pericardium is opened, such as with heart surgery, it can cause pain and fluid accumulation. In this example, this could occur days or weeks later, once again causing a possible diagnostic conundrum. Pericarditis, caused by heart attacks or heart surgery, is sometimes called "Dressler's syndrome."

Lastly, the pericardium can become inflamed without any primary heart issue. The most common is a viral infection of the pericardium. This is usually self-limiting but can raise concern about the possibility of heart attack. Most pericardial issues are called "pericarditis."

This could also occasionally be caused by a lung problem, such as pneumonia, or as part of an autoimmune condition.

Atrial Fibrillation

Atrial fibrillation has already been alluded to and is one of the most common of the so-called "arrhythmias" (irregularities of rhythm). The two most common are in fact virtually ubiquitous and thus not even considered abnormal. These are so-called premature atrial contractions and premature ventricular contractions. Some people do not sense or feel these, and they are noted incidentally on exam or EKG. Other people feel every single one. Sometimes, in these people, it can be emotionally disturbing and, if so, may require treatment (once again, "symptomatic treatment"). If innocent, as they usually are, they usually suppress with activity, as heart rate increases. "A-fib" (atrial fibrillation) is not considered normal, although it can be quite innocent. It is sometimes seen in the setting of some other acute illness, like pneumonia, and reverts as the illness wanes. It can be seen in people who appear to be well, and it definitely can occur in people with no other discernable heart disease. It can be "paroxysmal," occurring occasionally for widely varying periods of time, or persistent. It is an irregular rhythm, sometimes sensed by the person and sometimes not. It may allow cardiac pumping at a relatively normal rate. However, the rate tends to be somewhat accelerated and occasionally can be very fast, almost certainly causing symptoms. A-fib may be present in as many as 10% of people over the age of seventy.

There are three potential complications associated with atrial fibrillation. What is happening with A-fib is that instead of the atria contracting in response to an electrical stimulus from the sinoatrial node, usually set at about seventy beats per minute, in response to rapid, disorganized electrical impulses, they begin to contract virtually non-stop at about 300 per minute, but with minimal if any forward thrust. In essence, they are "quivering," instead of contracting. Potential complications emanate from this arrangement. First, although the atrioventricular node downstream in the conduction system is not set up to conduct at 300 beats per minute, it is common to see an accelerated rate at perhaps 100 to 150 beats per minute. This could cause an already weakened heart to decompensate. Secondly, the lack of atrial contractile force reduces overall cardiac output by up to 20%. This too could lead to decompensation in a weakened heart. Thirdly, with the atria not contracting well, blood can pool in certain areas of the atria, such as the so-called atrial appendages. Once it is pooled, or stagnant, it can clot. Should a clot break loose later, it is immediately pumped through the heart and goes out into the lungs or into the systemic circulation, and can cause trouble wherever it goes. The biggest concern is that there is a 25% chance that the clot will go up into the head, and cause a stroke, increasing the yearly risk of stroke by a significant measure.

So, there are three potential targets for treatment in atrial fibrillation. The first is rate control if the ventricular rate is fast. Secondly, there is treatment of decompensation (congestive heart failure) if that is present. Thirdly, there is long-term anticoagulation with Coumadin (warfarin) to prevent clotting and reduce stroke risk. Occasionally, a procedure called "cardioversion" is attempted, whereby after adequate sedation, an electrical current is delivered across the heart in an attempt to shock it back into rhythm. Less often, but certainly in younger people, several types of ablation techniques can be tried. In this situation, after appropriate "mapping" using an electrode in the heart, it may be possible to apply radiofrequency energy to one or several locations in the atria to permanently block the fibrillating rhythms. Atrial fibrillation is the most common indication for long-term anticoagulation with warfarin.

Concept of (Congestive) Heart Failure

Congestive heart failure is a descriptive term used to describe a very common state seen with any type of advanced heart disease. Recall that by far, the most common form of heart disease is known by various terms, including coronary disease, coronary heart disease, arteriosclerotic heart disease, and ischemic heart disease. The pathology (meaning abnormality) is the same—that being restricted blood flow to the heart muscle. By implication, this represents cardiomyopathy, i.e., heart muscle disease, although in many cases it is relatively mild. As it progresses, as it usually does over the years, it can eventually do so much damage to heart muscle that limitations begin to appear. The right ventricle might be weakened to the point where it cannot deal with the full load of incoming blood. This could result in increased pressure throughout the entire venous system, resulting in the appearance of edema everywhere. Edema is a term referring to leaking of fluid out of the vascular system into the tissues. When we see this in the extremities, we identify it as swelling. It is more prominent in legs than in arms because of the obvious fact of nature that water "rolls downhill" and tends to collect in the lowest parts of the body. When it occurs in the abdominal cavity, it could also be recognized by increased girth. In the chest, it could result in so-called pleural effusion, which is fluid in the space between the lung and the chest wall, and would cause shortness of breath. All of these types of fluid retention can come on very slowly, so as to be less obvious or noticeable than what might be expected. Perhaps a tip-off might be an unusually rapid weight gain, with no change in eating. In fact, as the digestive organs become progressively more congested, there is often a loss of appetite and even low-grade nausea.

Recall that the left ventricle receives blood from the lungs and pumps it all over the body. If one stops to think about what might be the symptom as the left ventricle begins to fail (your assignment now is to stop for a moment, and think about it), two prominent symptoms immediately emerge. Recall that on the back side of the circulation as the pressure in veins rises, fluid tends to leak out. In the case of the pulmonary veins, heading for the left ventricular pump, it can leak into the plural space, as already described, usually slowly bringing on shortness of breath. Worse than that, if it begins to leak into the alveoli, the air sacs of the lung, air becomes replaced by fluid, and we have the onset of a term you may have heard, called "pulmonary edema." This tends to come on more rapidly, and sometimes so rapidly that it is called "flash pulmonary edema." (Who said doctors aren't poetic?) This is sometimes dramatically described as drowning in one's own fluid. The second prominent symptom on the forward side of the circulation is weakness, as the left ventricle is unable to meet the needs of muscle tissue all over the body.

So, in summary, congestive heart failure is an umbrella term used to describe the inability of the heart to perform its function of pumping blood to meet metabolic needs. It represents advanced heart disease. Its appearance over months to years can be very subtle, at first only noted during times of increased activity or some type of physical or emotional stress. As the disease process continues, it becomes more chronic and can eventually be present at rest, with very limited ability to even walk. The best news is that this doesn't have to be you. It is, in most cases, a preventable disease. For those of you who already have it, the injunction to exercise, exercise, exercise, eat a good diet, keep your weight down, no smoking may no longer be fully implementable.

The three exercise components may have to be pared all the way down to very modest exercise. The others are still mandatory. If you remain obese, or keep smoking or eat the wrong foods, you will likely not recover.

Fortunately, as the pathophysiology ("patho" meaning abnormal and "physiology" meaning cellular function) has become more clearly defined in the last ten to fifteen years, the medical treatment of congestive heart failure has improved dramatically. It is now possible for people with severe congestive heart failure, who previously might have had a life expectancy of a few months to a few years, to live five years or more, within a restricted life style with appropriate medication, supplements, and life style changes. For people below the age of sixty-five, there may also be an option of heart transplantation.

Heart Attack

There are two terms intimately connected with coronary artery disease which are deserving of a few comments. The first is a term that I first became aware of at about age ten. That is about the time that I began to learn about the uncles and aunts and other sundry people in my large extended family having "heart attacks." This is a term which doctors continue to use in discussions with both patients and other doctors. If the doctor felt particularly professional at any point in time, he or she might try to impress others by calling the same thing "myocardial infarction." Although the term is still used, the third generation term that you might hear spoken is "acute coronary syndrome." Heart attack and myocardial infarction are vernacular expressions which likely mean the same thing. Acute coronary syndrome, being an attempt to improve communication between doctors, is likely slightly different.

The consequences of coronary obstructions have been known for over a hundred years, and the term heart attack quickly came into common usage. It was meant to detect a syndrome, whereby the victim would experience chest pain, with varying distribution, sweat profusely, vomit, gasp for breath, and possibly die on the spot. Or, the patient could make it to the hospital, where an EKG would be done, which could confirm the diagnosis. A heart attack is this syndrome, with the additional understanding that the coronary blockage resulted in death of heart muscle fed by that artery. So, heart muscle death is the sine qua non. Depending on the amount of muscle death, the spectrum could be anything between full recovery to invalid status, possibly with secondary complications and death occurring weeks to months later. The treatment was strict bed rest for the first two to three weeks. After that, there was a very gradual increase in activity such that after another three to four weeks, the person was ambulating slowly in the hallways of the hospital and could then go home. Hospitalization traditionally lasted six weeks, and then six more weeks at home before returning to full activity. Medications were available to assist with certain complications. This was the standard of care when I began medical school. Smoking was still allowed in hospitals, but I don't recall if people recovering from heart attack were allowed to smoke. Diagnosis was refined, as so-called cardiac enzyme studies came on the scene. These represent a family of chemicals which are released from dying heart muscle cells and make their way into the circulation, where they can be recovered and measured in the lab. These tests are still used every day, with great reliance placed on them. Analysis of these enzymes made it apparent that the full-blown syndrome need not be present for heart muscle cells to die. In fact, there could be only minimal symptoms and perhaps not even enough to disturb the EKG.

The term "acute coronary syndrome" has made its way into discussions of coronary disease in the last five to ten years and perhaps implies something slightly different regarding coronary disease and myocardial perfusion, with the emphasis on slightly. As mentioned above, so-called cardiac enzyme studies are now heavily relied upon and are very frequently done in many different clinical settings. In addition, a relatively newly arrived test is having an impact in clinical practice—that being the "BNP" level—standing for "brain natriuretic peptide." Just about the time that the heart had fallen from its lofty positions as having been considered the seat of the soul, and even a source of intelligence, to nothing but a simple pump like you might use in your basement after a flood, along comes the BNP. This shows that the heart itself can produce a substance which acts like a hormone, travelling through the circulation to distant locations and having an effect on those tissues. That is exactly what the "endocrine glands" do. In this case, when ventricular muscle fibers are stretched, as they would be if the ventricle is not contracting strongly and becomes overfilled with blood, BNP is released by heart muscle cells. This in turn causes blood vessels all over the body to dilate, thus increasing their capacity and taking the load off the heart muscle. In addition, it causes the kidney to excrete more sodium which pulls fluid along with it, reducing blood volume. This is another recently discovered, wonderful backup up system to limit or correct the negative consequences of congestive heart failure.

So now, we are concerned not only about the heart muscle cell death (heart attack or myocardial infarction) but also factors that are perhaps more subtle, causing muscle stretch, with or without death of some cells, as determined by the cardiac enzyme studies. Therefore, an "acute coronary syndrome" could be caused by eating too much pizza (salty), with subsequent fluid retention, with subsequent increased stretch of cardiac muscle fibers, with possible death of some of these fibers and release of cardiac enzymes, even if there is no change in the coronary blockages at that moment. Eating salty food is only one example of many, which could tip the balance and precipitate such an event. Other triggers could include smoking a cigarette, contracting an acute illness, pain, emotional stress, physical stress, etc. It might not seem too important that a person has a few cardiac muscle fibers die in one of these events. But if these events are occurring repeatedly, daily, even mildly, it can all add to the burden of gradually diminishing cardiac function. This is a good example why, in order to stay well, taking your pills is simply not good enough. Without meaningful attention to lifestyle, damage (disease) will progress.

Once again, one of our modern-day tragedies, talked about here and there, but not sufficiently emphasized, is that the spectrum of arteriosclerotic heart disease, so common and so dangerous, and so expensive to treat, is largely preventable.

Tobacco Use

Now, a few words about tobacco abuse, and more after our next section. Just as exercise is the very best thing healthy people can do for themselves, use of tobacco in any form is the very worst thing they can do for themselves. In the USA, the percentage of adults smoking has dropped remarkably since the first Surgeon General's report in 1969, linking tobacco usage with strongly negative health consequences. Unfortunately, this is not true for most of the rest of the world. Regardless, in the USA, we see a residual group of about 25% of adults who smoke regularly, even if not heavily. We seem to be leveling off, identifying this group as so addicted, or so in denial that they cannot or will not quit. I have dealt with large numbers of these people, who have survived lung cancer, emphysema, and heart disease of all types and continue to smoke. Many have cut back. Unfortunately, even one inhalation of tobacco smoke once per week is enough to keep body chemistry geared toward systemic inflammation and hypercoagulation. Cutting back is good, but not good enough. It is unlikely that most of these people will quit completely, but they must continue to try. Banning smoking would obviously only provoke the appearance of a black market, which would make the situation even worse. One puff once per week is bad enough that every smoker should envision a skull and cross bones on every tobacco product.

The Benefits of Cigarette Smoking (?)

Is it necessary to repeat my often-mentioned notion that it is generally inaccurate to say always or never? The oxymoronic notion of smoking to improve health likely applies to a very small number of people, but I think it may exist. It might be fueled by observations of this person that members of his or her kindred smoke and live to old age without smoking-related maladies. More likely, it emanates from an "incurable" addiction (if the tobacco is available, I will use it), which in turn may be generated by a rare type of brain biochemical arrangement. The alternative is that it may in some way improve neurocognitive or bodily systems, which might otherwise present major obstacles to full functioning in some way.

As is clearly apparent, I have gone to great lengths to come to grips with my encounters with countless intelligent, well-meaning people over the years, who, rather than say they cannot quit smoking, say that they will not, no matter what happens to them.

In summary, perhaps it is possible that in these people, smoking may be less harmful than not smoking.

Cardiac Testing Procedures

Before leaving the heart and vascular system, I would like to comment briefly on cardiac testing procedures, done frequently and heavily relied upon. The oldest of these is the electrocardiogram, which came into clinical usage in the early 1900s. It remains commonly used, but its utility is now rather circumscribed. As a technique begins to slide from its period of prominence to its eventual arrival at the trash bin of obsolescence, the enthusiasm which the bearer of expertise carries seems to wane simultaneously. Upon its inception in clinical medicine, electrocardiographs represented a huge breakthrough and were utilized to allow for a wide range of cardiac diagnoses. People avidly studied tracings trying to tease out bits of information. Even upon my entry into medicine, it was still the major diagnostic tool used to detect heart attack. Basically, the EKG is a pictorial representation of the conduction system of the heart, as just discussed. Therefore, it measures the electrical activity of the heart and all conclusions drawn were obtained from this single parameter. Even now, in the doctor's office, with a patient experiencing chest pain at that moment, it could indicate a high probability of what is now called an "acute coronary syndrome," which would mandate a call to 911 and a trip to the hospital.

However, just as many patients lie in their hospital beds hooked up with EKG leads, the main purpose it serves now is to give information regarding the rhythm of cardiac excitation. In this venue, it remains preeminent, and I do not see evidence for a quick relinquishing of this function. So, it is still an eminently useful tool for dealing with this very important part of overall cardiac function. A modification of the full EKG is a test called the Holter monitor. This is a portable device worn by the patient for twenty-four to forty-eight hours, with leads connected to a small computer to store the data in an attempt to get more information about cardiac rhythm and dysrhythmias. It is very commonly used and may provide crucial information. For instance, it is almost invariably used for people who are experiencing "palpitations" or for those who have had syncope (meaning sudden loss of consciousness). EKG and Holter monitor are very cost effective and "non-invasive" (non-invasive, an often used term which means nothing enters the body and implies a very high level of safety).

Another very common and cost-effective study is the so-called stress echo. This is a test which is restricted to people who are able to walk for at least a few minutes on a treadmill. For those who cannot walk on the treadmill, a modification of this technique can be used to obtain similar data from a "non-exercise stress test." On most occasions, a standardized protocol is followed, the most common being the "Bruce protocol," in use for over fifty years. This test is sometimes done as a "screening test" in a person felt to be at high risk for heart disease, particularly "silent" or undetected ischemic heart disease. It is also used for people who are experiencing chest pain, particularly if the pain is non-descript or not particularly suggestive of coronary disease origin. With this test, the patient first undergoes a standard echocardiogram, which in itself gives a wealth of information about cardiac structure and function. The echocardiogram is basically a cardiac ultrasound test. Sound waves are bounced off the various cardiac structures and, when returned to the transducer, give a visual, real-time image of the heart (real time, meaning as it is beating at that moment). The person then undergoes a standard exercise protocol, beginning with minimum energy expenditure and ending up with at least moderate to marked energy expenditure for their age, sex, and level of fitness. While they exercise, full EKG leads are in place, closely watched, and blood pressure is monitored. Oxygen levels can also be monitored as an addendum. Immediately upon completion of the exercise, the person lies down again, and another echocardiogram is done. A healthy heart will show augmentation of ventricular wall motion after exercise, implying increased contractility, implying adequate blood flow. If such is not the case, restriction of blood flow is suspected. Overall fitness can be observed and measured. Arrhythmias can be detected. Recall that a screening test should be safe, convenient and/or easy, and inexpensive. This study meets those criteria, although the full cost could be as high as $1,000. The test can also be used for evaluation of people with exercise intolerance or shortness of breath. It is a very useful test. If abnormal, depending on the circumstances, it may require a trip to the "cath lab" to further investigate coronary blood flow and other issues.

The cath lab, meaning heart catheterization laboratory, is the place where the cardiologist, and perhaps the cardiac surgeon, ultimately get the most accurate information about cardiac structure and function, with emphasis on the coronary arteries. In the lab, a catheter is threaded up to the heart, from an artery in the groin. Transducers can then be introduced to do direct pressure measurements from inside the heart, and the aorta, sometimes solidifying information gained from the echocardiogram. The key procedure involves injection of "dye" (contrast media which is easily seen on X-ray) into the coronary arteries, during which time a series of rapid sequence X-ray pictures are made of each artery and its branches. Blockages, or lack of such, can be identified. Angioplasty or stenting can follow. The subsequent images thus obtained can be used by the surgeon to strategize what type of bypass will be done. This procedure is also very commonly done and provides crucial information. It is infrequently done as a screening test because of high expense and the fact that it is "invasive."

Coronary calcium scoring using CT technique is a controversial study. Although it has been utilized for at least ten years already, it still has not found a uniformly accepted niche for its use. Many cardiologists have invested financially in such scanners, and facilities, raising familiar questions about its increased usage. It is always nice to have data, but is it really crucial in terms of directing treatment? This study uses cat scanning techniques to see how much calcium is embedded in the walls of the coronary arteries. There is some correlation between the amount of calcium seen and the likelihood of experiencing an acute coronary syndrome. The only indication I see for it is perhaps, when all the preceding information has not clearly indicated what a treatment approach should be, this study could be a "tiebreaker."

Peripheral arteries are studied with ultrasound and angiograms, just as is coronary disease. However, I don't think that these studies should be done by cardiologists, as is sometimes the case, as they rarely do the repairs. These are done generally by interventional radiologists, or vascular surgeons, and they should do the studies. In addition, since peripheral artery blockages rarely result in sudden death, the impetus to use these as routine screening tools by anyone needs to be tempered and combined with solid clinical data, otherwise obtained. The so-called peripheral vascular disease is caused by the same factors which cause coronary disease, and it needs to be treated aggressively just as would coronary disease to neutralize the effects or risk factors.

Pulmonary

As has already been mentioned, the lungs are functionally interposed between the right and left sides of the heart. Oxygen-poor blood returns from the tissues all over the body to the right heart and to then be pumped into and through the lungs. The project is to release one of the main products of cellular metabolism—carbon dioxide— and to replace one of the two main cellular fuels—oxygen—into the blood. Blood then returns via the pulmonary veins to the left side of the heart, where it is pumped throughout the body.

Basic Anatomy and Physiology

Recall that the structure of the lung is such that it brings blood and air into very close apposition so that this transfer can occur. The blood factor arrives as noted. Air arrives by a series of channels, beginning at the nose and/or mouth, which meet at the back of the throat, proceed downward past the larynx ("voice box") and into the trachea ("wind pipe"). The trachea, a semi-rigid tube supported by rings of cartilage, divides and divides again and again into a series of progressively smaller tubes called bronchi, continuing to divide into bronchioles before reaching the alveoli ("air sacs"), where air and blood are finally close enough (within a few millionths of a meter) that the diffusion of the two major gases, driven by respective molecular pressure gradients, can occur. Recall that oxygen is carried primarily in the red blood cell, bound by iron. Carbon dioxide is carried primarily in the plasma, the liquid element of the blood.

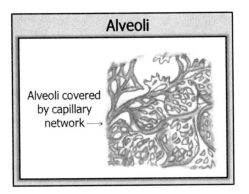

Alveoli

Alveoli covered by capillary network ⟶

We have some basic understanding about how the blood gets there. However, has anyone considered seriously how the air gets there? Clearly, it is not because of strong atmospheric winds. In fact, it takes an expenditure of energy to accomplish this, thanks to the "muscles of respiration." There are at least four muscles, or groups of muscles, involved. Basically, these are divided into the "accessory muscles," including muscles in the neck, back, and between the ribs, and the major muscle being the diaphragm. The diaphragm is a thick pancake-shaped muscle, which, when it contracts, changes from a dome shape, as it descends toward the abdomen, to a much flatter shape. The point is that it descends several inches, substantially enlarging the chest cavity. Also as a sidelight, the diaphragm, with several attached membranes, acts as a partition separating the chest from the abdomen.

In healthy people at rest, or with quiet activity, 80% to 90% of the power of respiration is generated by the diaphragm. This figure drops slightly with strenuous exertion. The role of the diaphragm drops significantly in certain disease states, notably emphysema, where usage of the accessory muscles markedly increases, because of the diaphragm being anatomically altered by the emphysema, much reducing its functional capability. The purpose of all the respiratory muscles is to increase the volume of the chest cavity. By doing so, according to Boyle's law, which we all learned in high school but immediately forgot (the pressure and volume of a gas are inversely proportional), as the volume of the chest cavity increases, air pressure in the cavity drops in reference to atmospheric pressure. The pressure differential, created by muscular contraction, causes air to passively rush into the chest (a very local atmospheric wind). Importantly, the act of expiration, or releasing air, takes much less effort in healthy people, as the built-in elastic elements of the lungs and chest wall literally squeeze the air out, using the stored-up energy generated by the contraction of the respiratory muscles. Please note that as air enters the lung, the bronchi dilate slightly, but importantly. As the lung contracts, the airways narrow slightly. This phenomenon has important implications in diseases of the airway.

So, we now know something about the raison d'etre of the lung, to bring air and blood close enough to exchange gases. The rest of the substances of the lung and chest wall provide support and protection.

Support is provided by the so-called interstitium, which carries blood vessels which nourish the lung tissue itself, nerves, lymphatic channels, and elastic and fibrous elements. Protection is provided by the chest wall, consisting of skin, ribs, breast bone, muscles, and the pleural membrane which is folded into a double layer. In addition, the bronchi and bronchioles are covered by a very thin layer of secretions, under which lie cellular elements with moveable parts, called "cilia," creating a moving stream of mucous, going up toward the larger bronchi and throat, where it can be coughed out.

The surface area of the respiratory membranes, from the mouth to the alveoli, is enormous, estimated to be the size of a tennis court. Once again, the only life-sustaining purpose of this is to bring air and blood into intimate contact. What comes into or onto this huge surface is everything else in the air and blood. The air contains particulate matter of all types, including inorganic (never living) or organic substances (living or having lived), including all of the usual air pollutants, allergens of many types, viruses, bacteria, and other "living" agents. An allergen, such as pollen can play an active role in common disease processes, such as hay fever and asthma. As mentioned before, we tend to think in terms of all or none, disease or no disease. We pay much less attention to the likelihood that inhaled substances can have subclinical (below detection) effects which may nonetheless contribute to the total burden on the body's immune system.

Immune System

What may now be coming into focus, in bits and pieces, is that the body (just like us as a whole) tends to be extremely xenophobic. It hates "other." It would do almost anything to protect against invasion. It has layers upon layers of forces designed to destroy invaders, whether they be living or not living. Invaders basically have three ways of gaining entry into the body. The first, and most obvious, is the skin. The skin provides a clearly visible boundary of "us" on one side and "them" on the other. Depending on the invader, the skin can be broached either by diffusion directly through (the same process that allows us to use transdermal medications of many types) or a frank rupture of the skin, such as a cut or penetrating wound. The implications and repercussions of this have been experienced by all of us.

The other two portals of entry are less obvious, but equally important, and in fact extremely important. The second is the gastrointestinal tract, from mouth to anus. Yes, you guessed it! We do use orally absorbed drugs and rectally absorbed drugs. This entire channel through the body, including esophagus, stomach, small intestine, and large intestine, is the recipient of all the food and liquid we might ingest, as well as whatever mucous from the respiratory tract that we swallow. Despite the fact that the water we drink is "treated" to reduce, but not eliminate, frankly dangerous infective agents, this water, and also "bottled water," is teaming with tiny little creatures, each carrying its packet of DNA (not us) and a variety of other handiworks. Some of this passes directly through, never being absorbed. Parts of it need to be dealt with by the immune system, which is abundantly stretched along the GI tract.

Please note a very important fact that is easily overlooked and underappreciated. While a substance sits in the lumen (channel) of the GI tract, although it appears to be "in" the body, it is not truly "in" until it crosses the first layer of cells, variously named, depending on the anatomic location. It is at that point that the invader encounters the full brunt of the immune system. Another way of looking at this is that the lumen of the GI tract is technically not in the body.

The third portal is (drum roll), you guessed it! The lungs! This is perhaps the most important in terms of the potential for exposure of "us" to "them." Whereas the skin has a surface area of a few square feet, the surface area of the pulmonary system is approximately 2,100 to 2,800 square feet, depending on whether the invaders are playing singles or doubles. Also, consider that in some days your skin stays intact and may not be called upon to do much in terms of battling invaders, besides staying intact. Consider that you may put two liters of fluid and food into your GI tract, and maximum three, or four, or... (?) liters of beer on a hot summer day. Compare that with the 4,300 liters of air that enters the respiratory tract on the same day that you are doing nothing but sitting around and drinking beer. As can be seen, the potential for invasion is much greater through the respiratory tract than anywhere else. Were it not for the elaborately layered and interconnected, and multi-potential capabilities of the immune system, our lives would be very stormy and very short. As far as the lungs and the GI tract are concerned, both have physical barriers, already mentioned, as well as both innate and adaptive portions of immunity, involving both cellular (solid) and humoral (liquid) components. In the respiratory tract, there exists the added layers of mucous with cellular components and their projections (cilia) moving this barrier constantly toward the mouth and out of the body. There are enzymes and other peptides dissolved in the mucous to kill invaders. In fact right at that level, which could be envisioned as the doorway into us, are awaiting a host of elements including white blood cells, including our highly trained, take-no-prisoners, natural killer cells. These cellular elements are ready and waiting to release or activate their interleukins, interferons, cytokines, prostaglandins, leukotrienes, and the complement cascade, the latter with the ability to instigate "rapid killing" of invaders. This is the immune system in its full battle regalia. They do their job so well that despite the 4,300 liters of air spread over 2,800 square feet of surface area, the respiratory tract below the larynx in healthy people is considered to be "sterile," meaning no bacteria or viruses grow when secretions are harvested experimentally, and attempts are made to grow them.

Stay tuned for a discussion of autoimmune disease, when "we" become overly aggressive and start to attack ourselves. Also, I lied about the portals of entry. There is actually a fourth, perhaps of lesser magnitude overall, but still with the potential for causing big trouble. That is the urinary tract, to be discussed soon.

Back to the respiratory tract. A common way of looking at the respiratory tract has been to divide it into "upper," above the larynx, and "lower," below the larynx. Both ENT doctors and lung doctors and others share the upper compartment. However, ENT doctors are forbidden by custom, and by pressure to preserve their referral patterns from lung doctors, from venturing below the larynx, except in one instance—that being performance of surgical tracheostomy.

Another way of evaluating the respiratory tract is to divide it into diseases of the airways and diseases of the lung itself. This division works very well from a conceptual context, as long as we add in the vascular component, meaning pulmonary arteries (diseases of the pulmonary veins are uncommon). The upper tract, consisting exclusively of the airway, has already been discussed in reference to upper respiratory infection. This includes pharyngitis (throat infection), rhinosinusitis (nose and sinus infection), and otitis externa, media, and interna (outer, middle, and inner ear infection).

Laryngeal Disorders

Laryngitis implies inflammation or infection of the larynx or voice box. This can be seen as a part of a full-blown upper respiratory infection (URI) syndrome, or it can be seen, less often, as an isolated entity. Basically, the only major or common symptom of laryngitis in adult patients is voice alteration. There are several ways the voice may be altered, but the most common is "hoarseness," meaning appearance of a rough or gravelly sound. When seen alone, one would have to differentiate it from some type of mechanical injury, such as overuse (prolonged speaking or yelling) or perhaps excessive dryness. Even acid reflux, if it refluxes all the way up to the larynx, can damage the vocal cords. In this case, be grateful that you have only laryngitis, as the implication is that you came very close to having a much more serious situation, either bronchitis or pneumonia, had the acid made it past the vocal cords into the lower airway. Please note also that just as the entire upper airway is susceptible to allergic insult, via pollen, so is the larynx. Rarely, because the larynx represents a relatively narrowed channel, should there be enough swelling from whatever the cause, this could narrow the channel through the larynx enough to cause "stridor." Stridor involves a marked alteration or complete loss of the voice and is usually associated with some degree of shortness of breath. In rare cases, this could be extreme and could mandate emergency treatment. There are some viruses that appear to be laryngotropic, meaning they go right to the larynx without going anywhere else. Significant narrowing of the larynx is more common with allergic phenomena than with infections.

Vocal Cord Dysfunction Syndrome

The last two laryngeal abnormalities to be mentioned are two sides of the same coin. Appreciation of these conditions, and especially the fact that they are relatively common, has come about within the last ten to fifteen years. They are both interesting and occasionally frightening

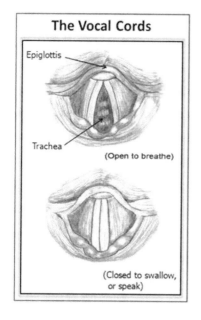

The Vocal Cords

Epiglottis

Trachea

(Open to breathe)

(Closed to swallow, or speak)

phenomena. The first is so-called vocal cord dysfunction syndrome. This condition can go undetected for many years and can masquerade as asthma. When masquerading, it tends to be an explosive type of "asthma" which can lead to many trips to the ER and usage of high doses of potentially toxic drugs to control it. It can even result in what appears to be "respiratory arrest," or cessation of breathing, which mandates emergency intubation (placing a large bore tube directly into the airway). The mechanism is as follows. Just as the airway tends to dilate with inspiration and narrow with expiration, the vocal cords tend to separate with inspiration and come together with expiration (see diagram). With vocal cord dysfunction syndrome, the opposite is true, with the cords approximating during inspiration. Obviously, this could result in stridor, with very abnormal voice and marked shortness of breath. The cause appears to be acquired, as a habitual, but unconscious process, often related to some type of stressor. The diagnosis can be suspected by the history rendered by the patient and the witness. It can be further suspected when there are sudden, dramatic swings in airflow capacity and confirmed by visual inspection of the larynx at the time of difficulty. The condition is corrected by speech therapy. Elucidation of this syndrome can be mildly embarrassing for the patient, but enormously embarrassing for the bevy of doctors who have been caring for this patient, supposedly asthmatic, using toxic drugs, and who are now considering the possibility of relocating to Tombouctou.

Laryngospasm

The second condition is that of laryngospasm. The larynx is surrounded by muscle, including the very important epiglottis, which contracts to close the larynx during the swallowing reflex so that the swallowed material is directed to the esophagus, rather than the trachea. As is always the case, when you or your new car are functioning well, you may take for granted the complex mechanisms occurring all around you, allowing you to silently cruise the highway, well above the designated speed limit. I can assure you that the everyday functioning of your body is enormously more complex than anything designated "vehicle." Swallowing is a perfect example of something that you do, without thinking about it, hundreds of times per day. For most of us, for most of our lives, the mechanism proceeds flawlessly. Eventually, and somewhat commonly, the ravages of aging catch up with us, and the very complex reflexes that have occurred in perfect synchrony for all those years resulting in the act of swallowing begin to falter. This may occur with aging alone, more commonly with a number of common neurological diseases, such as Parkinson's disease, multiple sclerosis, and stroke, and less often with many other disease processes. At that point, the most common threat is so-called aspiration, with the possibility of "aspiration pneumonia." What is happening in this situation is that the epiglottis is not closing perfectly so as to incompletely seal off the airway from the material (including simple saliva) directed downward. Thus, this material can enter the airway. In most people, this instantly precipitates a very strong cough reflex in an attempt to get the material out of the airway. In a person with a weak cough, or no cough (like unconsciousness from sleep, drugs, or alcohol), the material can make it all the way into the depths of the lung, with resultant pneumonia.

Laryngospasm is a forceful closure of the larynx, seen in a wide variety of circumstances including incipient aspiration. Rumor has it (I cannot find experimental documentation of this, and I don't advise trying this at home) that it is a primitive reflex, seen in babies when they are immersed in water. It occurs from gastroesophageal reflux and with dysfunctional swallowing. It can occur as a reflex in response to strong coughing. It definitely can occur transiently, with sudden immersion in cold water. It seems to occur most frequently in the setting of violent coughing. With this scenario, and others, the person is unable to breathe in or out and has a panicky feeling of impending doom. It invariably stops after fifteen to thirty seconds and allows breathing to proceed naturally, as if nothing had happened. The experience can be terrifying. It is almost invariably more troublesome than serious, and frequently, all that is required is treatment of the underlying conditions and reassurance.

Tracheostomy

Moving past the larynx, deeper into the chest, the airway is now designated trachea. As noted previously, this is the "territory" of the lung specialist, with one exception. There is a surgical procedure called "tracheostomy," which entails creating an artificial opening in the trachea exiting the skin at the base of the neck. Up until the last ten years or so, this was always considered to be a surgical procedure, done by a general surgeon or an ENT surgeon. There is now an option for doing this procedure using an endoscopic technique (bronchoscope), at the bedside in the intensive care unit, by a lung specialist. The procedure is occasionally done as an emergency, such as when the airway above is completely blocked, or when attempts to pass the large bore tube from the mouth or nose past the larynx are unsuccessful.

Much more commonly, it is done "electively," as a non-emergent procedure in a person who needs a very reliable opening to the lower airway during recovery from an acute lung illness. There are occasions when permanent tracheotomy may be needed. Surgeons may be called upon to perform this elective procedure.

As noted before, the multiple overlaying facets of the immune system work so well that the airway below the larynx is considered to be functionally sterile (no microorganisms), although it may not be absolutely so. The two major disadvantages of tracheostomy, temporary or permanent, have to do with the need to make accommodations to preserve voice (now that exhaled air comes out of the trachea rather than traversing the vocal cords) and the loss of the antiseptic barrier provided by the intact larynx. In other words, the trachea becomes invariably infected. Although this is often surprisingly well tolerated, at other times, it can be very problematic, leading to repeated bouts of clinical (recall that "clinical" placed in front of a word or phrase means "in the real world") infection, including pneumonia. Technically, infection of the trachea is called "tracheitis."

The term tracheitis is not commonly used because after ten to fifteen centimeters, the trachea divides into the left and right mainstem bronchi, and immediately by many more branches. It is virtually impossible to isolate symptoms of the trachea from those of the bronchi, and so, the term most commonly used is "bronchitis." The bronchi terminate deep in the lung contiguous with the bronchioles. These airways do not have cartilaginous rings, nor do they have glands under the lining membrane. They terminate directly into the air sacs, called alveoli, where the exchange of oxygen and carbon dioxide occurs. Inflammation (a normal and essential portion of the immune system) or infection in the bronchioles is called "bronchiolitis." This is somewhat uncommon, but very important, as it involves airways that are one millimeter or less in diameter. It is easy to see how it would not take much in the way of inflammation (recruitment of additional cellular elements, with tissue injury and appearance of edema, i.e., increased extravascular fluids) to narrow or shut down these airways. This process, when seen clinically, is usually viral in origin. It is particularly dangerous in children and can be fatal. Inflammation and/or infection of the air sacs can be called "alveolitis" but is more commonly called pneumonitis or pneumonia.

Infection and Inflammation

So, we have moved all the way down from the upper airway into the air sacs, which is the end of the line as far as ventilation is concerned. We have mentioned any number of conditions ending in "-itis," which always implies infection and/or inflammation. And, incidentally what is the difference between infection and inflammation, or are they the same? The answer is that they are not the same. They are closely interrelated. Infection can be dealt with relatively easily in terms of its definition. Basically, it means that some type of living (recall the debate as to whether or not viruses are truly living or not) organism, designated "them," is causing trouble in "us." The organism could be viral, bacterial, or "atypical," with features in between viral and bacterial (chlamydia). They could be fungal or yeast, or a particular type of bacteria called *mycobacteria*, responsible for tuberculosis or a spirally shaped treponema causing syphilis. Finally, although not a major problem in most of the so-called West, large parts of the world harbor parasitic infections with single-celled organisms called protozoa or multi-celled, and often very large, worms called helminths. These cause enormous amounts of suffering in poor countries that we almost never hear about.

This plethora of different types of infective agents, from submicroscopic viruses to large worms, do damage in many different ways. Please recall that healthy people harbor huge numbers of "infective," primarily bacterial agents, in and on their bodies at all time. These generally leave us alone and are content to stay out of the body technically, although in the body, as already described. The largest concentrations of these organisms, known as "germs" in the vernacular, are found in the nose, mouth and throat (as far as the larynx), colon and rectum, vagina, and over the entire body surface on the skin. Bathing or showering removes a small, but important, portion from the skin. Some of the germs are helpful by warding off more aggressive germs or by producing needed nutrients which might be difficult to get elsewhere. These organisms have lived in harmony with us for many thousands of years and show no major inclinations to change their behavior and get nasty. However, under many clinical circumstances, they can and will become nasty and cross a boundary, entering "us" and causing a clinical infection.

When this occurs, wherever it might be, unless the person is moribund, or their immune system is demolished by disease or treatment of disease like chemotherapy or radiation, this immediately incites an immune response, with inflammation being a potent part of this entire layered, choreographed counterattack. In a nutshell, inflammation involves the arrival of white blood cells en masse, bringing along their buckets full of chemicals which kill on contact and/or attract more white blood cells and activating the humoral mechanism in the hopes that previous contact with these germs will bring in ready-made antibodies which also kill on contact. This entire reaction to the infection is the "inflammatory response." However, recall that it is not activated solely in response to infection. As mentioned earlier, it can be activated by allergy. It will be activated by anything which irritates the body, whether it is mechanical like a broken bone, chemical like food poisoning or a chemical burn, or like too much ultraviolet light exposure (sunburn), and any one of thousands of different factors which simply injure the body in some way. Injury is the key concept. With or without an infection, the inflammatory response, with all of its complexity, is the first and most important step in repair or healing. In other words, with the arrival of all of the inflammatory mediators also comes a supply of all of the agents (cellular, proteinaceous, chemical, and otherwise) needed to put things back together as can be best accomplished. "Miracles" such as this are occurring all the time, every day, outside of our voluntarily control. The body is fixing itself. The inflammatory response, a miracle!

Here are a few last comments about inflammation before we get back on track with the lungs. On the surface of the body, the inflammatory response is easy to spot. There are four key clinical indicators, as were described by Celsus in the first century A.D. and taught to us in medical school, in Latin: (1) *rubor* (redness), (2) *calor* (heat), (3) *tumor* (swelling), and (4) *dolor* (pain). The more of these present simultaneously, the more likely that this is inflammation. The end product of inflammation is pus, which is a conglomeration of many elements, but mainly white blood cells and, in the case of infection, dead germs. The exact same changes occur inside the body, but in that case, the only clue might be the pain.

Alveolitis versus Pneumonitis versus Pneumonia

Okay. Now that we thoroughly understand infection and inflammation, and appreciate the similarities and differences, let's get back to the lungs and finish up with lung infections, appreciating all along how the lung goes about dealing with this. Recall that we have discussed all kinds of "-itis" conditions, including "alveolitis," which involves the deepest part of the lung, the air sacs, and we still haven't heard a word about "pneumonia." Although this term has been used for hundreds of years, it now has a somewhat indistinct or imprecise connotation. When the term is used, the unspoken implication is that there exists a lung infection. So, the term is useful in conveying this assumption. But what anatomic area is involved? Is alveolitis pneumonia? The answer to these questions is also more implied than definite. Although the infection could have arrived deep in the lung via the airway or the circulation (the capillaries blanketing the alveoli), it is likely that the alveoli are involved early on. However, once the immune system swings into action, which is almost immediately, and as it ramps up its counterattack, a large amount of fluid from the circulation leaks into the area. This essentially "drowns" that area of alveoli, with the terminal bronchioles that run into them and spreads across the septae (very thin membranes), separating groups of alveoli called lobules. So, the term pneumonia is not truly isolated to any one anatomic designation and comes to involve possibly large geographic chunks of lung tissue, with everything in it.

Alveolitis, on the other hand, implies that only the alveoli are involved. If you want to impress your doctor, use the term "pneumonitis" or "alveolitis." Pneumonitis is a slightly more erudite name than pneumonia and is somewhat interchangeable with it. However, both pneumonitis and especially alveolitis leave open the possibility that the cause of the inflammatory response (they both end in "-itis," meaning inflammation) may not be infection. Recall that the lung laid out flat has the surface area of a tennis court. It is easy to appreciate that with its exposure to a host of airborne agents, including fumes, gasses, pollen, smoke, and who knows what else, any one of these could independently damage the alveoli or trigger an immune response, similar but different than an inflammatory response, and cause alveolitis or pneumonitis, with lots of damage, but very little fluid and a different clinical picture. In fact, there are a larger number of such conditions, falling under the category of "interstitial lung disease" which involves the terminal parts of the airways, including alveoli, which are not infections, per se. This group of diseases can be acute or chronic. When chronic, they can be especially difficult to treat, cause considerable scarring, seriously damage lung function, and eventually lead to the need for lung transplantation.

Lung infections, whether called pneumonia or pneumonitis, are generally speaking easier to deal with. Viral infections usually do not respond to antibiotics, even those directed toward viruses. Most people, unless very debilitated from other conditions, respond well with supportive care and make a full recovery. Bacterial and atypical infections, with the exception of hospital-acquired infection which may involve germs which are highly resistant to most antibiotics, usually respond well to supportive care and selected antibiotics.

Adult Respiratory Distress Syndrome

There is a condition called adult respiratory distress syndrome (ARDS), in which either a lung infection or some other serious systemic (influencing large parts of the body) inflammatory condition sweeps the lung into the inflammatory reaction. This is akin to an acute alveolitis. Fluid pours into the alveoli, leading to frank respiratory failure and the need for assisted ventilation with a machine. Despite an enormous amount of research over the last 40 years since description of this syndrome, the mortality figures are still high, in the range of 50%. Global treatment consists of treatment of the underlying condition that precipitated the ARDS and of full respiratory and cardiovascular support.

As a sidelight regarding ARDS, I was involved in publication of a research paper in 1967, utilizing data of three women who had multiple pregnancies. Although we identified the clinical picture, and the immune response which caused it, we had only a fragmentary appreciation of the full spectrum of the disease. In 1972, when I began my pulmonary fellowship at the University of Colorado, my mentor was the head of the department, Dr. Tom Petty. He was a giant in the field of pulmonary medicine and cast a very long shadow. In 1967, he and his colleagues had also published a paper on acute respiratory failure, with a large enough number of cases of divergent causes to name the process adult respiratory distress syndrome. Sadly, after a glorious career and mentoring several hundred pulmonary doctors, Dr. Petty passed away in December 2009.

Infections involving fungi and tuberculosis are not very common and will therefore be mentioned only in passing. TB is no longer the scourge it once was, but it is still seen sporadically in developed countries. Treatment of this is now complicated by emergence of drug-resistant forms. The major problem is diagnosis. If it is thought of and diagnosed, treatment is curative in almost all cases. TB continues to be a huge problem in underdeveloped countries. Fungal infections are relatively rare. Unless one thinks about them, they can smolder for a long time. Once diagnosis is established, treatment with antibiotics is usually curative.

Diseases of the Airway

Diseases of the airway include bronchitis, already discussed, and a disease called bronchiectasis. In bronchitis, the walls of the bronchi may be inflamed and/or infected, causing damage to the cilia and mucous layer. The diagnosis is made clinically, with cough being the main symptom, productive or non-productive of sputum. The walls remain structurally intact. Bronchiectasis, caused by a number of factors including longstanding bronchitis or previous pneumonitis, is different in that the bronchi lose their structural integrity and begin to dilate as its cartilage support begins to disintegrate. This further compromises clearance of mucous and debris from the airway. Eventually, pockets and cysts may form, causing further stagnation of secretions, at which time the lower airway becomes chronically infected. Although less common now than in the pre-antibiotic era, it is still relatively common. It is characterized by recurring bouts of significant clinical infection with cough, mucous, fever, weakness, etc. Culture of secretions is necessary, as there tends to be the presence of unusual and/or drug-resistant germs. This can be a debilitating disease, which tends to wax and wane. The treatment involves "postural drainage" to help mucous get out of the lungs, so-called mucolytic agents to loosen secretions, and antibiotics.

The two other major diseases of the airway are asthma and emphysema. Both are very common. There is often considerable overlap, with elements of both present in a substantial number of people. There are also several notable differences. Asthma, in its pure form, is a genetically based disease, most often seen in young people. Emphysema, also called COPD (for chronic obstructive pulmonary disease), in its pure form is almost always smoking related and seen in older people. Let's look at the pure forms first and then discuss the overlap.

Asthma

Asthma is a disease characterized by marked variability in airflow, normal to severely reduced, brought on by change in caliber of the airway, in turn brought on by contraction or relaxation of the muscular elements wrapped around the airways. It frequently begins in children and young adults. It is now known that there are genetic factors which predispose the person to this condition. It is also known that it is a disorder which involves the inflammatory cascade, at least in part. It is felt that in a susceptible person, exposure to an environmental "trigger" activates the inflammatory reaction, with release of its chemical mediators and with subsequent constriction of airway muscle and subsequent airflow obstruction. Asthma is often very mild, and can go undetected for many years, if not a lifetime. The only symptom may be a sporadic cough. This can be an important clue to its presence in a youngster, or anyone else, particularly if the cough is brought on by exercise, cold air, or upper respiratory infection. Another clue might be a person who has prolonged cough which can linger from four to six weeks after a simple URI. The cough is generally dry. Presence of allergies, such as eczema or hay fever, is another clue, as allergies and asthma, both involving the airway, often go together. As the airflow obstruction becomes worse, shortness of breath comes into the picture and may eventually be a major problem.

Asthma tends to be a somewhat unpredictable condition. There may be long periods of remission, lasting for many years, punctuated by episodic difficulties, usually brought on by colds or allergic episodes. Or, it may be chronic and severe. The level of treatment depends completely on the severity. The object is to allow the affected person to experience a normal life style. Treatment is usually very effective. However, longstanding undertreatment, allowing for persistent airflow obstruction, can cause permanent damage, which eventually can look like emphysema. For those in whom the diagnosis is uncertain, there is a good test, generally called "methacholine challenge," or provocation, done in pulmonary function labs.

Reactive airway disease syndrome is a "new" diagnosis, which has been often discussed in recent years. In my opinion, it is nothing more or less than very mild asthma. It too is diagnosed during a methacholine challenge test. Often times, it is not severe enough to be treated. When treatment is necessary, the medications used are the same as those used for asthma.

Emphysema (COPD)

Emphysema, on the other hand, whether or not there turns out to be identifiable or reproducible genetic predisposition, is almost invariably seen in the setting of long-term tobacco abuse. Perhaps, the genetic factors will eventually be found to be the most important reason why "light" smokers may be seriously affected and heavy smokers not at all affected. Because of its connection with smoking, emphysema is generally a disease of middle-aged and older people. The pathology (abnormal findings on microscopic examination of tissues) is different than that of asthma. With emphysema, the alveolar sacs undergo dissolution, with rupture of their membranes, coalescing into larger and larger cysts. This causes two major physiologic (cellular mechanisms) derangements. First, the elastic elements of the lung are greatly reduced as the alveoli break down. Recall that the lung becomes inflated when the volume of the chest cavity is increased by contraction of the muscles of respiration and air passively rushes in. The air is then expelled by passive contraction of the elastic elements, like an inflated balloon. With loss of the elastic elements, this does not occur as efficiently, such that air cannot flow out, i.e., "airflow obstruction." The second physiologic derangement occurring as the alveoli break down is the loss of surface area of the alveolar membranes, in turn allowing for a much smaller area for critical gas exchange. In other words, one half or one fourth of a tennis court is simply not enough. The result of all this disruption is simply shortness of breath. It is relentless. It may fluctuate slightly, or even moderately, depending on a variety of circumstances (the "asthmatic component" of emphysema), but it never fully corrects. It will progress steadily as smoking continues. If smoking stops completely, it should stabilize after six to twelve months. If smoking continues even very "lightly," like "a few cigarettes per week," it will continue to progress. Since the disease involves anatomic disruption of the alveoli, and we do not have the technology to reverse that, the disease is incurable. It may respond somewhat to the same type of medication used for asthma, but the response is much less than that seen for asthma. Medications are utilized because victims of this disease are grateful for and appreciative of even minor levels of improvement. This is a very debilitating, systemic (all over the body) disease, which negatively affects muscles, nutrition, neurologic considerations, the heart, and the brain. People suffer tremendously with this disease, as they shrivel up over years. It is almost 100% preventable, by not smoking, ever.

Pulmonary Vascular

Pulmonary vascular issues of some types are common and relatively easy to deal with. The most important of them is a condition which really should not even be considered a lung disease, although it does occur inside of the lung. This is pulmonary emboli, or blood clots in the lung.

Recall that all of the blood, returning from all over the body, returns to the right side of the heart, to be pumped through the lungs, to get rid of carbon dioxide and pick up a load of oxygen. We have not yet discussed the coagulation system. When we speak of "blood," there are basically two elements that make up this liquid that you see filling up three test tubes in the lab, with the needle in your vein. Yes, it is a liquid. However, its status as a liquid is very tenuous. It needs to be a liquid in order to flow, through the arteries, capillaries, and veins. On the other hand, we are clumsy creatures always doing inadvertent damage to ourselves by banging this or smashing that. In addition, there are numerous common medical conditions which can cause blood vessels to become disrupted, with subsequent "bleeding" (escape of blood outside of the confines of the vascular system). This can be visible on the surface of the body as a bruise or a hematoma (a mass of blood—liquid, clotted, or both). It may also occur internally and/or "pseudo internally." An example of the latter would be an ulceration which forms in the stomach or duodenum (the first portion of the intestine receiving output from the stomach). This will be discussed shortly in more detail. If the ulcer is deep enough to encounter an artery beneath the surface, it can erode into the artery and cause it to bleed profusely. The bleeding occurs from the lumen (the interior space of a blood vessel or a tubular organ) of the artery to the lumen of intestine. I call it "pseudo internally" because since the lumen of the entire GI (gastrointestinal) tract is simply a hollow tube running through the body, at that point, it is already outside of the body. Were the bleeding to stop right then, as it could, you might never know about it. Truly internal bleeding occurs all the time, everywhere, such as into a muscle, into a cavity, or into the brain. If the bleeding does not stop quickly, you could be in very big trouble.

Coagulation

So, as mentioned above, we need the blood to be liquid to flow, but we need a mechanism to stop the flow when it becomes life threatening. Guess what? No need to put in on your wish list because you already have it! It is called the coagulation system. As we have all likely witnessed, the bleeding from the injury we just sustained stops quickly with a little pressure, just as the blood taken from the vein changes from liquid to solid in the test tube. Actually, if you watch the test tube long enough (don't try this unless you are really, really bored), or if you place it in a centrifuge, you would eventually see something interesting. The blood separates into several components. Recall that I just mentioned that there are basically two elements in the blood. These are the liquid medium, called the serum, and the solid or cellular elements, which include red blood cells (carrying oxygen), white blood cells (part of the immune system), and platelets, fragments of tissue no good for anything besides clotting. The heaviest element, the red blood cells, goes to the bottom of the tube. The thin layer of white blood cells layers on top of that, and the serum stays on top of everything. Normal blood is approximately 40% to 45% cellular, and the rest is serum. This percentage or ratio of cells to whole blood is called the "hematocrit," the most common term used to assess for anemia.

The system for regulating the level of blood clotting going on at any given moment is exceedingly complex. The proteins involved are mostly enzymes, which speed up certain chemical reactions. At some point in the distant past, the only two groups of people that could memorize the so-called factors (participating elements) of the coagulation cascade were medical students and hematologists (blood specialists). Now that we have learned so much more about the genetic mechanisms which produce factors which turn on and turn off coagulation, even they can no longer memorize this and need to resort to their pocket computers. Your good luck is that I will not even show you a sketch of the coagulation cascade. The main point is that it is exceedingly tightly regulated in health so that blood flows when it needs to, clots when it needs to, and may well be doing both at the same time, without you even needing to think about it. There are many diseases which induce imbalances in the system and demand treatment to avoid uncontrolled hemorrhage or uncontrolled clotting.

Phlebitis

Getting back to the pulmonary vascular system, as just mentioned, it receives all the blood returning to the body via the venous system. If the above mentioned delicately-balanced coagulation system has been upset, such that clots have formed within the veins somewhere in the body, either because of an overactive clotting system or an underactive anti-clotting system, these clots pose a major threat. They can become attached to the walls of the veins and set off an intense inflammatory reaction called "phlebitis." The inflammation can be so intense as to completely shut off the venous channels. If that occurs, other smaller veins may take over and try to act as conduits for getting blood back to the heart. These veins may dilate and become tortuous at which time they may become identifiable as "varicose veins." This may cause a permanent disruption of venous function in the area, leading to chronic congestion, with subsequent pain and formation of edema (extravascular fluid accumulation). This most commonly occurs in the leg veins or pelvic veins. When it does occur, it can create a "post-phlebitic syndrome," with chronic pain and swelling of the leg (or arm, or wherever it occurs).

Pulmonary Embolism

The other thing that can happen if a clot forms in veins is that it can dislodge and be swept up by the vascular flow. Next stop is the heart. Should the clots be small, they might go through the right atrium and right ventricle, into the pulmonary arteries and into the distal branches of these arteries. This is called "pulmonary embolism." If the clots are very large, they have potential to completely close off blood flow through the heart and cause sudden death.

Venous thrombosis, phlebitis, and pulmonary embolism are all very common. Many episodes likely go undetected, causing minor symptoms. They are all singly or in total capable of causing a large number of acute and/or chronic problems. Doctors have become aware of this huge threat, which is why so many chronically ill or hospitalized patients are given one or several different types of "blood thinners," which really don't thin the blood but interrupt the coagulation cascade at differing points, reducing the likelihood of clot formation. These drugs include aspirin, Plavix, heparin, and warfarin (Coumadin). The main danger of these very useful agents is, of course, excessive bleeding. Many of the rituals emphasized to patients in the post-operative state as part of the recovery scheme are designed to reduce the likelihood of pulmonary complications and/or blood clots.

Hemoptysis (Coughing Blood)

Hemoptysis is the medical term for coughing up blood. This is not very common, but just common enough to warrant mention. It can be extremely important in one particular circumstance. Obviously, the source of blood could be anywhere from the nose or throat, or larynx to anywhere within the lung itself. There is a very wide range of conditions which can cause this. Most of them are not serious, but a few are very serious. You likely can't tell whether it is serious or not, unless you are one of those rare people who experience massive hemoptysis, enough to saturate all the Kleenex you can find and to make a mess of the house while you are trying to find the Kleenex. In addition, if it collects in the lung faster than you can cough it out, it can cause severe shortness of breath. It is a terrifying event (for the doctor as well).

Even a trace of blood, alone or mixed with sputum, can be very important. Fortunately, by far, the most common cause is simple bronchitis, such as might occur with a typical URI. However, this harkens back to the dilemma as to whether the chills, fever, and weakness you experience is the flu, from which you will quickly recover, or sepsis from which you may quickly die. The small amount of blood that you noticed is potentially the first sign of lung cancer. There are other possibilities. It is a condition which warrants a trip to the doctor's office. A brief visit can substantially reduce your concerns about a potentially lethal condition.

The very interesting and important topic of lung cancer is discussed elsewhere.

PART V
DIGESTIVE/GASTROINTESTINAL

On the cellular level, the two major fuels needed for cells to be able to do what they are programmed to do are oxygen and glucose. We have just dealt with oxygen. Now for glucose, or sugar. In the cell, glucose and oxygen combine to form carbon dioxide and water as waste products and adenosine triphosphate (ATP), the pot of gold. ATP is the energy currency of the cell, a rechargeable battery. It is a nanomachine present in all living creatures, from bacteria to humans. It is estimated that the average cell in the body contains a billion of these intricate nucleotides.

It is the purpose of the GI tract to get ingested food, into a digested state, so that energy present outside of the body (in the lumen, of the GI tract) can be taken into the body to supply the glucose necessary for ATP production.

The organs included in the gastrointestinal system include the luminal organs, such as mouth, esophagus, stomach, small intestine, and large intestine. It also includes two other organs which are intimately involved in digestion, by emptying their digestive secretions into the lumen. These two are the liver and pancreas. As usual, the emphasis here is not on physiology, but on the names and causes of common diseases along the way in the tract.

Swallowing and Peristalsis

The first major common difficulty along the luminal tract involves the area between the mouth and the esophagus which is the area involved with the complex reflex of swallowing. This has been discussed already under the topic laryngospasm and with the potential for what is called aspiration pneumonia. I did not explain completely what the existing options are for someone who either cannot swallow safely or reliably, or who has a progressive disorder, which will obviously make the swallowing even worse.

In fact, the esophagus is perhaps not strictly a digestive organ, as it does not participate in digestion, which is preparation of ingested food for absorption, out of the lumen and into the body. The mouth does participate because of it salivary enzymes. The only purpose of the esophagus is to transport the swallowed material from the back of the throat to the stomach. This is not a passive act, with food dropping from the back of the throat into the waiting stomach, with a "plop" (as I envisioned it as a child). It is an active process requiring a sequence of contraction waves, which in fact characterizes all of the luminal digestive organs. These contraction waves are called "peristalsis." So, what I say about the contraction of the esophagus applies also to the stomach, small intestine, and colon as well, with some regionally unique niceties.

Esophagus

The esophagus being a vertically oriented organ is assisted in its contraction waves by gravity, especially with liquids. This is the explanation for those of you who have had the pleasure (?) to watch a prodigious beer drinker guzzle a liter down, without stopping to breathe. That is another activity I would not recommend trying at home, unless the 911 van is waiting in your driveway. That type of ability involving relaxation of the entire esophageal musculature is very unusual. Even liquids usually take one or two contraction waves to get the fluid into the stomach. Food, especially if poorly or quickly chewed, may take three or four contraction waves to get it into the stomach. So, what is this dysphagia (difficulty swallowing) all about?

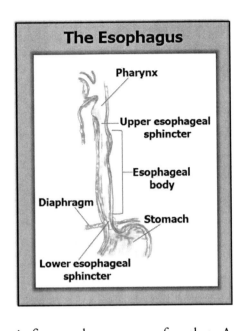

The Esophagus

Pharynx
Upper esophageal sphincter
Esophageal body
Diaphragm
Stomach
Lower esophageal sphincter

Remember the caveat, diagnosis first, and treatment after that. As always, diagnosis largely comes from a detailed, meticulously drawn history. The first major fork in the road is to decide whether the dysphagia is secondary to a motility (peristalsis) problem or to an obstruction. Or, both! Motility in the GI tract refers to adequacy, or inadequacy, of forward propulsion of ingested material. In this case, keep in mind that "forward" is ultimately headed for the back door, i.e., the rectum and anus (I apologize for the non sequiturs). Both issues, motility disorders and obstructions, are common, and progressively more common with aging. Motility is under control of the autonomic (automatic) nervous system. Obviously, the nervous system controls myriads of coordinated activities all over the body, including this. Just as the ability to walk or run (the so-called gait) of an older person is likely not what it was at age eighteen, so neither are the coordinated contraction waves of the esophagus. The most common form of motility disorder of the esophagus is called presbyesophagus, with a variety of discoordinated waves, including even waves going back up. Usually, the dysphagia associated with this is somewhat intermittent, and not severe enough to jeopardize health. When it is more severe, so-called pro-kinetic agents, fostering forward propulsion can be helpful.

Obstructions can occur at any point along the way in the esophagus, particularly malignant ones. Fortunately, benign obstructions are much more common and occur most often in one of three locations. The first is right at the juncture of the pharynx (back of the throat) and the esophagus, where lies the upper esophageal sphincter. Sphincters in medicine refer basically to luminal (hollow) organs and specifically to circumferentially oriented muscle fibers, which, when they contract, act to pinch closed the lumen.

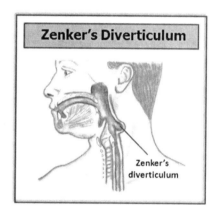

Discoordinated swallowing, in this area of the pharyngoesophageal junction can also account for development of a diverticulum (out-pouching) of the esophagus, appropriately named Zenker's diverticulum by the humble doctor who first described it. This diverticulum can be large enough to contain perhaps an ounce of material, which could be later discharged and cause cough, feeling of choking or bad breath, depending on whether it is discharged upward or downward. In most cases, these diverticula are asymptomatic (without symptoms). When symptomatic, there are endoscopic or surgical techniques to close the pocket.

Farther down, and just above the diaphragm, is an area where a ring-like narrowing can occur, called Schatzki's ring, named after himself by the equally humble Dr. Schatzki. These ring-like structures usually have normal lining membrane over them and extend for only a few millimeters. Many are asymptomatic. If sufficiently symptomatic, they can be dilated using an endoscopic procedure, with a balloon, to physically stretch it open. With obstruction in the mid- to lower esophagus, people generally complain that things seem to get "stuck," rather than a feeling of "choking," or inability to initiate a swallowing reflex, which more likely emanates from the upper esophagus.

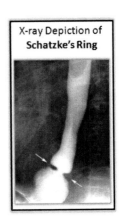

X-ray Depiction of Schatzke's Ring

Also, in the lower esophagus, there are two other types of strictures which can occur, one benign and one malignant. Again, the benign type is much more common. This can be easily differentiated from the ring structure by its endoscopic appearance because the lining membrane is usually irritated, and possibly even ulcerated. This abnormality is generally thought to be the result of long-term acid reflux, with sufficient inflammation set up to result in scarring and stricture. These too can be dilated endoscopically, with initiation of lifetime usage of strong acid-reducing medication.

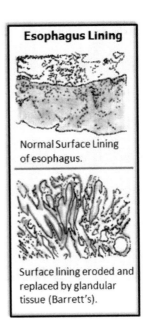

Esophagus Lining

Normal Surface Lining of esophagus.

Surface lining eroded and replaced by glandular tissue (Barrett's).

Barrett's Esophagus

This lower esophageal area is also the most common site for so-called Barrett's esophagus, named after the humble Dr. Barrett. This is thought to be a premalignant lesion (another difficult term, as discussed in the case of colon cancer), treated with lifetime acid-reducing medicine, and lifetime, frequent (every three years) endoscopic surveillance. By implication, excess acid in the esophagus is likely a predisposing factor for those genetically susceptible to esophageal cancer.

Acid Reflux

So, acid reflux, or as it is now called GERD (pronounced like "herd," and standing for gastroesophageal reflux disease) is a big deal. In fact, a very big deal. The most common symptoms of acid reflux are often described as "heartburn," or "acid indigestion," particularly if the latter is felt in the lower chest. It is the factor behind a high level of morbidity (trouble) when mild and can even lead to strictures and possibly cancer. Besides popping a pill, which is what the pharmaceutical company wants because they make money, and which is what your doctor wants because you have already used up your ten minutes, before the days of potent acid reducing medications, there were a host of good, free, side effect free, and healthful tips, which were given to people with symptomatic acid reflux. Here they are, resurrected from the dust bin of medical practice.

First, avoid substances which are known to stimulate the stomach to secrete more acid. Also, avoid substances which cause relaxation of the lower esophageal sphincter, which when relaxed offers no impedance to material going backward or upward into the esophagus. This list includes commonly ingested foods and

Archaic Non-Medicinal Treatment of GERD

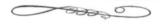

- o Limit acidic foods (vinegar, citrus).
- o Limit foods that stimulate acid production (alcohol, fatty meats).
- o Limit foods and meds which cause relaxation of the lower esophageal sphincter (alcohol, coffee, theophylline).
- o Limit intake of fluids with meals.
- o Avoid cold liquids with meals.
- o Avoid lying down for 4 hours after eating.
- o Eat more during the day and less at night.
- o Consider elevation of head in bed 4-6 inches.

commonly used medications, such as alcohol, theophylline (breathing medicine), nitrates (commonly used in heart disease and hypertension), and calcium channel blockers (very commonly used in hypertension), coffee (even decaf!), chocolate, orange juice, mints, and estrogen. Alcohol includes red and white wine. In general, fatty foods are more likely to produce problems.

Lastly, and very importantly, are cultural or habitual patterns which need to be assessed and possibly changed. This would include avoidance of large amounts of liquids with food, as this creates increased volume and pressure in the stomach, with higher chances for reflux. Strictly avoid cold liquids, which cool off everything in the stomach, including the enzymes and acid which is necessary for the first phase of digestion, which ends when the valve blocking egress of food from the stomach to the intestine, opens, and food gets pushed into the intestine. This will take much longer to occur if the gastric contents are repeatedly cooled by cold beverages, temporarily inactivating the enzymes. The evening meal should be eaten as early as possible or at least allowing four hours before lying down. Lying down neutralizes the effects of gravity and makes reflux more likely to occur. One could also consider eating a little more in mid-day and less in the evening (see chart).

In summary, GERD or acid indigestion, or whatever you call it, is a message being given to you by your stomach and esophagus, this being the main way they transmit bad news. The bad news is that you are doing something wrong. There is an "imbalance" somewhere. Either too much acid is being produced, or it is being made too easy for this acid to get up into the esophagus, where it does not belong. The body is very forgiving most of the time, allowing you to abuse it in a variety of ways, with little in the way of problems. But, we know about the innate "wisdom" of the body through our discussions of incredibly complex healing and protective processes such as inflammation and immunity.

No doubt that the body is trying to deal with the "imbalances" of digestion. However, when it is overwhelmed after you eat a late-night fatty meal, washed down with ice water, and topped off with chocolate, mints, two glasses of wine, and coffee, it cries, "Help!" See this not as a punishment or an annoyance, but as an important message.

Does intention have anything to do with health? Does it ultimately matter whether you intend to be healthy or simply look for another pill to take? Perhaps, the answer to these kinds of questions is not yet known with certainty, but I do believe that intention, the mental/emotional part of us, acting through the brain's limbic system, into the hypothalamus, into the endocrine system via the pituitary gland, and through the autonomic nervous system, does matter, very much.

Hiatus Hernia/Stomach

As we just barely enter into the stomach, we pass through the hole in the diaphragm that allows the GI tract, great vessels, and assorted other tissues to leave the thoracic cavity and enter the abdominal cavity. It is right here at this juncture that a commonly encountered entity is found—that being the "hiatus hernia." I called it an "entity" rather than a disease. This is a structural abnormality which perhaps arises because the hole in the diaphragm is too large. There can be several other possible explanations. Regardless, this allows a portion of the stomach to move upward alongside the esophagus, into the thoracic (chest) cavity. This herniated portion may move up and down, depending on circumstances, or it could stay "fixed" in the chest. It may be small or quite large, perhaps even the size of an orange. Remarkably, most of them seem to cause little if any trouble. GERD/heartburn occurs with or without hiatal hernia. It is diagnosed on X-ray or endoscopy. Most are left alone. Occasionally, if strongly symptomatic or very large, they may need to be surgically corrected.

By entering the stomach, we have entered the working portion of the GI tract, with the work being digestion and eventual absorption of glucose and other nutrients, eventually ear-marked for cells all over the body, to supply the raw products for cellular metabolism to occur. Interestingly, the GI tract is more of an "endocrine gland" than the endocrine system (classically described as pituitary, thyroid, adrenals, and ovaries or testes). These are now identified somewhere between ten to fifteen true hormones, released by GI tissues, travelling to distant sites and affecting function of widely divergent body tissues. A few of these will be mentioned, but the emphasis will remain on digestion and common diseases (see Table).

The major hormone, which stimulates acid secretion in the stomach, is gastrin through its action on the parietal cell with its production of hydrochloric acid. The ability of the stomach to produce acid is prodigious. We already know that too much acid can be harmful. What about too little? The answer is definitely yes. This can result in impaired digestion and absorption of protein, bacterial overgrowth with malabsorption of other nutrients, and diarrhea; and even "heartburn" from bile. Regarding incidence (how common) and prognosis (eventual outcome) of low acid production, there are gaps in our knowledge. It is thought to be possibly associated with increased stomach cancer and gastrointestinal "carcinoid tumors," which can become malignant. It does increase

(Very) Partial List of Gastrointestinal Hormones	
1. Gastrin / cholecystokinin	• Acid production • Pancreatic enzymes • Gall bladder contraction
2. Secretin	• Bicarbonate production
3. Ghrelin	• Appetite stimulation • Growth hormone production
4. Vasoactive intestinal peptide	• Decreases Acid • Increases Insulin
5. Somatostatin	• Inhibits growth hormone production
6. Enkephalin	• Decrease motility
7. Glucagon	• Increases blood sugar level
8. Motilin	• Enhances peristalsis

morbidity. It can be associated with so-called pernicious anemia, in turn caused by vitamin B 12 deficiency, in turn caused by absence of "intrinsic factor," produced by the same stomach cells that produce acid. One of the main causes of destruction of parietal cells is thought to be an autoimmune reaction, i.e., the immune system having been too aggressive in its surveillance in the stomach.

And what about medication, including commonly used OTC meds for acid indigestion? Can they cause a dangerous reduction in acid production? The answer, remarkably, is not known, although it seems it should be known. As mentioned above in discussing heartburn, we tend to see this as a disease needing to be stamped out with pharmaceutical agents, rather than a message to change our ways. Although it is easier to take a pill, we truly do not know what the domino effects of frequent medication usage might be.

There is an amazing story regarding stomachs and acids and ulcer disease which has emerged in the last fifteen to twenty years. The initial tellers of the story were awarded the Nobel Prize in medicine. There are still many crucial unanswered questions. Although we have known about acidity and "ulcers," or "peptic ulcers," or "acid peptic ulcers," or "gastric ulcers," or "duodenal ulcers," or "gastritis" for well over 100 years, it has been only recently that we became aware of the connection between a bacterial infection of the stomach or duodenum, and this condition with all of those names. The name of the bacteria is *Helicobacter pylori*, or "*H. pylori*." It is very commonly found in the lining membrane of the stomach, more common in older people and more commonly in underdeveloped countries. Although it definitely seems to be associated with low-grade chronic gastritis, most people are asymptomatic. When symptoms become severe enough to warrant investigation, if *H. pylori* organisms are found on biopsy of the stomach lining, it is generally recommended that both acid-reducing meds and antibiotics be given to eradicate the infection and prevent further problems.

Things are never that simple. Some researchers feel that *H. pylori* is part of the "normal flora" of the stomach and should be left alone. Up to 40% of people harbor the germ, and yet, most of them have no symptoms. One can say that as interesting as it may be to think about a bacteria being involved with such a common set of diseases of the stomach, it is safe to say that the final chapter regarding *H. pylori* has not been written (perhaps, another Nobel Prize?).

I will briefly mention another hormone, produced in the stomach, and elsewhere, including the hypothalamus (the brain). This hormone is called ghrelin, and very likely is involved in obesity, at least in some people. Ghrelin stimulates hunger. It was noted shortly after bariatric surgery (surgical approaches for obesity) came on the scene that appetite was often dramatically reduced immediately after such surgery. Subsequently, it was found that ghrelin levels are much reduced. In thin people, ghrelin levels are highest between 12:00 midnight and dawn, during sleep, when excessive eating is not an issue. It is not yet known for sure whether or not there is an aberration of circadian rhythm (day–night fluctuations) of ghrelin in obese people.

Stomach cancer is a common disorder, more common above the age of fifty, and twice as common in men as in women. Prognosis is poor, unless discovered very early, "accidentally." There are only sketches of what might be factors involved in its genesis, including most of the conditions mentioned above, including chronic gastritis/gastric atrophy, pernicious anemia, and *H. pylori* infection. Certainly, genetics play a role, as does cigarette smoking and nitrosamines in cured meat.

The pylorus and pyloric valve mark the distal end of the stomach. The most dramatic event involving the stomach is vomiting, which represents forceful contraction of the stomach muscles, often times aided by contraction of abdominal muscles, greatly increasing intra-abdominal and intra-gastric pressures. When the thick pyloric valve at the distal end of the stomach is closed, as part of the vomiting reflex, stomach contents are propelled outward. Although this is a common event, seen in a large number of systemic or local diseases, in frail or obtunded (not completely alert) people, this can be a somewhat dangerous occurrence. Besides the potential for injury to the esophagus, throat, and mouth from acid, there is the real possibility that the first deep breath after emesis (vomiting) could result in aspiration of vomit into the airway. This too, rather remarkably, usually does not result in serious consequences. However, the tracheitis, bronchitis, and pneumonitis, which are potential complications, can all have very serious consequences.

Motility disorders of the stomach are relatively common. When severe enough to be symptomatic, this is understandably called gastric stasis. It can be part of the picture of autonomic dysfunction of the entire intestine, or it could occur in the stomach alone. The most common cause of gastric stasis is diabetes, seen as part of the autonomic neuropathy sometimes present. It can be very problematic, with recurrent vomiting, nausea, destabilization of diabetes, and all the dangers of recurrent vomiting. Medication and dietary changes may be somewhat helpful.

Acid Protection

The final comments regarding the stomach are fascinating from the standpoint of evolution. Our physiology is set up such that acid is necessary for digestion of protein, as well as other possible functions. Gastric secretions are acidic enough to burn the skin. Nevertheless, most of the time, it does not appear to cause any damage to the stomach lining membrane. This is because of a particular arrangement of the way hydrochloric acid produced egresses through specific channels in the mucous layer. There are actually two very thin layers of mucous, the top being loosely attached and the bottom, adjacent to the lining membrane, being very tightly adherent. Acid escapes into the lumen of the stomach through specific channels carved out of this mucous layer, so that in essence, the acid never really contacts the lining membrane. In addition, the lining membrane also produces bicarbonate, which can neutralize any wayward acid molecules in the lining membrane, so that the pH at the lining membrane remains very close to neutral.

Once passed the pyloric valve, into the first part of the intestine, called the duodenum, the lining membrane looks grossly (meaning with the naked eye) similar to that in the stomach. However, it is very different microscopically. It has no acid-producing cells. In fact, the mucous layer described in the stomach is greatly reduced in thickness and increased in permeability such that the duodenum is very susceptible to damage from acid, hence the common "duodenal ulcer." In addition, whereas stomach cancer is relatively common, cancer throughout the duodenum and the remainder of the small intestine is rare.

What you would notice is a prominent pimple-like structure, with an opening in it, called the sphincter of Oddi. This opening is a channel which usually represents the combined channels of the drainage ducts coming out of the liver and carrying bile, as well as drainage from the pancreas, carrying important digestive enzymes. Importantly, besides being critical for digestion, this fluid is strongly alkaline, neutralizing the acidic contents coming from the stomach. Everything is just so beautifully orchestrated!

Liver

The liver is a large, dense organ located on the right upper side of the abdomen, with its dome sitting right under the diaphragm, with lung just above. There are membranes on both upper and lower sides of the diaphragm, contiguous with the same membranes going to the top of the lung and to the lower part of the abdomen. This is one of the reasons why lower lung conditions can be felt in the abdomen and certain abdominal conditions can be felt as high as the neck (recall "referred" pain).

The liver has always seemed a curious thing to me. Certainly, it is crucial for digestion, and its drainage channels empty into exactly the right spot in the intestine to accomplish this. Not wishing to be accused of anthropomorphizing too much, I see the liver as being "the little engine that could." Over the course of evolution, as our early worm-like and then tadpole-like ancestors became increasingly more complex, demanding all kinds of new physiologic processes, such as storage of food energy, release of such energy when needed, manufacture from scratch, the ambrosia of digestion, none other than *glucose*, manufacture of cholesterol and other components of every cell membrane in the body, production of coagulation factors, production of all kinds of crucial proteins—there was the little engine that could, saying "I can do it." If that wasn't enough, who is going to join the emerging immune system producing cellular and humoral components to participate in this joint effort? No one asked the liver to act as a sieve, accepting all the blood from the intestines, filtering it, and dealing with unwanted detritus and all kinds of intoxicants, but the liver took on that task as well. Later, it even took on responsibilities regarding hormone production and blood pressure control. So, that is our selfless hero, the liver, much more than the simple digestive organ that you thought it was.

The Prevestigial (?) Gall Bladder

So, although digestion occurs only sporadically, the liver is working around the clock. The main product for digestion produced by the liver is bile, which is essential for breakdown of fat in preparation for absorption. When produced in between meals, bile comes out of the liver and is diverted into a storage facility, waiting for release during the next meal. That storage facility is the gall bladder. Although this structure is found widely in the animal kingdom, it appears to have seen better days. At some point in our development, it might have been more important than it is now. Because of symptoms which are attributed to the gall bladder, it is frequently removed. The majority of these people without a gall bladder have no obvious short- or long-term disability. A small number have some type of digestive disturbance, with diarrhea being the most common. Others develop specific food intolerances which were not present before. Overall, it is somewhat surprising that so few people have noticeable problems after gall bladder removal, and that itself is the most compelling evidence that perhaps the gall bladder has gone the way of the appendix and is on the evolutionary road toward becoming a vestigial organ.

In general, one can legitimately raise the question as to whether or not too many gall bladders are removed unnecessarily. Abdominal pain is very common. Gallstones are very common. Please recall the dictum that two facts about a related topic may or may not be part of a cause-and-effect arrangement. Many people with gallstones have no discernable digestive problems. It is also known that the presence or absence of gallstones can be a dynamic process, with stones appearing and disappearing from time to time. The point is that the gall bladder should not necessarily be removed just because it has stones. Investigation of abdominal pain and "indigestion" is always challenging. In difficult situations, gall bladder removal is justified, in my opinion, if the following criteria are met: (1) There are symptoms present "compatible with" gall bladder dysfunction. (2) After careful evaluation, no other obvious cause for the symptoms has been found. (3) The patient is in good enough condition to undergo the operation. (4) The patient understands that the possibility exists that the problem will persist, even after the gall bladder is removed. Sometimes, the patient's "vote" is the tiebreaker ("I understand, Doctor. I want you to take out my gallbladder"). Occasionally, we hit the jackpot, and following surgery, the patient states, "this is the best I have felt in years!" Is that subjective or objective? In other words, was the gallbladder chronically inflamed and/or infected and thus seeping "toxins" into the body, or is this just a big, grand placebo effect? I suspect that it is "real," but we need to discuss this hugely important topic.

Placebo Effect

The classical placebo effect is described in terms of the time-honored "sugar pill." Shortly after basic scientific criteria were applied to medical research, it became apparent, accidentally, that sometimes people undergoing experimentation had a predictable or anticipated response, when nothing was done. Eventually, experiments were designed to take this phenomenon into consideration, culminating in the often-mentioned, double-blinded, randomized *placebo-controlled* studies involving sugar pills, or reasonable facsimiles. The most unbelievable study ever done in the history of medicine using a placebo group was at the beginning of the cardiac revascularization era, in the 1950s. After experiments in dogs, investigators in Montreal began to use a procedure whereby the internal mammary artery, running under the breast bone, was implanted or tunneled directly into the heart muscle with the thought that it might relieve angina by increasing blood flow to the heart muscle. A control group was used, in which the chest was opened and then closed, but no implantation was done. In fact, the placebo group showed a marked reduction in angina, which was used to compare with the results of the implantation. Obviously, such an experimental protocol would never be allowed at this time because of the risk to the patient. However, it does point to the power of the placebo response. Numerous studies have documented that the placebo response is very substantial and, in some studies, is as high as 30%. This is where we learn the lesson of humility. It is humbling to acknowledge that the mind is so powerful, i.e., "mind over matter," that it appears to be able to affect cures by intent. *Cures by intent!*

So, the placebo response is a great teacher. It tells us that biologic systems have a level of complexity which extends beyond anything which would be statistically or mathematically predicted. Biologic responses, especially when the whole organism is taken into consideration, with its genetics, its life experience, the continual interaction between these functions, and its magnificent limbic system, the seat of our emotional responses may eventually escape formulaic explanations no matter how sophisticated the computer simulations may be. In a way, I hope so. That may be the last bastion that may perpetually separate us from the coming of our robotic peers, intellectually far superior to us. Recognition of the placebo effect, with its powerful ability to heal, is beyond our intellectual grasp and deeply humbling. Incidentally, more about our robotic family, later.

Back to the gall bladder. There are two very nasty conditions which can affect this possibly vestigial organ. Both are relatively unusual, to rare. The gall bladder can be the seat of primary malignancies. They are rare, except in certain widely separated ethnic or geographic groups, particularly northern India and Central and South America. Gangrene of the gall bladder is uncommon, but seen sporadically, and represents the breakdown of the walls of the gall bladder, with spillage of infected and caustic material into the abdominal cavity. Both of these conditions are potentially life threatening and require prompt surgical attention to improve chances of survival.

The prodigious list of activities in which the liver is involved has been mentioned. It is easy to appreciate that chronic liver disease could result in widespread cellular dysfunction, subtle or overt, with many different possible avenues causing such dysfunction. Clinically, occasionally, one can identify one major area of dysfunction, which could be life threatening, with many other areas of function appearing flawless. So, there is a great deal of individual variability in how liver disease expresses itself. In addition, diseases may occur very precipitously and quickly prove to be fatal, or serious problems such as viral or cancerous conditions can smolder for years. Once again, there appears to be built-in marked individual variability, a common keynote in complex biologic systems.

The liver gets its blood supply from two sources. One is arterial blood having come from the left side of the heart, just as most other tissues receive theirs. However, it is useful to envision the liver as a large venous sump. It is estimated that at certain times, up to 25% of all the blood in the body may be in the liver. The second supply of blood is venous blood, all of it coming from the intestinal tract. Therefore, all of the materials absorbed from the gut, whether it be drugs, nutrients, water, and everything that was in it, including viruses, bacteria, parasites, alcohol, and environmental toxins filters through (not just flows through) the liver. As daunting as this may seem, the liver is prepared to deal with most of it, especially if the exposure is not excessive. The Kupffer cells in the venous sinusoids of the liver are functionally part of the immune system as a first line of defense.

In addition, the liver cells themselves are genetically programmed to deal with the onslaught.

Hepatitis A

However, as always, depending on the balance between "us" and "them," the defenses can be overwhelmed. It is the interposition of the liver—between the gut and the heart—that makes it so vulnerable. Venous blood leaving the liver drains directly into the inferior vena carva and then into the right side of the heart. Inflammation of the liver is called "hepatitis." There are many different forms of hepatitis, including several common and serious forms. There are three viruses which are especially likely to cause hepatitis, conveniently named A, B, and C (there are others of lesser frequency). Hepatitis A has been a common infection in childhood and is generally so mild that it may not be detected as such, with diagnosis identified years later as a positive antibody titer. The illness can be moderately severe in susceptible adults, but recovery always occurs spontaneously, although the illness may last four to eight weeks.

Hepatoma and Hepatitis B and C

Hepatitis B and C are more serious in nature because of their tendency to become chronic. This chronicity can result in intermittent or even continuous low-grade symptoms and also predisposes the person to eventual chronic liver failure or hepatoma, which is the primary cancer of the liver. Please note that cancer in the liver is a very common finding in many types of cancer originating elsewhere in the body. When a cancer at any site spreads by the vascular system to a site physically separated from the primary site, it is said to have metastasized, with the area of spread called metastasis or metastases. Since the liver has such a lush blood supply, it is frequently the site of metastases from many divergent types of tumors. When this occurs, it always presents major challenges in terms of "cure" and, depending on the size and number of metastases, may make a cure impossible. Primary cancer of the liver that is arising in the liver cells when present nowhere else is an unusual tumor and is usually associated with chronic hepatitis B or C infection. It is also seen in end-stage liver disease, called "cirrhosis," of many causes, with chronic alcohol toxicity being the most common. As can be surmised, it tends to be seen most commonly in geographic areas where hepatitis B and C are most common, such as Africa and China, where it is relatively common. It is relatively uncommon in most parts of the world. Prognosis is very poor. Surgical removal, or liver transplantation, at this time represents the best chance for cure.

Back to hepatitis B. It is a very common infection in endemic areas, with 10% to 15% of infected people becoming chronic carriers, i.e., not spontaneously cured. In endemic cases, transmission usually occurs at the time of birth or in childhood. In areas with low prevalence of infection, intravenous drug abuse and/or unprotected sex are the most common modes of infection. Fortunately, there is an effective vaccine available, highly recommended for susceptible populations and for people traveling to endemic areas.

Hepatitis C is the most dangerous of the viruses infecting the liver, as only about 25% of those infected spontaneously clear the virus and 75% to 80% remain infected. No vaccine is available. Treatment is available but with two significant limitations. The course of treatment is long and arduous, with patients feeling poorly during treatment, even though they may have no symptoms before treatment. In addition, treatment is effective in eradication of the virus only about half the time. The propensity toward development of cirrhosis is high, as it is in hepatitis B, although the possibility of liver cancer is less. Symptoms of chronic infection without cirrhosis may be subtle or may include joint pain, fatigue, itching, and chronic flu-like illness. Transmission occurs by contaminated blood products, intravenous drug abuse, tattooing, and sharing of personal items.

There are other forms of "hepatitis," including acute and chronic, several of which are quite common. There is a very common entity, rather unglamorously called "fatty liver." In fact, that seems to be the basic problem, with an increase of fat deposition in the liver. It is sometimes seen in people with diabetes and sometimes in obese people as well. Occasionally, it is seen with no obvious association with any other disease process. It usually comes to attention "accidentally," when minor aberrations of liver tests are found with blood testing, done perhaps as part of a routine examination. When tracked over several years, it often shows some degree of fluctuation, with tests occasionally normal and usually only slightly out of line when abnormal. Generally, people with this condition have no symptoms. It is necessary to check for hepatitis B and C. When seen as an isolated phenomenon, there is no specific treatment. When related to diabetes and/or obesity, if those issues can be successfully treated, it usually resolves or improves. There is a low level of concern about this condition. However, because of the fact that we can "never say never," a small percentage of people appear to have a progressive disorder, which can lead to cirrhosis.

There is also a form of hepatitis associated with alcohol intake. Recall that alcohol is metabolized by the liver. This can occur in a person who is not a regular drinker of alcohol but perhaps drinks substantially the day before a blood test is done. In this person, the blood tests are usually back to normal in a few days. It can also be seen in people who drink alcohol "socially," but regularly. In this case, unless they reduce or eliminate alcohol consumption, the hepatitis, as documented on blood testing, may persist. Once again, it is necessary to check for hepatitis B and C. This may be the precursor of alcoholic cirrhosis.

With the finding of hepatitis, it is always useful to think about the possibility of a drug-induced injury. Acetaminophen (Tylenol), alone or in any combination, is likely the most common. Other commonly used drugs can inflame the liver, including antibiotics like amoxicillin and furadantin (used for urinary tract infection), antibiotics used for skin infection, antituberculosis, and antifungal agent (toenail fungus), and cholesterol lowering drugs.

Lastly, there is an unusual form of hepatitis called autoimmune, with the presumption that there is either something slightly unusual about the liver cells or the immune system itself, such that the immune system detects "other" when there may not be any other. This form of hepatitis has a strong predilection for young and middle-aged women, sometimes seen in conjunction with other suspected autoimmune conditions and sometimes with a blood test picture including auto-antibodies, which is highly suggestive of the diagnosis. Confirmation of diagnosis is made by liver biopsy. Treatment is available, albeit not without some danger in itself.

Generally speaking, the diagnosis of hepatitis is made on blood sampling. Liver biopsy is not always needed. Although done with a needle and not requiring surgery, since the liver is such a vascular organ, the major risk of liver biopsy is excessive hemorrhage. Because of this, doctors need to carefully select who are those people with hepatitis, in whom the information gained from liver biopsy, whether it be for prognostic or therapeutic reasons is sufficiently important to warrant a possible major complication.

Cirrhosis/Alcohol Ingestion

The term cirrhosis has been used a number of times already. It is an important term implying that there has been severe damage of the liver, with the appearance of scarring. Recall that "scar tissue" is often the end result of an inflammatory condition which is, in turn, the end result of the body's attempt to respond to something causing irritation. We have already discussed how this "irritation" can be part of "them," such as infection or cells turned cancerous. It can be the result of an autoimmune reaction (possibly a mistake by the body). Now, we see that it can also occur from toxic substances, such as alcohol or medications. Alcohol intake is the most common cause of cirrhosis, with viral hepatitis a distant second. There is a truism which is perhaps most apparent with liver disease—that being that we generally enjoy major organ function with built-in huge surpluses of functional capability. Most of the major internal organs, with a notable exception being the brain, do not alert us with symptoms until approximately half of the organ has been destroyed. In some cases, such as with the kidney (to be soon discussed) and the liver, function may have to be reduced by 75%, i.e., only 25% of function remaining, before we get the message via symptoms. This is true for the liver. Even though the liver may be severely damaged, if the cause of the damage is identified and eliminated, the person can remain reasonably healthy and possibly live out a full life span.

Regeneration

Lastly, the liver is truly remarkable and unique in one way. It is the only major organ in the body that has the potential for substantial regeneration. This applies to both a diseased liver, if the disease can be arrested, and to a liver which has been partly surgically resected. For instance, with cirrhosis, if the cause of the cirrhosis, perhaps alcohol, is eliminated, within the interstices of the heavy bands of scar tissue, liver cells can begin to regenerate. Alternately, occasionally as part of a comprehensive approach to treatment of cancer in the liver, either primary or metastatic, a large portion of the liver may need to be removed. In this situation also, the liver is likely to partially regenerate. In fact, changes of gene expression can be identified within minutes of resection by the appearance of transcription factors (proteins that bind to specific DNA sequences, controlling the transfer of genetic information from DNA to messenger RNA), mitogens (substances promoting mitosis, i.e., cell division), and growth factors (putting the pedal to the metal). Each of these is responsible for a separate cell type, such as hepatocytes (liver cells), vascular tissues, and bile ducts. Needless to say, observations such as this have provided medical scientists with abundant fodder for further research in how to stimulate growth of tissues other than the liver.

We began the discussion of the liver remarking about the huge array of functions that it fulfills. We finish on its unique abilities. Quite a story for a brown, heavy, blood-soaked appendage of the intestinal tract!

Pancreas

Recall that the pimple noted just beyond the stomach, into the duodenum, usually carries products for digestion both from the liver and the pancreas. The pancreas is a much smaller organ, behind and below the stomach, just in front of the spine, whose digestive products deal mostly with carbohydrate metabolism. In addition, it produces several hormones of major importance, including insulin, going directly into the bloodstream, to act at distant sites, as is typical for hormones. The digestive enzymes from the pancreas are strongly alkaline, neutralizing acidity from the stomach. This "exocrine" function, meaning excreting substances into the lumen of the intestine, is crucial for digestion and for maintaining the integrity of duodenum. Were it not for the strongly alkaline pancreatic secretions, the duodenum would be "toast," perpetually ulcerated, and eventually scarred and blocked. Historically, this was a common occurrence, resulting in the frequent need for surgery to assist in management of ulcer disease. Over the last twenty to thirty years, however, with usage of two generations of potent acid-reducing types of medication, the need for surgical intervention for ulcer disease has dropped dramatically.

Insulin and Glucogen

In addition to its crucial "exocrine" function, the pancreas also has equally crucial "endocrine" functions, meaning production of hormones which directly enter the blood stream. The best known of these is insulin, whose complex action basically facilitates transfer of glucose from the blood into the cells, where it is utilized as fuel, through its linkage to ATP. Insulin and its companion hormone glucagon are both released from clusters of specialized cells scattered throughout the pancreas. The vast majority of pancreatic cells are involved with exocrine (digestive) function. However, a tiny portion of cellular material found in these clusters, perhaps one million clusters in all and widely dispersed in the substance of the pancreas, produces insulin and glucagon. These clusters appearing grossly and microscopically as islands of endocrine cells scattered in a sea of exocrine cells are called the islets of Langerhans, which is named after the medical student who first described them. (Quite a feather in the cap for that medical student!) There are three cell types in the islets: the first two are the alpha cells secreting glucagon and beta cells secreting insulin, both into the blood stream. Eating, and subsequent digestion, allows glucose to be separated out and absorbed. Glucose entering the beta cells via the circulation triggers release of insulin, which in turn opens the cellular gates of the rest of the body, especially liver and muscle, so that glucose can enter easily. As glucose levels begin to fall, insulin release drops and eventually stops. This sequential dance between glucose and insulin is very, very tightly choreographed. If slightly too much insulin has been released, this is sensed by the alpha cells in the islets and glucagon is released, causing the liver to break down the storage depot of glucose—that being glycogen—and thus releasing glucose.

Feedback Loops and Gut Feelings

Many metabolic and neurologic processes in the body are controlled by these kinds of delicate feedback loops, with many diseases resulting from improper sequencing in the feedback loops. The autonomic nervous system, just to make things a little more complicated, also has some influence on insulin release, obviously tying insulin release, at least somewhat, to the brain!

Somatostatin

The third hormone released by the islets, specifically from delta cells, is somatostatin. In some ways, it seems to be the most interesting of the three perhaps because its most crucial functions, if there are any, are shrouded in complexity. It is generally considered to be an inhibitory hormone. Perhaps, that is all that needs to be said, as we know how important the brakes are on any vehicle. Besides the pancreas, it is also produced in the stomach, small intestine, and most notably in the hypothalamus (brain). Notice the number of *gastrointestinal* (GI) hormones which either have receptors in the brain, or affect the brain, or share production with the brain. This is especially interesting in reference to the commonly used expression about having a "gut feeling."

In the gut, we do know that it decreases many other GI hormones, with the net effect being delayed gastric emptying, reduced peristalsis (contraction waves through the luminal GI tract), reduced pancreatic exocrine secretion, reduced hunger, and reduction in production of its islet mates, the alpha and beta cells, with less glucagon and insulin secretion. Which of these is the most important? Not known.

In the hypothalamus, somatostatin is shunted right down to the pituitary gland, where it inhibits growth hormone secretion. Now that seems quite interesting in view of the fact that growth hormone has numerous functions, mostly anabolic, placing it at the top of the "anabolic steroid list" of abused substances. So, it is all very intricate, difficult to study, and thus still somewhat mysterious. Perhaps, as the basis of its role becomes better understood, it may one day be in the spotlight…somatostatin.

Diabetes

After beating around the bush for several paragraphs, it appears to be the appropriate time to discuss a contemporary "epidemic." Even doctors are calling it an epidemic, although, medically speaking, that term is usually saved for infectious diseases. The disease is diabetes. Is it caused by an infection, particularly a contagious one, or are we simply getting sloppy with our terminology?

Most people have at least some notion about there being two different kinds of diabetes, type I and type II. In fact, these two types are radically different diseases, sharing abnormalities of insulin availability. They are just about as different as benign and malignant tumors (technically both called "neoplasms," meaning "new growths"). Type I, sometimes called "juvenile" diabetes, although it can come on later in life, is an autoimmune disease, whereby the islet cells of the pancreas are destroyed by the immune system and insulin production is permanently abolished. Glucagon production is gone understandably, as with insulin loss, there would appear to be no reason for a need to have the liver increase glucose production. Somatostatin production, produced in other areas of the body and once again giving it an aura of importance to have several back-up systems, appears to be intact.

Prior to the development of insulin supplementation in the 1920s, people with this condition, mostly young people, were doomed to die. This was known since antiquity. What is not quite as clear is whether type II was also present. Likely, it was. Regardless, the only treatment, which could prolong life, was that of extremely low caloric intake. Observers in the 1920s considered the cure by use of insulin injections to be truly miraculous, as people who had been dwindling away, at the brink of death, rapidly recovered. The cause for the sudden destruction of islet cells remains unclear, except that it involves autoimmunity. As with other autoimmune diseases, there are speculations as to what the trigger mechanisms might be. The usual suspects are viruses, possibly other infections, toxicity, genetics, and combinations. Perhaps none of those is correct. It seems that as long as people with this condition will take their insulin and regulate it as best as possible, in some ways— because they may not have the full-blown "metabolic syndrome" of type II diabetes—they may do better than type II diabetics. Type I diabetes is found scattered throughout the world, with clusters in certain ethnic groups, usually inbred, suggesting genetic mechanisms in those cases. I don't think that the "epidemic" involves type I.

Type II or "adult onset" diabetes is epidemic in the world. In my opinion, its prevalence is greatly underestimated. It is now very, very common, much more than the reported 18% of people over the age of sixty. I would guess that the 18% figure would apply to people at forty-five years of age. By age sixty, it's likely 25% to 35% of the population. It is assumed that the rapidly rising rates over the last twenty years are secondary to lifestyle changes centering on obesity and low energy output, i.e., indolence, or the "couch potato syndrome." In support of this notion is the theory that for the minority of people who significantly change their lifestyles, the diabetes goes into hibernation, becoming invisible. However, against this logical theory is that I am not convinced that the differences in our lifestyle over the past twenty to thirty years is sufficiently different now to explain this explosion of type II disease. Since it is well known that our genes are constantly interacting with the environment, the nature versus nurture debate is over; both nature and nurture, and the nature–nurture interaction, are crucial. Perhaps, we have simply entered a stage of rapid genetic change. (Recall that the wolf became the dog in approximately fifty years.) Perhaps, both explanations are correct, allowing us to use the safety net of the "multi-factorial" denomination. Even scarier, maybe none of these current speculations are correct.

In stark contrast to type I, type II diabetes is not an autoimmune disease. In fact, at least early on, there is not even a lack of insulin. Although I have never seen it quite described this way, perhaps we can look at "adult onset" diabetes as consisting of types II-A and II-B. Type II-A would be then early on, particularly in the obese, underactive people, with A1C under ten. (A1C is the current "standard" for assessment of severity of type I and type II diabetes. Levels up to 6.0, or 6.5, are considered normal.) In this situation, we do actually see the terminology that was attached to the metabolic syndrome in the late 1980s, i.e., "insulin resistance," as part of the problem. There is also what could be called "glucagon–insulin desynchrony." Recall that in a healthy person, rise in blood sugar after eating immediately triggers release of precise amounts of insulin to reduce the blood sugar, with glucagon ready to make corrections if slightly too much insulin was released, and blood sugar is heading down too much. In type II diabetes, release of insulin in response to rising blood sugar may be slightly delayed. Maybe this is part of the "insulin resistance." Then, when it is finally released, which may be off by only a matter of minutes or ten to twenty points of blood sugar, the beta cells may release too much insulin, making it possible for blood sugar to drop too fast and too much. Although many people without a diagnosis of diabetes describe themselves as being "hypoglycemic" (low blood sugar), without documentation of this, this is the clinical situation in which documentable hypoglycemia can unequivocally occur, even though glucagon release tries to obviate this possibility. This is why it has been known for a long time that hypoglycemia may be a very early sign of diabetes.

After adding up all the insulin released in twenty-four hours in a type II-A diabetic, it may be that normal or even excessive amounts are being released. Some doctors speculate that constant overproduction of insulin causes islet cells to "burn out." There is no proof for this, but this could be a tie-in with type II-B. In this condition, there is a gradual drop-off of islet cell numbers and function, so that eventually insulin deficiency is seen. So, early on, we have desynchronization of glucose metabolism. Later on, we may have persistent elevation of glucose levels, as islet cell numbers and function decline. Some doctors think that in genetically predisposed people, this islet cell drop-off is a function of senescence (aging). This may be correct. What about drugs? Could the drugs we use to treat type II-A diabetes lead to type II-B, with the need to add insulin? Obviously, we don't know.

So now, we have the background and knowledge to have some understanding as to how non-insulin drugs work, alone or in combination. I agree that the chemists who named these drugs should be severely punished or, at least, threatened with such.

(1) Sulfonylureas—the oldest class, and still widely used, stimulate the beta cell to produce more insulin. Since they do this even in the setting of normal blood sugar levels, there is always a chance for hypoglycemia. We have fifty years of experience with these drugs, examples of which are glipizide or glyburide.

(2) Biguanides—such as metformin, which is perhaps the most widely used of all oral diabetic drugs. They inhibit the liver from breaking down glycogen, which is the storage form of glucose. They have a very long track record and low likelihood of causing hypoglycemia.

(3) Thiazolidinediones (TZD)—reduces insulin resistance, making what is available, more effective. Several of these have been pulled from the market because of side effects, with Avandia and Actos still available.

(4) Alpha-glucosidase inhibitors—block enzymes in the intestine which break down starch, which leads to less glucose available for absorption. Popularity of these drugs (and possibly of patients using them) is limited because of increased flatulence and diarrhea.

(5)   Meglitinides—stimulate beta cells to produce insulin, only when glucose levels are high. Prandin and Starlix are examples.

(6)   Dipeptidyl peptidase IV inhibitors—both stimulate beta cells and reduce liver glucose production (Januvia).

In people with type II diabetes, there is substantial resistance to the use of insulin, as islet cell function degrades. Some people have true needle phobia. Insulin needles are remarkably fine (small gauge) and short (one half inch). Sometimes, I tell people that the only way to hurt themselves is to trip and accidentally poke their eyes.

There are a number of what sounds like other varieties of diabetes, including gestational diabetes and steroid-induced diabetes. These conditions are the result of temporary hormone imbalances. These people may be another example (along with documented hypoglycemia) of people who may be "pre-diabetic." The same type of situation is seen in people who develop high blood sugars in response to any significant illness, such as flu, pneumonia, trauma, need for surgery, etc. Once again, in these situations, there is a temporary increase in a stress hormone production, precipitating a temporary diabetic state. The punch line is that patients such as those should consider themselves to be diabetic and should invoke all of the lifestyle choices necessary to keep themselves "pre-diabetic" rather than flagrantly diabetic.

Lastly, the basic end result of dysregulation of glucose metabolism has a domino effect, causing widespread metabolic dysfunction and involvement in a condition of widespread vascular inflammation. There are other culprits in this scheme, but diabetes and tobacco abuse are likely the most incendiary. What we therefore see clinically for the most part is vascular compromise, involving both large arteries and tiny arterioles. The distribution seems to be peculiar to individual patients, as is so often the case in this very complex biologic machine we call the body. It is the location of the part of the body involved, and whether the damage is mostly in large or very small arteries that determines what symptoms arise, and what treatment options are available. The list of complications is known to most people with diabetes, including kidney failure, with the need for dialysis or transplant; hypertension; heart disease of all types, possibly leading to heart failure; cerebrovascular disease, leading to strokes and dementia; peripheral vascular disease leading to impotency, muscle loss, gangrene, and amputations; vision problems, even leading to blindness; and neuropathy which can occur anywhere, and result in perpetual pain. This is truly a horrible litany. However, of course, there are some people who live to a ripe old age with no complications. There will be more said about this puzzling randomness in the concluding comments about preparing for the end.

Metabolic Syndrome

You don't want your doctor ever to tell you that you have metabolic syndrome or, even worse than that, you are a "metabolic syndrome patient." If he or she does, it is just about the same as your schoolmate in sixth grade calling you a "fat slob," and it is obviously time to find a new doctor—hopefully a fat one.

The term metabolic syndrome was first used in the 1950s, underwent clarification in the 1970s, and too much clarification in the late 1980s, when it was proposed that "insulin resistance" was the key element. Recall that "syndrome" refers to a constellation of symptoms. It is not usually expected that a given person will have every element of the constellation. After all, constellations are big (consider the Milky Way). "Insulin resistance" is a term which is not really different from pre-diabetes, which may be only two pounds different than diabetes. Most biologic phenomena occur on a continuum, hence the bell-shaped curve. The attempt to define the metabolic syndrome as being a state of "insulin resistance" is too restrictive, in my opinion. The constellation includes obesity, sedentary lifestyle, insulin resistance/diabetes, low high-density lipoprotein, high triglycerides, high blood pressure, fatty liver, and increased systemic inflammatory markers.

Obesity is not a uniform finding in metabolic syndrome. Then, what is meant by obesity? Unfortunately, the body mass index (BMI) has come into vogue, particularly with people who may be candidates for bariatric surgery, as insurance companies may use the BMI to decide if they will or will not pay for it. Most of the patients who come to my office cannot relate to "30 kg/m²." There are other attempts to define obesity. There are ratios between circumference of the body at the waste and hip. There are calipers measuring thickness of skin. You can be immersed in water and be told your percentage of body fat quite precisely. Personally, I subscribe to the Justice Potter Stewart method. That is, "I know it when I see it" (whether it is pornography or obesity). I usually ask a person to reflect on their lives. How much did you weigh in high school? When you graduated college? When you went into military service? When you were married? Most of the time, people remember those numbers. Assuming the person has not been grossly obese all of their life, that figure is the figure to start with, regarding (1) an ideal weight and (2) a real-life acceptable weight.

Remember the story of John Doe—gifted athlete to obese amputee. Here is a fact that you will resent and resist. That's OK. It is still a fact. (Please don't attack me, as I am only the messenger.) In ideal circumstances, a person should weigh less in their fifties or sixties or beyond than they did in high school or when they were married.

This is because muscle mass, a water-logged dense tissue, normally diminishes during the aging process. Exercise may slow the process, but it does not stop it for most people. Muscle mass is usually maximal at about age twenty. Therefore, in the ideal world, not the real world, a person weighing 160 pounds at age twenty, should weigh 150 pounds at age sixty, and 140 pounds at age eighty (loss of twenty pounds of muscle). So, that same person weighing 190 pounds at age sixty is forty pounds overweight. Split the difference, and set a goal to lose 20 pounds over the course of one year. That turns out to be a caloric deficit of only 150 calories per day. This is very achievable by most people. The two main instructions are to be patient and be consistent. Overdoing it by 1,000 calories for one per day in a week negates the whole process! Slow and steady.

Not intending to sound sadistic, I love to see patients with newly diagnosed diabetes. Incidentally, as of this writing, it is recommended that the diagnosis be based on the hemoglobin A1C level, specifically greater than 6, or more recently suggested 6.5. So, technically, if your level is 6.1, you are diabetic. I am happy to see them because I have nothing but good news for them, and to use the vernacular, I can "empower" them. The formula is self-evident: (1) Lose weight (ten to twenty pounds, depending on level of A1C), (2) Eliminate table sugar (3) Proportionally, reduce carbohydrate intake somewhat (4) Exercise (any type, but preferably thirty minutes of aerobic activity five times per week). Any of these individual factors are effective. When all four are utilized, results are virtually guaranteed. No medication. "This is not cancer… you are not helpless at the feet of your doctor…you can fix this yourself."

I send them out the door and tell them to return in three months for re-evaluation. Many people do not return voluntarily. Those who are successful do return. The unsuccessful ones are begged to return to see what the problems with initiation of this fool-proof method might have been. Another pep talk, and one more three-month trial. If they fail again, as many do, they get the pills. Walking out the door with pills represents a sad failure. Most diabetics cannot do what they need to do, i.e., use the message of diabetes to develop a healthy lifestyle. Please recall the multitudes of hormones which have receptors in the hypothalamus, which connects with the limbic system (the "emotional" brain), the pre-frontal cortex, and other areas of the cortical, "thinking" brain. Where is the breakdown? It has the appearance of apathy or dysthymia (on the road to depression) so pervasive in society. Or perhaps, it is the false notion that pills are as good as intention. Lack of willpower? But maybe, it all has to do with receptor function or dysfunction. In that sense, maybe for some, diabetes is hopeless. Ultimately, those who are given and use medication appear to be at a distinct advantage over these who do not use it. Pills are better than nothing, but fall short compared to intention.

Diabetes is a terrible scourge. It has an element of randomness about it, just like the shooter walking into a building or climbing to the top of the tower. Although there is some correlation between level of diabetic control and incidence of complications, the correlation is not tight. That is, even people who are well controlled can develop terrible complications, and occasionally, even these poorly controlled may escape complications. Right now, the reasons for this remain obscure. Perhaps, it has something to do with the "co-morbidities" (other accompanying diseases frequently seen) in any given diabetic. Likely, answers to this seeming paradox will be forthcoming. But, there is some correlation. Don't forget about intent. The brain, including the cortex, is involved in the course of all chronic diseases. Trying to be well, even if not fully succeeding, may be the missing link.

Pancreatic Cancer

Thus, we have spilled much ink defining one common disease of the pancreas. We will now discuss a few others much more quickly. First, let's discuss quickly cancer of the pancreas. It too is a horrible disease. It is somewhat common and very difficult to diagnose. By the time definitive symptoms arise, the disease is usually incurable. There have been several heroic surgical procedures devised to try to save people. In terms of risk factors, there is little known. Family history of pancreatic cancer, cigarette smoking, obesity, and chronic pancreatitis appears to predispose. Light to modest alcohol intake does not seem to predispose. Some studies have pointed to helicobacter infection, but that is not conclusive. Less than 5% of people with this disease appear to be permanently cured, with life expectancy of six months to two years after diagnosis.

Pancreatitis

Acute pancreatitis, an inflammation of the pancreas, at least diagnosed clinically, is not very common. We know that it can be part of a mumps virus infection and likely caused by other viruses as well. Very high triglyceride levels can precipitate an attack. Some cases are caused by blunt injury to the abdomen. A few types of drugs, including diuretics and anticonvulsants, are linked to acute episodes. Cigarette smoking (surprise!) increases the risk. It can rarely be seen as part of a widespread autoimmune reaction. Many isolated cases appear to be truly idiopathic, meaning no definite causative factor can be found.

Because of the potent digestive enzymes manufactured in the pancreas, there is a fine line between acute and chronic pancreatitis. It is not hard to imagine that with acute pancreatitis of any kind, enzymes may leak from the pancreas, damaging pancreatic architecture by digestion of pancreas instead of digestion of food and setting the stage for further episodes.

By far, the two most common causes of both acute and chronic pancreatitis are gallstone disease and alcoholism. In most people, the biliary duct from the liver and gallbladder and the pancreatic duct combine just before they jointly enter the duodenum, at the sphincter of Oddi. Gallstones that make their way to the sphincter, but are too large to pass through, can block the pancreatic duct, perhaps sufficiently to cause spillage of enzymes into the pancreas itself. Once damage is done, as noted above, even if the gallbladder and stones are subsequently removed, recurrent pancreatitis is a possibility. I do not think that the presence of asymptomatic gallstones is sufficient to warrant gallbladder removal to protect the pancreas alone, although that may be one consideration.

Alcoholism is an addictive disease. In fact, despite the severe pain and danger associated with pancreatitis, the person may continue to drink alcohol. If so, it is likely the bouts of pancreatitis will continue. Islet cells are also destroyed, and diabetes ensues. In some people, the pancreas may be damaged so severely that there is no longer enough tissue to produce enzymes, and the disease may thus "burn out." Unfortunately, after years of alcohol abuse and with diabetes, these people are usually doomed to chronic illness.

ERCP

Before moving on to the small intestines, I will briefly mention a diagnostic procedure which has become relatively common. It is called "ERCP." As noted before, the ampulla of Vater can be easily identified at the time of endoscopy. This punctuate opening can be relatively easily entered, at which time contrast material can be inserted into the biliary and pancreatic ducts, followed by a series of X-ray pictures. This can be very helpful in the diagnosis of jaundice, which may involve blockage of the biliary channel, backup of bile in the ducts and blood, with subsequent

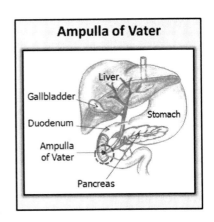

Ampulla of Vater

yellow discoloration of the skin. The common things causing such obstruction include stones and tumors of various types and strictures. At times, the procedure can be therapeutic as well as diagnostic, in that the sphincter opening can be enlarged to allow for the passage of stones. Strictures can be dilated. Biopsies can be done. As with any other invasive procedure, there is some risk, which is generally higher with this type of endoscopy than with most others. There is now a technique using MRI which may give comparable diagnostic information, with a lesser degree of risk.

Intestine

By the time intestinal contents leave the duodenum, almost all of the crucial materials needed for completion of digestion, with subsequent absorption into the blood, have been supplied. The small intestine comprising the short duodenum, and then the much longer jejunum and ileum, extends to approximately seven feet. All along this course, with contraction waves moving digestive products forward, digestion is continuing while absorption begins. The surface area of the small intestine is greatly increased by a series of foldings of the lining membrane, not necessarily appreciated from a casual glance. The image of a tennis court is once again borrowed, as a representation of the possible surface area, this time with the products of digestion on one side and the blood vessels (capillaries) on the other. The actual absorption takes place on villi and microvilli, which are outpouchings produced by the folding of the lining membrane, like an accordion.

Although there are many systemic processes which can affect intestinal function, for the most part, there are relatively few primary small intestinal disorders which would be considered common. For instance, malignancies are less common than in most other internal organs. Since it is absolutely essential that things move along and through the intestine, one might guess that disorders of motility might be important. In fact, motility disorders are seen in acute illnesses, such as viral syndrome, or after surgery, but chronic motility disorders are uncommon with one exception. In the ensuing paragraphs, I will attempt to sketch out the relatively common diseases (primary) and conditions (secondary).

IBS and the "Diagnosis of Exclusion"

Beginning with motility, the one common disorder seen is "irritable bowel syndrome" (IBS). This is another of those diseases whereby we think we know what it is, but there is no single or definitive diagnostic study that clinches the diagnosis. Therefore, it becomes a "diagnosis of exclusion." This term represents an important concept in medicine and is relatively easy to understand. It refers to the fact that a diagnosis of IBS or any other disease without a diagnostic "clincher" cannot be made confidently without considering several to many other potential diagnoses. In other words, once the other diagnoses are excluded, one can more confidently presume the diagnosis under consideration. Depending on many different circumstances, the "excluding" part of the algorithm can occur along different pathways. One of the considerations might be how easy or difficult it may be to exclude other issues. If only one imaging study or one blood test suffices to exclude most or all serious problems, most doctors would order that test. However, if the exclusion process is going to be arduous, with many different types of diagnostic studies, including invasive studies, which always carry a risk of adverse reaction, or if the evaluation is going to be exceedingly costly, and especially if the patient is not adequately insured, the diagnostic algorithm at some juncture will likely be truncated.

With irritable bowel syndrome, there are generally not systemic symptoms (involving the whole body), but a list of potential symptoms which involve the abdomen and/or pelvis, and "sound" like they may be digestive-related. At its core, we think that IBS represents dysfunctional motility. The clearest notion of this might be the concept that instead of the beautifully orchestrated waves of contraction, sweeping evenly all the way from esophagus to anus, there are areas of disordered contraction. For instance, if two segments close together are contracting simultaneously, and the downstream contraction is not moving forward as it should, pressure will quickly build up in the intervening segment and cause pain. Delayed peristalsis may be occurring off and on at a number of points at any given time, setting the stage for excessive fermentation of digestive products with subsequent production of gas and bloating.

Emphasizing again, the precise mechanisms are not known. We think that the autonomic nervous system, which controls peristalsis, is involved. Recall again that the ANS has connections with different parts of the brain, including the limbic system and the cortex, so emotional and "thinking" states are involved.

As always, and especially in a condition representing a "diagnosis of exclusion," meticulous history taking is the key to proper diagnosis. In fact, getting back to the concept of how much of an investigation should be done, that is, the abovementioned three different pathways of investigation, the first might be history alone. The symptoms of IBS are usually multiple. The possibilities include bloating, increased gas, which could be belching and/or flatulence, and/or distention, diarrhea and/or constipation, "indigestion," acid reflux, nausea, and abdominal pain, often migratory. When this history is obtained in an individual who looks well, is relatively young, whose symptoms are somewhat intermittent, who has not deliberately lost weight, whose physical exam and basic laboratory profile are unrevealing, and in whom the symptoms are linked to stressful situations, the diagnosis may be relatively assured, and no further investigation may be needed, particularly if the person is underinsured. On the other end of the spectrum, in a person who looks ill, has lost weight, and has abnormal exam and lab findings, even with the same symptoms, they will likely need a full investigation to exclude truly serious issues.

This is a dilemma facing doctors and patients every day, having to do with how far to go with testing before a tentative diagnosis is made. There are many personal and societal forces pushing both parties back and forth. The doctors role, as biased as it may be, is to give advice, hopefully preceded by a discussion of pros and cons. Obviously, the doctor should recommend what is best for this individual patient, at that particular time. The roadblocks impeding this approach and potentially leading to violation of the Hippocratic Oath, have already been mentioned.

Diarrhea and constipation.

Understandably, the speed at which material moves through the GI tract, from esophagus to anus, will ultimately determine whether a person's bowel habits are normal or not. The "or not" basically revolves around two topics that perhaps are better described as "conditions" rather than "diseases," much of the time. A condition implies a state of affairs perhaps more subject to lifestyle factors. The topics are diarrhea and constipation.

In industrialized countries, diarrhea is often a nuisance associated with a brief illness. In underdeveloped countries, it can sweep through, killing many people, especially children, along the way. This discussion revolves around conditions in industrialized, technically advanced societies.

As mentioned, chronic or recurrent diarrhea in our society is not a very common problem. There are many potential causes of it. Here are some of the most common causes of chronic or recurrent diarrhea. Diarrhea is likely better characterized by the type of stool, loose to watery, rather than by the frequency (more than two or three movements per day), although both may be taken into consideration. The corollary of this is that a long period of two or three stools per day, without other symptoms, is likely a normal variant.

Celiac Disease

Celiac disease perhaps is more common than previously suspected, now that there is a simple blood test which can afford a diagnosis in a high percentage of cases. As with many other disease entities, at times the symptoms may be so mild that the disease goes otherwise undetected. The disease is considered to be autoimmune, in this case with an intolerance to a protein called gluten, found in wheat and other grains, including rye and barley. An enzyme called tissue transglutaminase alters the protein in such a way that the immune system (T cells) reacts with the small intestine lining, with inflammation and eventually partial or complete loss of the multi-layered folding, called villi. Chronic diarrhea is probably the most common symptom. Fatigue is also common, but is so common in general, as to be not terribly helpful with diagnosis. There can be a number of differing metabolic disturbances, depending on the severity and location of the inflammation and villous atrophy.

Lactose intolerance is caused by a reduction in the enzyme lactase in the intestinal lining cell. In this case lactose, a sugar found in milk and milk products, cannot be absorbed properly and passes intact into the colon where bacteria act on it to create gas and pull fluid into the colon, with subsequent symptoms, including diarrhea. Lactase deficiency is usually partial, and many people with this arrangement can tolerate small amounts of lactose-containing foods. In others, the deficiency can be severe and mandate the need to completely exclude all lactose. The disease can occur at any age. There is a transitory form, such as seen after viral enteritis. It is also linked with celiac disease, in that celiac disease can cause enough villous atrophy to severely limit lactase availability. Diagnosis can be "clinched" by strictly avoiding all milk products, which should promptly result in resolution of diarrhea.

Inflammatory bowel disease

Inflammatory bowel disease is a term used to encompass Crohn's disease and ulcerative colitis. Several "newer" or more recently recognized diseases, such as collagenous or microscopic or lymphocytic colitis, are included in this category. Historically, attempts have been made to separate Crohn's disease and ulcerative colitis, with Crohn's occurring anywhere in the luminal GI tract and characterized by inflammation through the entire bowel wall, whereas ulcerative colitis is restricted to the colon and involves only the lining membrane. It is possible that these are two variants of the same inflammatory reaction, with the cause being unknown. Both can have diarrhea as a major manifestation, particularly ulcerative colitis. With these conditions, it is common to have at least trace amounts of blood in the stool, and occasionally, the bleeding can be heavy. The Crohn's disease variant has a potential for causing small intestine strictures (blockage) and/or perforations, any one of which may need surgical intervention. The ulcerative colitis variant increases the risk of colon cancer quite significantly, such that frequent colonoscopic surveillance is indicated. Since these diseases are of unknown cause, perhaps autoimmune, they are not considered to be truly curable, although extended remissions, with or without medications, are possible.

Regarding the more recently described inflammatory conditions, under the label of "microscopic colitis," it is thought that perhaps these are further variants of the Crohn's–ulcerative colitis model. In this case, on direct inspection of the colon with the colonoscope, the lining membrane appears normal. Multiple random biopsies may be done to establish the diagnosis. There may be a link between usage of non-steroidal anti-inflammatory drugs, or anti-depressant drugs in this variant.

As already suggested, chronic diarrhea may be one of the "systemic" symptoms of a disease that does not primarily affect the intestine such as diabetes or overly active thyroid gland. Carcinoid tumors (benign, but with malignant potential) occur in several areas of the body and cause diarrhea. Overly active thyroid activity can cause diarrhea, as can anxiety from any cause.

As can be appreciated from this brief overview of chronic diarrhea, establishing a definitive cause can be quite daunting. As stated, it all begins with the historical details. Extent of workup should be influenced by the clinical circumstances and should be mutually agreed upon by doctor and patient. In the proper setting, with no other diagnosis found, that is with multiple other diagnoses excluded, a diagnosis of irritable bowel syndrome can be tentatively established. A diagnosis of exclusion, in a sense, is always tentative, as a truly definitive diagnosis can make itself known later at any time.

There are a few final points to be made regarding diarrhea. Obviously, the discussion might look remarkably different if we were discussing diarrhea in a so-called third-world country. Travelers to such countries can return with whatever endemic diarrheal illnesses exist in that country. Travel history should always be reviewed.

Clostridium Difficile Colitis

Lastly, there are two types of diarrhea which can be seen in the setting of antibiotic usage. The first is simple alteration of bacterial flora in the large intestine, as some bacteria are killed off while others are not. This type usually subsides promptly with cessation of antibiotic and possibly with addition of "probiotics" to repopulate the colon with normal flora.

The second is quite interesting, in that it almost has the appearance of a new disease, even though it was first observed about twenty years ago. It is now very common and can go on for a long time if not specifically identified and treated. This is so-called *Clostridium difficile* colitis, a response to previous antibiotic usage and caused by overgrowth of *C. difficile* bacteria, which produces a toxin, damaging the colon lining membrane. This is a much more troublesome disorder, which can present with both systemic and local symptoms, and may occur weeks to months after the last antibiotic usage. People with this infection generally feel ill. They have varying manifestations, including fever, loss of appetite, abdominal pain, indigestion, and varying severity of diarrhea. Diagnosis is usually easily made on a sample stool specimen, whereby the specific toxin produced by this kind of bacteria can be identified. Treatment is with one or several other antibiotics which are specifically designed to reduce the population of the offending bacterial overgrowth, with treatment effective in most cases.

Constipation, Epidemiology, and Dr. Burkitt

We have just contrasted the topic of diarrhea in the industrialized world, where it is a symptom of many diseases and a relatively uncommon nuisance, and the underdeveloped areas, where it is a very serious disease, responsible for the deaths of millions of people. In some ways, constipation is a mirror image of this epidemiologic scenario, very common in the industrialized world, a source of great distress for many people and perhaps a much more serious disorder than has been previously recognized. Alternatively, we don't hear much about constipation from the underdeveloped parts of the world.

As with most medical topics, as much as we may know about them sometimes, there is likely much more that we don't know, particularly on a genetic, cellular, and subcellular level. Ultimately, keeping the world running smoothly might be much easier if we knew the precise cellular and subcellular mechanisms of disease. Thus far, after thousands of years of "medical science," we have arrived at the cusp of the motherload, at the event horizon of this great medical black hole. It is likely that in the next twenty to thirty years, we will understand disease more deeply than was ever imagined and hopefully with increased ability to intervene positively. Up until now, over these millennia, where the images of disease causation have been blurred (if not outright foggy), we have greatly relied on gross correlations made between any given disease process, and other diseases, prevailing situations and events, and tried to view disease in the macroscopic milieu in which it is seen. These types of investigations, creating correlations, are the essence of epidemiology. Actually, this type of epidemiologic sleuthing has taken us a long way. Or, at least we think it has.

Obviously, there have been a number of tragic misconceptions which have held sway even in highly developed countries, whereby the appearance of disease was felt to be a punishment for the individual or society, for impiety or consorting with the devil. Despite the fact that enlightened people in ancient Greece, such as Hippocrates, tried to move us away from deeply held prejudices, these persisted in a widespread manner up until pre-modern times even in the most educated members of society. It may never be known how many women lost their lives for having been accused of witchcraft, but estimates range into the millions. Such denigration of women continued flagrantly until the middle of the twentieth century, where one would frequently hear the diagnosis of "hysteria," almost never in men, followed by confinement in an asylum for months to years, stripped of all rights. Vestiges of this belief system still persist even today.

Some of the greatest minds of the day, including Descartes, put forth the notion that animals were merely sophisticated machines, without a soul. Therefore, we need not to worry about their suffering. It is reported that the last free act of Friedrich Nietzsche in 1889, whose writing frequently dealt with the topics of prevailing cultural values and the objectivity of "truth," was to intervene in the public beating of a horse, at which time he collapsed and was confined in an asylum or at home for the rest of his life! Unimaginable cruelty to living creatures is with us today, sometimes overt, and often covert, and usually resting on deeply held beliefs regarding the invalidity of their lives.

Long before disease mechanisms were deeply understood, epidemiologic concepts moved medical science along, utilizing knowledge and techniques drawn from such disciplines as sociology, anthropology, biology, and more recently psychology and statistics, examining disease in the context of environmental influences on large populations, constantly looking for causal relationships. Seen against the backdrop of prevailing thought in his day, Hippocrates's delineation of the concepts of "endemic," regarding why certain diseases are seen in some places and not others, and "epidemic," why diseases are seen some times and not others, is stunning. Epidemiologic concepts have been alternately utilized and ignored for centuries since then. In contemporary medicine, epidemiology has ascended to lofty heights, with most medical schools having established departments, with both MDs and PhDs from many disciplines participating on observational and experimental levels, still looking for those difficult to discern causal relationships. Epidemiology is highly regarded by proponents of evidence-based medicine. This fact, and the fact that whatever may be going on at the level of the cell, with its genetic instructions, which are constantly affected by environmental influences, makes it likely that epidemiology is here to stay, even as we experience an explosion of knowledge in cell biology.

Here is an interesting recent tie-in involving epidemiology, which will bring us back to the almost forgotten topic of constipation. During World War II, an Irish-born surgeon, Denis Burkitt, was part of the Royal Army Medical Corps and was stationed in Africa. After the war, he returned to Africa, where he made two remarkable epidemiologic observations. The first had to do with the frequent appearance of tumors, especially tumors of the jaw seen in children. He mapped the geographic distribution of this form of tumor and published an article regarding his findings in a medical journal in 1958. He gradually accrued much more knowledge about the disease and published a book about it in 1970.

What he, and others, had determined was fascinating. It was determined that the tumors were actually a form of lymphoma, technically called "non-Hodgkin's lymphoma." Eventually, strong epidemiologic evidence emerged which appears to show tight linkage of this lymphoma with the Ebstein–Barr (EB) virus. This is the same virus which in "the West" produces a very common infection in young people, called infectious mononucleosis. In the "West," this disease has been dubbed "mono" and is a contagious infection of the upper airway and its draining lymph nodes, and perhaps distant lymph nodes, and even the spleen. Increased lymphocytes are seen in peripheral blood, including atypical (genetically altered) lymphocytes. The disease is often very mild, although it may be protracted, particularly if there is an associated hepatitis. Importantly, this is a benign disease in the West, with no malignant behavior.

So why does EB virus cause lymphoma (a cancer) in parts of Africa and a very common relatively mild disease in the West? The difference appears to be the malaria parasite. The areas in Africa in which Burkitt's lymphoma has been endemic are the same areas where malaria is endemic. As malaria comes under better control in Africa, including attempts to reduce the mosquito vector, as well as use of netting over bedding at night and other interventions, the incidence of Burkitt's lymphoma drops. The thinking is that malaria infection in children causes an alteration in B lymphocyte surveillance and subsequently increased numbers of B lymphocytes. This increase in B lymphocyte population makes it statistically more likely that there could occur B cell mutations, particularly if these cells are also exposed to Ebstein–Barr virus. As bizarre and convoluted as this may all sound, this is the current thinking regarding a largely regional African tumor, Burkitt's lymphoma, and the world-wide Ebstein–Barr virus and infectious mononucleosis. This is an example of epidemiologic principles revealing how geography can greatly affect the expression of disease.

Denis Burkitt was not finished yet! Upon his return to England, where he had not practiced surgery for many years, he was stunned by the differing incidences of diseases he had seen in Africa versus diseases he saw in England. His last major publication in 1979 outlined his own feelings about the epidemiologic causes of common gastrointestinal diseases in the West. He proposed that many common diseases such as gall stones, other gall bladder diseases, diverticulitis, colon cancer, hemorrhoids, appendicitis, constipation, and others (including cardiovascular issues and obesity) were caused by low fiber diet. He proposed a notion, likely somewhat tongue-in-cheek, that in a given society, there exists an inverse relationship between the size of the stool and the size of the hospital. That is, the bigger the stool, the smaller the hospital. The smaller the stool, the larger the hospital. The book he published was titled, *Don't Forget Fiber in Your Diet*, and it was his most notable commercial success. In it, he proposed that the amount of fiber recommended in the Western diet, perhaps thirty to forty grams per day, is woefully inadequate in terms of producing the kind of stools which would allow us to greatly reduce the size of our hospitals. In conclusion, what can be said confidently is that his proposal has never been proven. However, it has never been disproven.

Pages ago, I mentioned that whereas diarrhea in underdeveloped countries is a very serious health problem, we never hear about constipation in those countries. Constipation in the West is big business. Although Justice Stewart might know it if he saw it, what is it medically? As commonly as people complain about it, it may even be more common than that. Perhaps, the most widely accepted medical definition of constipation has to do with the type of the stool itself, rather than its absolute frequency or infrequency. Stools that are hard and/or compacted are likely the most widely accepted as representative of constipation. Hard stools occur because they contain a paucity of water, the water having been absorbed during passage through the luminal GI tract. This could occur from decreased fluid intake or increased fluid reabsorption because of improper diet (ala Dr. Burkitt) and possibly slowed transit. Such stools are hard to pass and may require considerable straining. The straining may in turn be involved in the genesis of abdominal wall and inguinal hernias, hemorrhoids, and diverticula (to be discussed soon), and perhaps even pelvic floor descent, which changes the configuration of the colon, and could secondarily make passing stools even more difficult. So, passing a stool every day, or even more than once daily, could still represent constipation if the stools are hard, round, compacted balls, which are also low in total volume.

Ideally, stool should be passed every day. However, as with all other biologic processes, as has been repeatedly emphasized, there is a bell-shaped distribution of virtually everything. Stool character depends on many factors, including dietary character, water intake, amount of food and water ingested, medications being used, stress, travel, time allotted for evacuation, and others. I do not think that there is a widely accepted frequency of bowel movements to define constipation. The number "three" is often mentioned, meaning less than three times per week. I think perhaps that is too low, with four or five per week being more acceptable. It seems that the size and consistency of the stool are more important. Ideally, the stool should be soft, relatively large, and easy to pass.

There actually are some physical signs of constipation. Occasionally, particularly in thin people, hard stools can be felt on palpation of the abdomen. On occasion, during the course of rectal exam, similar hard stool can be felt in the rectum. Occasionally, a simple abdominal X-ray film, particularly when someone comes in because of abdominal pain (or bloating or nausea), may demonstrate the colon to be fairly clearly outlined by a large amount of retained stool.

There are many possible explanations for constipation, besides simply lifestyle decisions, and a thorough investigation may be needed. Regarding treatment, it has already been implied that a generous intake of fiber and water may be very helpful. Fiber not only adds bulk to the stool, but since it is not absorbed, it also helps to keep fluid in the colon. I don't think one can easily overdose on fiber, but too much could cause diarrhea. Many people have a particular food which acts as a cathartic for them. This tends to be very individual, but more often is a fruit product of some kind. It seems to me that using natural food products, including bran, fruits, and water, is best. Otherwise, there are many different types of commercial laxative products which act in different ways. Basically, most of them either add bulk or pull water into the colon. A lesser number actually irritate the lining membrane so that the membrane puts fluid out. Once again, these products, and the amount needed to be successful, tend to vary greatly in effect from person to person.

Colon (the Large Intestine)

As we move through the colon ("large intestine"), and the end of the GI tract, it should be pointed out that there are several common and important disease processes which can affect the small and large intestine singly or jointly. Some of these have already been discussed and will only be briefly mentioned as they relate to the colon. There are a few diseases which are specific to the colon, and they will be mentioned in more detail.

Digestion, that is preparation of ingested food for absorption and the process of nutrient absorption, is virtually complete by the time that peristaltic contraction waves push material from the terminal ileum into the colon. There is a very small amount of "digestion" which continues in the colon, compliments of the resident colonic bacterial population. Importantly, vitamin K, a requisite member of the team which balances between blood coagulation and blood flow, is produced and absorbed in the colon. The remaining water, which has escaped absorption by the small intestine, is substantially absorbed. Lastly, a number of critical substances, such as sodium, magnesium, and potassium, are absorbed there. Otherwise, the last remaining colon function is storage of feces (but hopefully not for too long), before defecation can be accomplished conveniently. An interesting mind game to play during a storm, with a power outage and nothing else to do, would be to imagine how differently society would be shaped, both physically and culturally, if we lacked storage capacity and shared similar bowel habits to horses or cows! Needless to say, it would look and smell remarkably different.

Some of the shared diseases and conditions involving other organs of the terminal gut include irritable bowel syndrome, diarrhea and constipation, and inflammatory bowel disease, such as Crohn's disease. Ulcerative colitis is considered part of the spectrum of inflammatory bowel disease but, as the name suggests, is restricted to the colon. Intestinal bleeding is a very common finding and is always considered to be important, as there are a number of serious potential underlying causes. It is stated, and rightly so, that bleeding can occur in one or several locations all the way from mouth to anus.

GI Bleeding

Of the diseases considered already, several can be associated with bleeding. This would include esophagitis (from reflux). With end-stage liver disease, called cirrhosis, there can be development of very large venous channels in the stomach and esophagus, called varices. As venous blood is partially blocked through the liver en route to the inferior vena cava and the heart, these large venous channels assisting blood back to the heart, being added on and not evolutionarily planned for, tend to be fragile and can bleed massively. Perhaps, the single most notable reservation we have about the use of non-steroidal anti-inflammatory drugs ("N-SAIDS"), such as ibuprofen and naproxen (both over-the-counter) and many prescription varieties, is their known potential for causing sudden, massive GI bleeding, with no antecedent warning, caused by ulcerations usually in esophagus, stomach, or small intestines. Aspirin, although it can cause bleeding, is less likely to cause such sudden, massive bleeding which can be life threatening. Cancers from esophagus through stomach and colon can bleed.

What has not been mentioned so far, as a major cause of bleeding, is a condition called angiodysplasia. Although this is occasionally seen in healthy people, it is more common in the elderly, particularly with heart or lung problems. In this condition, the cause of which is not definitely known, there is development of vascular malformations, veins and/or arteries, in or just below the lining membrane in whatever organ it may be. These may be multiple and located over widely disparate areas. They usually cause chronic bleeding, off and on, although sudden substantial bleeding can occur.

As can be seen or inferred, GI bleeding is always a concern. Please note that bleeding may be slow and intermittent, thus unknown to the person involved. It may go undetected for a long time. Diagnosis may be hinted at by the finding of anemia, with symptoms consistent with that, such as fatigue, loss of energy, or even shortness of breath. Bleeding can be confirmed by finding traces of blood in the stool which are invisible to the naked eye ("occult" bleeding). In situations with heavy bleeding, in the upper tract, perhaps as far as the colon, "digestion" of blood causes the stool to become dark brown to black. As heavy bleeding gets closer in origin to the rectum and anus, it may appear as "bright red blood" mixed in with or layered on the stool. The first step in diagnosis of the bleeding site will likely be "panendoscopy," meaning colonoscopy and upper GI (esophagus–stomach–duodenum) endoscopy. If that does not reveal the source, "capsule endoscopy" may be done to evaluate the small intestine, whereby a capsule containing a tiny camera and attached to a string is swallowed and then is followed through the small intestine and retrieved. This is a remarkable technique. In cases of heavy bleeding, a number of radiographic and imaging studies have been developed to help ascertain the source of bleeding. Most often, with one or all of these sophisticated interventions, the cause or causes can be found. Even blood from the mouth or nose can be swallowed and appear as blood in the stool.

Ileus

Another situation which is common to stomach, and small and large intestine, is a condition called ileus. Simply, this is a reduction or cessation of peristaltic activity of the entire GI tract. This invariably occurs after abdominal surgery and is the reason why people are unable to eat for several days to a week after such surgery, requiring intravenous fluids. This condition can also occur in the setting of any acute, severe illness or injury, once again explaining the dietary restriction seen.

GI Obstruction

Dietary restrictions are also necessary whenever there is an obstruction in the GI tract. This situation is different than ileus, in that peristalsis continues. Depending on where in the tract and how complete the obstruction is, these people can be very ill and may have to go to surgery quickly to relieve the obstruction. There are many potential causes of obstruction, both benign and malignant, and these may occur anywhere along the tract. One of the more common causes is "adhesions" from previous surgery. This is a particularly unfortunate circumstance, as it may be recurrent. Abdominal surgery always induces scarring in the abdominal cavity. Scarring can pinch off areas of the intestine. Hernias can do the same. So, once the abdominal cavity has been entered, this is always a possibility. Sometimes, with bowel rest, and good luck, the obstruction self-corrects. At other times, it requires surgical intervention, of course setting the stage for more scarring. If the obstruction occurs in the colon and surgery is needed to relieve it, it is likely that a temporary colostomy will be needed, with the option of reconnecting the colon later. A colostomy is created by surgical redirection of the colon so that it empties from the left lower abdomen, rather than from the rectum, into a collecting bag. Making the right decisions with intestinal obstruction requires the guidance of an experienced surgeon.

Appendicitis

There are a few diseases or conditions which are unique to the colon. One of these is *C. difficile* colitis, caused by usage of an antibiotic and which was already discussed. The appendix in a finger-like outpouching is found coming off the first part of the colon called the cecum. Although it may contain lymphoid tissue, this does not suffice as a pass to get into the Essential Organ Club. It truly appears to be vestigial and is a troublemaker at that. Appendicitis is a common inflammation, likely secondary to infection of the appendix, typically causing pain in the right lower abdomen, along with prominent systemic symptoms, and mandating its surgical removal. If left too long, it can rupture, causing peritonitis, or infection of part or the entire abdominal cavity. This is a serious and potentially fatal disorder, as it was for film star Rudolph Valentino in 1926. Rarely, the appendix can be the site of a carcinoid tumor, or a cancer.

Diverticulosis/Diverticulitis

Diverticula are outpouchings. Although they can occur in other hollow organs, when used alone in medical parlance, they refer to outpouchings of the colon. Diverticula better represent a condition rather than a disease. They are exceedingly common and usually found incidentally at the time of some type of imaging study or with colonoscopy. Most people do not have problems with diverticula. They are thought perhaps to be a result of increased luminal pressure in the colon and likely at least partially caused by constipation. However, infection in these outpouchings is a common complication and is then a definite disease, called diverticulitis. People are ill with this infection. Some can be treated at home, with bowel rest and antibiotics, but some need to be hospitalized. Recurring diverticulitis can permanently narrow the part of the colon involved, causing a permanent obstruction. This will likely need a surgical resection of the narrowed portion. Should the diverticula rupture, like an appendix, this can quickly cause the person to be desperately ill, and a surgical approach will likely be necessary because of the appearance of peritonitis. Recall that the colon is filled with bacteria. When they gain access to the abdominal cavity, such as with a perforation, the situation is dire. Survival is still likely, but recovery will be prolonged. A colostomy, permanent or temporary, will be necessary.

The Remarkable Anus and Hemorrhoids

Lastly, at the end of the GI tract is the anus, which is basically a thick, circular sphincter muscle, allowing us to keep the opening closed until convenient evacuation is possible. Colorectal specialists and other have marveled at how this obscure little muscle can with 99+% accuracy tell the difference between gas, liquid, and solid, and how much of each lurks inside, adeptly releasing only that which is safe to release and in a culturally acceptable way to boot! This is the site of hemorrhoids, which are veins, fairly substantial in size, and representing an alternative route for local tissues to shuttle blood back upstream. These veins can become visible and/or palpable, should they become irritated or should a clot form in them. They may protrude out of the anal canal (external hemorrhoids) or remain within the anal canal or rectum (internal hemorrhoids). They can become problematic with pregnancy, with increasing pressure on them from the enlarging uterus, impeding blood flow. The same can occur with severe straining, irritation from itching, or constipation. It is said to be an occupational hazard of long-haul truck drivers. Hemorrhoids, occurring at least once in a person's life, or present off and on, are exceedingly common. Most of the time, they can be left alone or treated with OTC products. They can become problematic if they bleed (anemia, messy) or if they clot (painful). Recurrent major problems may require one of several different surgical approaches, with varying complexity. Fortunately, this is not frequently required. The definition of "minor surgery" is surgery being done on someone other than you! I have had one young woman who died twenty-four hours, after routine hemorrhoidectomy, from sepsis.

Abdominal Hernias

This is as good a place to discuss hernias, as there will be. We have already discussed hiatal hernia, a common and usually innocuous condition of the stomach and diaphragm. It will also be mentioned that with significant swelling of the brain, the base of the brain may herniate into the foramen magnum and kill you. So, as can be inferred, a hernia seems to imply that a tissue of some type moves to a different place and may cause problems. Although hernias can occur almost anywhere in the body, most of them refer to movements of tissues within the abdominal and pelvic regions. Hernias are known to slide back and forth into their appropriate and inappropriate places.

In actuality, by far, a majority of symptomatic hernias occur in the groin regions and are called inguinal hernias, namely direct and indirect inguinal hernias, and femoral hernias. They are usually noted as a bulge or swelling. They usually migrate back and forth. They may first be identified by as unpleasant discomfort or even pain. They can vary in size from very small to perhaps the size of an orange. Most people find them to be "unpleasant" in some way. For those who are absolutely not bothered by them, there is the option to leave them alone. There is a small chance, perhaps 5% to 10%, that at some point they could move to where they are not supposed to be and get stuck—so-called "incarcerated" (another example of medical poetic prose). At that point, it is likely that an urgent surgery will need to be done and that semi-urgent repair will be much more complicated than had it been done electively. For the most part, they are not difficult for experienced surgeons to repair, with most done as outpatient surgery and back to work in a few days to a week, depending on the type of work.

Hernias also commonly occur anywhere in the abdomen wall, most commonly in the midline. The "belly button," or umbilicus for a more sophisticated term, is the place where in fetal life, the umbilical cord from your mother's placenta, entered your body to nourish you. Although it usually seals over tightly after birth, it may not. Abdominal contents may pouch into it, just as with inguinal and femoral hernias.

The rectus abdominis muscle is the thick muscle running from the base of the rib cage to the pelvic bone, one on each side. It is the muscle that allows you to do those 300 sit-ups in the morning and gives you that "washboard" or "six-pack" appearance of your abdomen. These two muscles, one on each side, are held together in the center by a relatively tough membrane. Unfortunately, with the ravages of aging and with increasing intra-abdominal adiposity, the membrane can weaken and eventually split, very much like unzipping a zipper. The most common area for this to happen is between the rib cage and the umbilicus. This may make its appearance as a prominent bulge in that area. However, with obesity it may not be noticeable to the individual, and it seems to produce fewer distressing symptoms than the inguinal variety of hernias. Finally, since the opening is usually so wide, the chances of incarcerating are much less. Because of all of these factors, many people, with or without their doctor's advice, leave these alone. Depending on the size, they can be more difficult to repair and may involve one or several nights in the hospital. Umbilical hernias do have a significant chance of incarcerating and thus are more frequently surgically repaired.

PART VI
GENITOURINARY

T he genitourinary system, as the name implies, in both males and females, includes the kidneys and the urinary bladder and their respective drainage systems, namely one ureter, on each side, and one urethra. In males, the reproductive organs include the penis, testicles, prostate, and seminal vesicles. This entire system is bound together in the specialty of Urology or Urologic Surgery. In females, the reproductive organs including external genitalia, vagina, uterus, fallopian tubes, and ovaries are medically managed by gynecologists, with urologists more or less confining their efforts to the urinary system. There is some degree of overlap, depending on personal physician interests, availability of specialty care, and regional customs.

The major purpose of the urinary system is to cleanse the blood of toxic materials, whether they are natural products of metabolism or toxins which have made their way into the body. The kidneys are the functioning elements in this arrangement. The kidneys are also critically important in regulating the chemical balance of body fluids. By the time that fluid has filtered through the kidney membranes into the collecting apparatus, called the ureters, the work of cleansing the blood is done. The ureters transport this fluid, now designated urine, to the urinary bladder, which is simply a holding tank. The bladder is a dome-shaped collapsible structure, whose walls are made largely of muscle, which repeatedly fills and empties. The tube leading out of the bladder is called the urethra, generally much longer in males because of its traverse through the penis. This urinary drainage system is another of those luminal structures, which is technically outside of the body, even though it is surrounded by the body.

Male Reproductive System

In males, the reproductive system includes the testes, which are the site of generation of sperm cells, in turn the carriers of the male contribution to the genetic makeup of future generations. Formed within tiny tubules, the sperm migrate out to a holding area, outside of the testicle called the epididymis where they complete their maturation. Interestingly, sperm cells are immunologically different than other cells and could theoretically incite an autoimmune reaction. The so-called blood–testes barrier prevents this from happening. For whatever reason, generation of sperm occurs more efficiently at temperatures slightly lower than normal body temperature. Many different mechanisms have evolved in different animal species to accomplish this. In humans, and in many other animals, the final solution was to have the developing testes migrate out of the abdominal cavity during fetal development, eventually being external to the abdomen in the scrotal sac. Although it apparently accomplished the goal of reducing testicular temperature, it also set the stage for a number of potential abdominal and testicular problems, such as direct hernias, twisting of the testicle called torsion, and injury. Scattered in between the seminiferous tubules are cells which produce testosterone, in turn under some control by the pituitary gland.

Semen is the fluid containing mature sperm cells during ejaculation. This fluid is a composite of several structures. So-called Cowper's gland provides pre-ejaculation lubrication. The majority of semen originates in the seminal vesicles behind and below the prostate—and to a lesser extent from the prostate gland.

Female Reproductive System

The ovary, in female vertebrates, is the counterpart to the male testes, producing gametes called eggs. Eggs carry one-half of the genetic information, and upon fertilization, with fusion of the nuclei of the sperm and egg, the full genetic compliment is re-constituted. Ovaries are located in the very lower-most portion of the abdominal cavity, tethered to the pelvic wall, fallopian tubes, and uterus by ligaments of various types. Just as the testes, the ovaries are both reproductive organs, so-called gonads, and endocrine organs releasing hormones, acting at distant sites. Whereas sperm are produced in the lining of the seminiferous tubules of the testes during the entire life of the male, eggs are "produced" within nests of follicles in the cortex of the ovary for a limited number of years, from menarche to menopause. A female is born with all the eggs she will ever have. This fact, coupled with the fact that hundreds of millions of sperm are seemingly endlessly produced during the life of the male, has been used to explain the obvious differences in mating behaviors in humans and most other vertebrates. Generally speaking, males are always ready and willing to copulate, whereas females are much more selective when and with whom they will engage. Although the human female may have somewhere between 200,000 and 500,000 eggs at the time of birth, a vast majority of them are destined to never see the light of day, degenerating into scars during their migration, in follicles, through the cortex of the ovary toward the surface. In fact, only one each month, or a total of perhaps 500 or less, makes it to the surface. This is under complex hormonal control, whereby the follicle literally explodes, releasing the treasured egg.

It is fascinating to speculate about this possible biological-behavioral link, and it seems possible to me that a complex organism could have inner knowledge or intuition about this type of arrangement. It is also appreciated through a number of different types of research endeavors that when it comes to reproduction, organisms do not reliably act altruistically but appear to act selfishly, wishing to pass on as many copies of their genes as possible. Ultimately, the kinds of questions being asked regarding this issue do not seem to be the type that will ever yield some type of incontrovertible evidence. Therefore, we may be forever left with speculation.

Fertilization

Regardless, in humans, the egg is swept up by the fimbriae of the fallopian tube, and the ciliated lining membrane attempts to sweep the egg in the direction of the uterus. The journey is a long one for a structure barely visible to the naked eye and likely takes a number of days. In the meantime, flagellated sperms, capable of forward and upward propulsion against the current of the ciliated lining membrane, are furiously fighting their way upstream, like salmon getting ready to spawn and die, hoping to get to the egg, not only before they die but first. Only one sperm out of the millions provided has the privilege of penetrating the much larger egg. Once this penetration occurs, the wall of the egg immediately hardens and becomes impenetrable to other sperms, which then do die. The meeting of sperm and egg usually occurs within the fallopian tube with the preparation for cell division beginning immediately. Meanwhile hormones such as progesterone, produced by the same follicles that released the egg now called a corpus luteum, begin to best prepare the uterus for implantation of the fertilized egg, now called a zygote.

At five days, a cavity appears in the zygote, separating what will become the embryo, from its surrounding supportive membranes. The zygote is perhaps 250 cells in size at the time of implantation in the uterine wall, facilitated by chemical reactions in both the zygote and uterus. Within ten days, the zygote is fully embedded in the uterine wall, and within a few more days, it begins to produce hormones which can be detected in the mother's urine as a positive pregnancy test. At about fourteen days, the "primitive streak" appears, destined to become the nervous system. This is just about the time that the open-door ability of the zygote to duplicate itself, by twinning, closes. By twenty days, a heart beating is visible in what is called the embryo. By ten weeks post-fertilization, the embryo gives rise to the fetus, with a distinctly human-looking face. All during this time, the developing zygote–embryo–fetus is especially sensitive to perturbations in its environment which can strongly influence the developing organ systems. At this level of development, it is both awe-inspiring and intimidating to appreciate that both physical and emotional factors of the mother's life can have a lasting impact on the developing fetus, for better or for worse.

The question as to when this "structure" can be considered to be "human" is at the heart of the debate regarding abortion, with opinions ranging from the moment of fertilization to the time of birth. The above description of the developing entity is factual. Beyond that, the debate may rage forever, based on elements which have nothing to do with the facts regarding the physical nature of the events just described.

Adjacent to the anatomy lab in medical school, there stood a series of book cases, in which were kept "specimens" of these very creatures mentioned above in various stages of development, from barely visible to full term, housed in bottles and containers of increasing size, swimming in formalin, so as to keep them preserved. I recall as a 21-year-old, first-year medical student standing mesmerized for long periods in front of those bottles, pulled in by these lifeless creatures, looking at the faces, the tiny fingers with the discernable finger nails and feeling intense sadness. I could never know why those little beings never had a chance to experience the richness of life. I could only know that for whatever reason, I stood there, looking at them and wondering why I did and they didn't.

Female Genital Disease

At a time when many infectious diseases described back into antiquity have come under control by the use of vaccines, antibiotics, and hygienic measures, the same cannot be said for venereal or sexually transmitted diseases. Herpes simplex virus type II, called genital herpes or just "herpes," is a ubiquitous infection thought to be present in 30% to 40% of adults in the USA. Many of these people have been previously unaware of the infection, with diagnosis made on blood testing. Even as little as twenty years ago, before reliable and commonly used blood testing was available, this was thought to be a terrible scourge, symbolic of the nasty nature of "unprotected" sexual activity, being performed by people who were not married and/or married to someone else, and/or too young to be having sex and/or unable to control their sexual impulses. Now, with the knowledge of its true incidence, it seems wasteful, to say the least, to castigate the many millions of people who harbor this virus for a lifetime.

In females, the disease may be truly hidden, occurring in the deep recesses of the vagina, not symptomatic enough to warn the person that something is wrong—and yet fully transmissible and very contagious. More commonly, lesions are located somewhere on the external genitalia and present as stinging or burning pain, or itching, followed by the appearance of one or several small blisters, which are likely to ulcerate. The course extends up to two weeks, although healing to the point of invisibility may take considerably longer. In the worst-case scenario, these lesions can be very painful, and be associated with systemic symptoms such as fever and fatigue, and may occur four to six times per year. This is the type of person who would likely greatly benefit from chronic anti-viral treatment, which usually significantly reduces the frequency and severity of episodes. In the best-case scenario, the person may have only one or a few episodes in the course of a lifetime, only mildly symptomatic. Very interestingly and unfortunate from the standpoint of control of this condition, viral shedding, which is contagious potential, can exist long after lesions have presumably completely "healed."

Taking all of these factors into consideration, every sexually active person needs to consider how important this issue is to them and then take appropriate action. Action could appear to be somewhat radical if absolute minimization of risk is the goal. Please note also that herpes simplex type I, causing "cold sores," and type II are somewhat interchangeable, based on sexual practices. That is, type I can cause genital lesions and type II can cause facial lesions.

Vaginitis

Vaginitis, an infection or inflammation of the vagina, is a common disease. There are three major types of infections involved, including candidiasis (yeast), bacterial (including gonorrhea), and trichomonal. Symptoms are somewhat predictable, being mostly itching and discharge. Pain is a variable symptom but is usually not severe and usually associated more with specific activities, such as sexual intercourse. The most common form of bacterial vaginitis is called, appropriately, bacterial vaginosis, caused by an overgrowth of normal vaginal bacteria. There is little doubt that experienced doctors, seeing a large number of patients with vaginitis, can tell what the infection is specifically on the basis of description of symptoms as well as observation of two crucial sense organs, being sight (appearance) and smell of the discharge. Nevertheless, the standard study for confirmation of diagnosis is to do smears and cultures of secretions. Once identified, treatment modalities with a variety of antibiotic agents, depending on the causative organism, are usually curative. Sporadic recurrences are common.

The type of vaginitis seen especially in post-menopausal women is usually caused by estrogen deficiency. Depending on severity and chronicity, topical vaginal estrogen replacement is usually very effective.

The "cervix" is a thumb-like downward protuberance of the uterus, entering into the vaginal space for up to several inches. Although it is a firm structure, it does contain a so-called os, a very small opening which is the distal end of a canal, which opens to the uterine cavity. The cervix obviously functions as a means of withholding something in the uterus, most importantly a fetus, supplying an obvious major obstruction to the gravid (pregnant) uterus. It is only at the time of early labor that the cervix begins to dilate, eventually opening widely to allow egress of the baby.

Whereas vaginal cancer is relatively rare, cervical cancer is relatively common and is the raison d'etre for the "PAP smear," which is performed on and in the cervix. Dysplastic or premalignant lesions are common. Carcinoma in situ or non-invasive cancer is primarily a disease of young women, whereas invasive cancer is more common in older women. These cancers are more common in black people compared to white and more common in certain geographic areas, including India and South America. Cervical cancer is particularly interesting from a scientific standpoint, as it is definitely linked to the human papillomavirus (HPV). This is the same virus associated with so-called genital warts, found in clusters over the external genitalia of both men and women. Knowing that a virus can cause a cancer opens questions about the role of viruses in other types of cancers and subsequently would lead to questions about vaccines to protect against cancer (recall the Ebstein–Barr virus in Burkitt's lymphoma). Other factors seemingly related to cervical dysplasia include the number of different sexual partners (again, with increased viral exposure from males, especially uncircumcised males, who may carry HPV) and cigarette smoking.

Uterus

One could pose the questions as to whether or not the uterus is of any value to the female who makes a decision early in life that she will not bear children. This mind game does seem to have some relevance in the sense that with the exception of that reproductive function, considered to be a benefit for most people, the uterus on surface evaluation seems to be heavily weighted toward problems rather than benefits. One would speculate that the uterus may have a role in the orgasmic response, in fact a particular role, logically dubbed "uterine orgasm." This variant of orgasm has been studied enough to reveal that it is not coincident with rhythmic contraction of pelvic musculature, so commonly appreciated with the most common orgasmic response. Uterine orgasm appears to stimulate the part of the brain called the hypothalamus to produce increased amounts of a hormone called oxytocin, which is generally stored in the posterior part of the pituitary gland (along with anti-diuretic hormone), for release during labor, to stimulate uterine contraction and nipple stimulation, to facilitate breastfeeding. This stored oxytocin released into the circulation cannot re-enter the brain because of the blood–brain barrier. However, there are oxytocin receptors scattered throughout the brain, reached by central projections from the hypothalamus. Effects of oxytocin on the brain are coming under increased scrutiny and have been found to be involved in a variety of behaviors, including lovingness, maternal instincts, trust, generosity, learning, and memory. There also are some evidences that it is related to autism. Most of these studies are very preliminary. Nevertheless, they raise enough questions to suggest that a great deal more needs to be known about the effect of oxytocin on the brain before we do anything to permanently alter oxytocin production, such as what would occur with hysterectomy. Incidentally, both the hypothalamic production and central projections are seen in males as well.

Otherwise, as noted, the uterus is the site of a number of common and a few vexing problems. Uterine cancer is fairly common, but uncommon in young women. Most cases are seen in post-menopausal women, ages fifty-five to seventy-five. The diagnosis is often made early, as the most common symptom is a reappearance of vaginal bleeding, predictably called "post-menopausal bleeding." When diagnosed under these circumstances, and thoroughly evaluated, most women are found to be in stage I of the disease. Surgical removal of the uterus as well as fallopian tubes and ovaries at this stage affords a woman a 75% to 95% chance of surgical cure.

Fibroid tumors are benign tumors arising from the muscle layer of the uterine wall. These tumors are very common. They can be single or multiple, small or quite large. Some people have no symptoms, even with fairly large tumors. Others have alterations in menstrual periods, typically heavier. Fibroids can be associated with female infertility.

Lastly, in some people, they definitely seem to be associated with pelvic pain of one or two types. Once again, related to menstruation, people can have much more painful periods. Secondly, separated from menses, they may experience dull, chronic pelvic pain, perhaps accentuated by menstruation.

Endometriosis

In some ways, the last disease entity to be discussed, although not a cancer and generally not life threatening, is the most problematic. Endometriosis is unfortunately common and appears to be increasing in incidence. This is a mysterious disease in several major respects. A number of theories have been advanced to account for this, including changing patterns of childbearing and breastfeeding, all the way to environmental toxicity producing estrogen-like stimulants. No uniformly accepted theory appears to be reaching a majority opinion. There is a general rule of thumb that the more debate there is about any disease entity, the more and differing types of treatment options will be promoted. As can be surmised, there are many treatment options regarding endometriosis, both surgical and medical, all showing effectiveness some of the time, but not often enough for a consensus to arise. As can be further surmised, many women continue to suffer despite having subjected themselves (sometimes repeatedly) to the best treatment available.

We do know some of the basics. For instance, it involves the appearance of endometrial tissue, which is the lining membrane of the uterus, outside of the uterus. These "implants" of tissue can attach themselves throughout the pelvic and abdominal cavities. Recall, of course, that these lining membrane tissues are very sensitive to the hormonal environment, especially estrogen, and swell and then slough and bleed monthly. The endometrial implants can do the same. Wherever they do this, they incite an inflammatory response, as the body's immune system tries to cope with abnormal irritation. Recall that inflammation (a protective response) can be, and in this situation is, linked to formation of fibrous scar tissue. This scar tissue itself can then become part of the problem, by binding structures together which are meant to slide across each other, pinching and pulling on nerve endings, and even narrowing or blocking bowel channels. The end result is pain, pain, and pain, generated in a number of ways and often accentuated at the time of menstruation. Although many people do have "spontaneous" improvement at the time of menopause, with ovarian failure and reduction of estrogen production, please recall that estrogens are also produced in the adrenal glands. Also, the role of aromatase has been implicated in the perpetuation of endometriosis after menopause, aromatase being the enzyme which enhances the production of estrogen, even environmental proto-estrogen compounds which make their way into the body.

So, endometriosis can be a huge problem, affecting women in the prime of life. Sometimes, after multiple combinations of surgical and medical treatments have been tried, with less than satisfactory results, we are left with usage of strong pain killers, which sometimes make the difference between being functional or not. There is a country and western song with an opening stanza that declares, "Sometimes it's hard to be a woman." This song wasn't written about endometriosis, but it could have been.

Ectopic Pregnancy

The fallopian tubes are conduits for the pinpoint-sized egg to make its way to the uterus. As mentioned previously, fertilization of the egg usually occurs within this channel. If, for whatever reason, the fertilized egg is slowed or blocked along its journey, it is possible that implantation will occur within the fallopian tube, rather than the uterus. The embryo burrows into whatever tissue it can, looking for a blood supply. Needless to say, this can do tremendous damage to the tube. This process is called "ectopic pregnancy," and the vast majority of these occur in the fallopian tubes. Diagnosis is usually made between five to seven weeks of gestation, with the appearance of pain. Ultrasound can confirm the diagnosis. Spontaneous abortion may occur. Drugs can be successfully used to enhance this possibility. Ultimately, surgery may be necessary to remove the ectopic tissue. Sometimes the tube can be preserved, but often it must be sacrificed.

Pelvic Inflammatory Disease

The other common problem affecting the tubes is a condition called "pelvic inflammatory disease." This is an infection, presumably arising in the vagina and ascending into the uterus and the fallopian tubes—and even up to the ovaries. The most common infective agents causing this are gonococcus (gonorrhea) and chlamydia. Often, the person is quite ill, with systemic symptoms, and, if with the gonococcus, can even have sepsis syndrome. The treatment involves prompt diagnosis, appropriate antibiotic usage, and may even require surgery if abscess is present.

Ovarian Cysts and Cancer

The reproductive function of the ovary in terms of producing eggs has been discussed. As was mentioned before, the egg moves toward the surface of the ovary, with the vast majority dying en route, involuting, and leaving small scars. Some follicles persist and remain functional in terms of affecting menstruation for variable lengths of time. A few can enlarge, anywhere from pea-sized to very large. The very large ones can cause pain symptoms, just from size alone. Most eventually involute. A few may rupture. When so-called ruptured ovarian cyst occurs, this may be heralded by sudden sharp pelvic pain. Even at this stage, the situation usually self-rectifies as the fluid from the cyst is reabsorbed. The major threat is that during the course of rupturing, an artery may be torn. This could cause substantial hemorrhage into the pelvis and require a surgical procedure to stop the bleeding. Ovarian cysts are generally followed along in their course by repeated physical exam and ultrasound.

Ovarian cancer is an entity which is often feared by patients, perhaps more than it need be. This high level of concern stems from the general knowledge that it is so difficult to diagnose. In addition, many people are aware of its genetic susceptibility. So, with a family history of such or with certain types of breast cancer, concern is heightened even further. This concern can be so intense that it sometimes prompts such people to request elective ovarian removal after childbearing is completed. It affects approximately one in fifty people (2% lifetime chance). It is generally a disease of older women, beyond fifty-five years of age. It is, in fact, very difficult to diagnose, so difficult that routine screening for it is not recommended. This concept is difficult for many people to accept but has a parallel in the previously noted lung cancer situation, whereby timing of diagnosis, early versus late, does not appear to affect survival. It seems that everything about ovarian cancer is sneaky. Early symptoms, which theoretically could afford a better chance of treatment success, are entirely non-specific and usually mild. Diagnosis and staging are usually accomplished at the time of exploratory surgery. Stage I implies confinement to the ovaries, while stage II is confined to the pelvis. Stage III is widespread in the abdomen or elsewhere. Treatment with surgical removal and chemotherapy can be surprisingly effective. Survival at five years after diagnosis is approximately 45% for all stages combined.

Sexually Transmitted Diseases in Males

Diseases of the male genital tract are overall substantially less common than those for females. As might be expected, all of the sexually transmitted diseases (STDs) of females are seen in males but with slightly different presentations. Whereas the infectious causes of vaginitis are relatively easy to diagnose on vaginal culture, in males, the only symptom may be burning in the urethra, i.e., within the penis. If there is a urethral discharge, this can be cultured in the same way that a vaginal culture would be assessed. Often, there are no obvious discharges. Sometimes, in such a case, secretions can be "induced," by the doctor performing rectal exam to get access to the prostate by firmly rubbing on the prostate. This mildly to moderately uncomfortable procedure is called "prostatic massage" and may produce just enough secretion to culture. If no secretions are produced, the only other option is to insert a dry culture swab into the urethral orifice at the tip of the penis. Besides being uncomfortable, the yield of meaningful results is low. If the sexual partner of this male has a known vaginal infection, sometimes it is simply best to treat the male for whatever the partner has and hope that this suffices.

On the other hand, some of the STDs are easier to diagnose in males because they are clearly visible, whereas in females, they could be hidden in the vagina or on the cervix. This would include the common venereal warts and herpes lesions. Syphilis, although much less common, usually shows a clearly seen lesion, usually on the penis. Incidentally, circumcision, which is removal of the penile foreskin, has become somewhat of the norm in Western culture and commonly practiced elsewhere. There are at least theoretical reasons why this might be desirable, largely related to concerns about hygiene and risk of penile or cervical cancer. Very rarely, there are mechanical problems such as incomplete retraction, which could interfere with erection or even urination. However, for the most part, as long as a person practices reasonable hygiene measures, there is no compelling reason to have circumcision. A subculture of uncircumcised males advocates against it for a number of reasons, most of which have nothing to do with health.

Testicular Tumors, Infection, and Torsion

As mentioned previously, the two structures which supply the majority of semen are the seminal vesicles and the prostate. The third and fourth major structures involved with male reproductive capacity are the testes and the epididymis. Recall that sperms are produced in the seminiferous tubules of the testes and then migrate through a relatively long tube called the vas deferens which empties into another channel which drains the seminal vesicle, just before it, in turn, enters the prostate. Of these four, only the seminal vesicles are virtually disease free. We have already discussed testicular function. Infection of the testes is somewhat rare, except for mumps (and perhaps a number of other viral insults) which causes "orchitis," with pain and swelling, and which can ultimately cause significant reduction in size and function of the affected testicle. Organisms associated with STDs can infrequently cause orchitis. The testicle can undergo several types of malignant degeneration, depending on the cell type involved. This too is usually accompanied by pain and perhaps enlargement of the testicle. Despite the potential aggressive nature of these malignancies, similar to what is seen in ovarian cancer, aggressive surgical and ancillary treatment can result in prolonged remission and cures in up to 90%, given particular circumstances. Lastly, the testicle can twist on its "stalk," called testicular torsion. This may be announced by sudden onset of intense pain, with no antecedent injury. Surgical correction is needed quickly in order to preserve blood supply to the testicle. Both testicular malignancies and torsion tend to occur in young people. Just as females are advised to do breast self-exam monthly, young males are advised to do self-exam of testes once per month. Testicular cancers are uncommon, occurring about one-fourth as often as ovarian cancer.

Epididymitis Equals Prostatitis

Both the prostate and the epididymis are subject to infections. The diagnosis of epididymitis can be made clinically by the basis of fairly sudden onset of pain within the scrotal sac. The testicle itself should feel normal, but the epididymis on the back side of the testicle may be exquisitely tender. There are a number of bacterial organisms which can be implicated, including those that cause STDs. The most common cause of urinary infections, *Escherichia coli*, may also be causative. Infections can occasionally occur in the setting of a urinary infection due to backflow of urine into the ejaculatory ducts. If this is not the case, that is, no identifiable urinary infection with positive culture, then antibiotic treatment must be somewhat empiric (meaning chosen by an educated guess), as there is no other simple way to culture the epididymitis. The bacteriology of prostatitis is more or less the same. Occasionally, prostatic secretions can be obtained by prostatic massage. Otherwise, the same guidelines regarding empiric treatment for prostatitis apply. Prostatitis, even low grade and without symptoms, can cause elevation of the prostate-specific antigen. Obviously, in a person above the age of forty, this could raise concern about the possibility of a prostate cancer.

Prostate Cancer

Prostate cancer is a common disease which warrants considerable attention. It is a scientifically interesting disease, from a number of standpoints, not the least of which includes a very broad spectrum of opinion as to what constitutes the best treatment. Unfortunately, there is enough subtle variability case to case such that consensus is often lacking. This should cause concern amongst the lay public, who should demand that medical scientists do a better job in stratifying risk. This would involve extricating personal bias and personal favorite treatments based on what the doctors do, rather than what is best to do. With this disease, it is justified to get second and third opinions and to aggressively question the treating doctors about facts and figures.

Another interesting feature of this disease is the often quoted dictum that if a man lives long enough, he will have prostate cancer. Although this may be true, rather than reflecting a scare tactic, it is designed to point out (a) how common the disease is and (b) that there is a huge biologic variability in tumor behavior, substantially dependent on the age of the person at the time of diagnosis. In general (never say never, and never say always), the dangers of this disease are inversely related to age at time of diagnosis. That is, the younger the patient, the more aggressive the disease can be, and the older the patient, the less aggressive it tends to be. A man in his forties with prostate cancer needs the best advice and the best insight.

Should the focus be on preservation of life or on preservation of erectile function? Now that the chuckles have died down, the fact of the matter is that this question is pondered seriously all the time. In a person considered to be a "candidate" for aggressive and hopefully corrective therapy, my own personal bias is to go for surgery, perhaps "radical prostatectomy" as front line treatment. I say this because any of the varied radiation therapy approaches, although they can be curative, could leave the person with lifetime debilitating side effects such as pain, rectal bleeding, diarrhea, and fecal incontinence, representing side effects of radiation proctitis (rectal inflammation caused from radiation).

Another interesting feature of this disease is the fact that for whatever reasons, unknown to me, the surgical approach regarding radical prostatectomy quickly lent itself to the possibility of robotic assistance. With the potential now for doing such robotic-assisted laparoscopic surgery, the operation appears to be safer, more effective, and with fewer side effects.

Prostate cancer in older men, as noted, tends to be less aggressive, particularly beyond the age of seventy-five. In fact, screening for prostate cancer is no longer recommended for people beyond the age of eighty. Once again, these are "guidelines," which can be and should be adapted and modified to meet the realities of the given situation. Treatment options at any age are still dependent on the stage of the tumor burden (confined to the prostate versus spread outside the prostate and to the location), the "Gleason score" (a means of estimating aggressiveness of tumor based on appearance under the microscope), and general health or so-called "co-morbidities." In reality, most men at age eighty have a life expectancy of five years or less. In these people, the best treatment may be very modest, such as medication to block testosterone activity, or none at all. Obviously, this approach might be completely inappropriate for an eighty year old, who has no serious illnesses, is physically active, and still has potential for living many years. Once again, this is an area where doctors must put their own egos and pocket books behind them and must advise patients based on the real politik. Consider also that despite the horror which most people respond to the concept of "rationing care" for financial reasons, if the will of the people manifests itself in that direction, in future years, the option of doing very expensive care for chronically very sick people may have already evaporated. Time will tell. I believe that "we" will get what "we," as a society, want.

For those of you who may be agonizing over discussions needing to be made regarding prostate cancer, Mukund Sargur may be able to advise you. He is a retired oncologist who has thoroughly studied the disease without bias. He can be reached best through Google.

Benign Prostatic Hyperplasia

There is another type of prostate growth which is very common and much less onerous. This is called "benign prostate hyperplasia" or BPH. It is the excessive non-malignant growth of the glandular elements of the prostate, often beginning at age forty or fifty and possibly culminating in a gland which is four times its normal size. Remarkably, in many instances, this creates little or no symptomatology. In fact, the only major common risk of this condition is that it can pinch off the urethra which flows through the prostate, causing a significant reduction in urine flow and possibly inability to completely empty the bladder. The condition is very common. The diagnosis is usually made on digital rectal (the doctor's finger) exam of the prostate and the appropriate history. Many people simply endure the nuisance of frequent, slow urination. Medications can help increase flow and/or shrink the gland. For those in whom this burden is too much—or who experience a complication such as a complete (agonizing) shutdown of urine flow, mandating a trip to the ER, sudden substantial urinary bleeding, or declining kidney function as urine backs up to the kidney—an operative procedure to relieve the obstruction may be necessary.

There are a number of relatively new operative techniques, which have appeared on the scene within the last ten to fifteen years, each claiming to be superior to the previous operative technique. The grand daddy of them all, however, has yet to be declared obsolete. In fact, transurethral resection of the prostate, affectionately dubbed TURP, and rhyming with burp, having been devised seventy-five years ago, is still widely performed. To a non-surgeon (me), it appears to be a very good operation. It is performed in the operating room, usually with a general anesthetic. It sounds ghastly. A large bore tube is inserted through the urethral meatus, at the tip of the penis, and advanced up to the level of the prostate. Resection can be carried out in several ways, but usually the prostate is literally scraped out. Most people spend one night in the hospital. There is remarkably little postoperative pain. A catheter is left in place for three to five days, at which time it is easily removed, and the process is completed. Results are predictably good in a high percentage of people.

If nothing else, medical practitioners are charged with the challenge of reducing suffering. In fact, it says so in the Hippocratic Oath. The names of the doctors who devised this operation may be lost to history or, at least, to common knowledge. The technique that they left behind has relieved an enormous amount of suffering, which stands as a milestone event. One could argue that those types of medical and surgical breakthroughs only occur every twenty years or so. This one has truly stood the test of time. Several others are coming, perhaps even bigger and better, to be discussed at the end of this book.

Female–Male Genital Complementaries

Close scrutiny by anatomists and physiologists has shown that the male and female genital organs share representative parts, either vestigial or crucial with a very few exceptions. Obviously, the ovaries and testes, although going about their work differently, have a similar gross (visual) appearance and both produce items containing half of the full, human, genetic compliment. The similarities between the penis and clitoris are slightly less obvious, but both share erectile tissue and both are important for orgasm. The correlation between Cowper's glands in the male, just below the prostate, and Bartholin glands, at the vaginal introitus, is discernable, as both provide lubrication. Finally, perhaps the most debatable or controversial correlation might be between the prostate gland and Skene's glands in the female, located along the course of the urethra and which some researchers call the "female prostate," both producing fluid which can be ejaculated (both women and doctors who have studied the female orgasmic response concur that female ejaculation appears to be real and a relatively common phenomena). The one very notable exception is the vagina, for which there is no male correlate. Incidentally, vagina derives from "sheath."

Having said all of that, in contrast to the genital tract, the urinary tract in males and females can be appraised jointly, as the differences between the two are relatively minor and the diseases shared are basically the same. It is relatively easy to divide the urinary tract into four parts. Three of these four have only one function. This in itself is slightly unusual, as it can be recalled that the major organ systems studied so far have a significant amount of built-in redundancy, with different members overlapping somewhat in function. Nevertheless, the urethra, extending from the bladder to the "outside," the bladder, and the paired ureters, extending from the kidneys to the bladder, can all be considered to be luminal (hollow) organs, similar to the GI tract, and are technically outside of the body, although surrounded by it. In contrast to the GI tract, in which materials are entering and leaving the inside-outside interface all the way through, the same is not true for urethra, bladder, and ureters. Their only purpose is to convey urine out of the body, or more accurately whereby it is no longer surrounded by the body, and to do it at an appropriate time. The kidney's job, as mentioned previously, is to filter the blood and regulate its chemical constituency.

UTI

The urethra and, to a lesser extent, the bladder are the two structures in which there are noticeable differences in disease profiles. The urethra in females is considerably shorter than in males. In addition, its terminus is enclosed by the labia minora and majora, thus just outside of the vagina with its relatively indolent bacterial population, but relatively close to the anus/rectum with its relatively nasty residential bacterial population. Having said all of that, including all of the "relatively," it is easy to appreciate why "urinary tract infections" (UTIs) are much more common in women than in men. When doctors use the term UTI, the unspoken implication is that they are referring to bladder infection. Urethral infections can occur as isolated entities, but they are usually related to STDs, not involving the rest of the urinary tract, which have been discussed already. The symptoms of urethritis and UTI may overlap considerably, with burning, worse with urination, urinary frequency, and even itching being all very common. Visible discharge, however, should not be seen in UTI and is much more common with urethritis/STD.

Doctors have been accused, and rightly so, of having warped senses of humor and appreciation. After all, who else but a doctor could marvel at the intricacies of urinary infections? Here is another example. For most people, primarily women, a UTI is a nuisance, a day or two of burning and frequency, a quick trip to the doctor or lab to pee in a cup, a few days of the appropriate antibiotic, and it is all over. Digressing for a moment, is a culture necessary? The answer is that it is highly desirable. The bacteriology of UTI seems to have changed in the last twenty years such that a large number of previously considered oddball bacteria are now showing up in cultures. In addition, we all know about the so-called indiscriminant use of antibiotics, much of which is demanded by patients and provided by doctors fearful of demanding patients, and which has lead to considerable resistance patterns in bacteria that were previously sensitive to everything. I may occasionally make an exception, in a very few cases. First of all, if the person has no insurance and not much money, since cultures are expensive ($40 to $60), I might do an educated guess first. Secondly, if the person lives in a remote area or has a chronic catheter system of some type, ensuring that they are likely infected chronically by a number of germs, I might do the educated guess. In the person without insurance, a simple $10 urinalysis should be done to at least confirm that it is a urinary infection and not urethritis. Since almost all urinary cultures are done by commercial labs, I am happy to say that asking for a culture does not financially reward the doctor in any way.

Back to the innocent little bladder infection. Two very bad things can transpire, particularly in the elderly and/or chronically ill. You have heard enough about "sepsis" by now, previously called "blood poisoning" to guess that even though the bladder is a luminal organ, and technically outside of the body, the infection can make its way into the bloodstream and produce the full-blown sepsis syndrome and possibly result in a fatal outcome. Although this is not common with bladder infection, it can occur. The second bad thing which is frequently seen in the elderly is altered mentation. This occurs most often in people who previously have been thought to have some evidence for mild cognitive dysfunction. However, sometimes it can be the sentinel, first event. In fact, if this looks like a typical bladder infection (not ascending into the kidneys), with no fever, normal or slightly elevated white blood count, "negative" blood culture, no back pain (where the kidneys are), etc., I consider cognitive dysfunction or confusional state to be the first sign of an emerging dementia. So, everyone should be aware that if granny, whom various family members have previously noted, could be showing just a little bit of "memory" problem, suddenly becomes quite confused, although many would think first of a stroke, it could be a simple bladder infection. We don't really know why or how this brain–bladder connection works. Recall, that the full-blown sepsis syndrome involves a variety of signs and symptoms, including confusion or even coma. Does this mean that a few bacteria have slipped into the bloodstream and poisoned the brain?

Back to the bladder infection in otherwise healthy people. Given the anatomy, perhaps it is a more surprising fact that some women go a lifetime with no bladder infections than to the fact that some women have occasional bladder infections. Women should pay a little more attention to genital hygiene than men. I had one female patient who became ill enough to be hospitalized at the time of her second, sequential UTI, having come through the ER, with its multiple layers of care. I came in to see her. As I entered the room, she sat bolt upright in bed, pointed her trembling finger at me and shouted, "If you tell me to wipe from front to back, I'll scream!" Since then, I have never told a patient to wipe from front to back. No one has yet screamed at me when I suggest that they pee after intercourse rather than before, which is an effective way to wash the urethra naturally.

UTIs in males, particularly relatively younger males, are so uncommon compared to females that when definitely identified as such, one is obligated to at least question why that might have happened. For instance, could there be infected stones in the urinary system, particularly bladder stones which may be immobile? Could the prostate be partially obstructing such that the bladder does not empty completely, thereby creating stasis? Recall that the body does not like stasis. Most of the time, stasis is related to mild depletion of body fluids and low urinary output. The body is like the Everglades, which is functionally a very shallow, very wide river, very slowly moving south to the Gulf of Florida. We too have a similar need to flow and cleanse our tissues and enclosed spaces.

This leads to perhaps the most common reason for UTI in both males and females. Personally, I don't think that everybody needs to drink eight glasses of water every day, everywhere. However, I think that some people may need to do this, or even more. Some may need to do it all of the time, and some only some of the time. How many times have I emphasized that to my way of thinking globally, although we are remarkably similar, there are abundant subtle factors creating dissimilarity, such that we have our particular little needs, likes and dislikes, which are not really diseases? As we go through life, I think we figure out these little subtleties, perhaps unconsciously, which come to constitute our habits, which give others fodder to take potshots at us. The point is that low fluid intake with subsequent low volume urinary flow may be the common denominator for UTI in people who have no other obvious explanation.

In summary, UTIs are very common in females. They are unusual but not rare in males. Drink enough to produce 1,500 cc (1½ quarts) urine per day, for an average-sized person. Keep the wide river that we are, inching along.

Dysfunctional Voiding

Thank goodness for our bladders, with the same level of gratitude, and for the same reasons that we feel for our colons. Had we evolved in a way whereby urine consistently had egressed from us, somehow, society would have evolved in remarkably different ways. Bladder infections are not the big problem. There are bigger prices that we have to pay for the luxury of having our bladders. There are three other common diseases or processes to consider. Once again, since pelvic anatomy and physiology are more complicated in females, they tend to have more difficulties with structural issues. Ultimately, those issues tend to lead to problems with voiding, either inability to void easily or inability to not void easily.

Likely because of the childbearing process, females have problems with pelvic support, so-called pelvic floor problems, much more often than males. This can involve alteration in the lowermost portions of the urinary and bowel systems, which need certain angles to function properly. As the pelvic floor sags, these angles are altered, such that evacuation of urine and/or feces may become difficult. Recall that the bladder is in front of the vagina and the rectum in back. Loss of anterior support can cause the bladder to sag and may be visible in the vagina as a "cystocele," pushing down and from front to back. Loss of posterior support causes the rectum to sag, can make bowel evacuation difficult, and can be seen as a downward and back to front bulge in the vagina, called "rectocele." Often, they are both present. Occasionally, the situation can be so severe that either one or both of those can physically pouch enough to protrude outside of the vagina.

These can be very vexing problems. I have seen them take over a person's life such that the person spends hours daily trying to evacuate bowels and bladder. Echoes of that Tammy Wynette "Hard to be a

Woman" song return. There is really no medical treatment for this, except for attempts at keeping feces soft, so that they have a better chance to be evacuated. The situation regarding the bladder is actually more complicated in some ways, in that, with loss of pelvic support, there can be either inability to empty and/or inability to withhold urine in the same person, at differing times. There is no medicinal treatment for this. There are a number of surgical procedures devised to deal with these problems. In my experience, they offer tantalizingly variable results. The best advice I can give is to approach the decision to have surgery deliberately and thoughtfully. Be inquisitive and direct. Ask the right questions of the doctors you choose to see. How many of these operations have you done? What percentage of patients have good results? What is the worst complication you have had? Etc.. Perhaps, this might be the type of undertaking where you might want to go to a different city, to a "tertiary referral center" where they do these operations every day. Perhaps you want to have a doctor who specializes in "female urology." Lastly, perhaps this is the type of surgery which will eventually lend itself to robotic assistance.

Another "bad" condition, again much more common in women, will be mentioned in passing, as it is not very common. This is called interstitial cystitis. This is a disorder generally affecting middle-aged to elderly women. The major symptom is continuous, intense "urgency," meaning a very strong feeling of the need to urinate, even minutes after urination of a small amount of urine. This intensely unpleasant feeling may be very briefly relieved by urinating. This does not appear to be caused by infection. The diagnosis tends to be confirmed at the time of cystoscopy, which is a procedure whereby an instrument is advanced through the urethra and into the bladder. With instillation of fluid into the bladder to distend the walls, a pinpoint array of hemorrhage can be seen. Or if a solution containing potassium is instilled, this can cause an inordinate amount of pain. Many different approaches have been used to address the problem, including medications by mouth and meds instilled directly into the bladder. Recall the rule of thumb that the greater number of options available to treat a condition, the lesser likelihood that any one or a combination of options will help. Sometimes pain-relieving medicine helps. The cause is unknown. When there is nothing else to offer, avoiding the four Cs (carbonated beverage, citrus, caffeine, and vitamin C) may help.

Hematuria

Bladder cancer is more common in men by a factor of two or three to one. Symptoms can be very non-specific and overlap with infections and other diseases. However, there is a very notable tip-off which may push the diagnostic workup to a conclusive result. This is urinary bleeding. The bleeding can be sudden and substantial, or it can be microscopic and intermittent. Blood in the urine is called hematuria. Once this is definitely established (eating beets can make the urine red; a breakdown of red blood cells in the circulation, called hemolysis, can do the same), by seeing excessive numbers of red blood cells under the microscope, it is necessary to thoroughly investigate this finding. The most common cause of hematuria is UTI because UTIs are so common. Kidney and bladder stones are common, and both are usually accompanied by, at least, microscopic hematuria. Ureteral and kidney tumors can cause hematuria. Inflammation of the kidneys, called "nephritis," of which there are several varieties soon to be discussed, causes bleeding into the urine. Some of these kidney diseases are not usually progressive, and not much feared, but can still show a continuous appearance of hematuria. Lastly, when the workup is completed, a certain number of these conditions are caused by our handy-dandy garbage can term "idiopathic," i.e., cause unknown. For those of you who feel that with the training they receive and the fees they charge, doctors should do better, inserting a "T" into idiopathic gives a better term, i.e., "idiotpathic."

So, what is the "workup?" As always, the diagnosis may lurk in the history. A detailed history, including occupational history, history of trauma, length of time the hematuria has been present, and family history (cancer, urinary tract stones), could truncate the workup. If no hot clues are forthcoming, physical exam probably will not add much. Nevertheless, exam of genitals, including urethral meatus (opening), could reveal something important. Abdominal exam could reveal a "mass," just above the public bone for bladder or in either upper outer abdominal area for kidneys. Women should likely have a full pelvic exam to reduce the possibility of a vaginal source of bleeding. Blood testing may not yield much but should give information about kidney function and possibly regarding the question of nephritis. All of these, so far, have been relatively easy and consuming only one office visit.

If nothing is forthcoming at this juncture, as is often the case, there remain three bigger and more expensive undertakings ahead. As is the norm, "invasive" studies are usually reserved for the end of the evaluation. Imaging studies would probably come next, such as a CT scan of the kidneys, ureters, and bladder, so-called "CT-KUB" or "CTIVP," looking for stones, tumors, or whatever. If that is unrevealing, then an invasive study, cystoscopy, mentioned already, will likely come next. During a cystoscopy, a flexible scope is inserted into the urethra, advanced past the prostate in males (and please recall that enlarged prostates are somewhat prone to spontaneous bleeding), and into the bladder, where a careful direct examination is carried out. Biopsies can be done, if indicated, and the ureteral orifices can be identified, with samples of urine taken from each side. If there is still no answer, the last decision, made perhaps by the urologist, your PCP, and you, might revolve around the question of whether to proceed with the most invasive and last study—that being a kidney biopsy—looking for nephritis or nephropathy. Sometimes these are done by kidney specialists and sometimes by "interventional radiologists." Have it done by the most experienced person if it is being seriously considered.

Please recall that doctors generally subscribe to the notion that if a diagnostic study is unlikely to change decisions regarding therapy, then it probably should not be done. This is where you come in, by agreeing to live under the veil of not knowing versus doing every possible test which could culminate in a knowing. It may be helpful to play out mind games, before the answers are in. For instance, if the biopsy shows kidney disease "X," requiring potentially dangerous drug "Y" to slow it down, will I accept that or simply wait and watch? On the other hand, what would I do if the biopsy shows normal tissue, implying that we might have a sampling error, having missed an area of pathology with the needle? Would I consent to the biopsy again? Kidney biopsies, as is true for many other types of needle biopsies, are "blind" in the sense that although it is known that the needle is in the organ, the pathology deep in the organ may be inhomogeneous and thus missable by the needle tip.

Bladder Cancer

Getting back to bladder cancer, there is a good chance that the first major symptom could be hematuria. Bladder cancer is relatively common, more frequent in males, usually middle age and older. There are certain occupations which appear to predispose to this condition, possibly accounting for the male preponderance. These include metal fabrication, rubber manufacture, and textile work. There is a definite connection with cigarette smoking. There is a weaker connection in people with habitually low intake of fluids.

The lining membrane of the urinary system, from urethra to the collecting ducts in the kidney, shares the slightly peculiar ability to deform significantly, without splitting, and is called transitional (cell) epithelium. Most of the urinary tumors in these areas have the same appearance under the microscope. So, finding malignant cells in the urine may be very important but doesn't necessarily pinpoint where the tumor is. Statistically, since the bladder is so relatively large, and bladder cancer relatively common, most often it represents bladder cancer.

As with many other luminal organs, depth of penetration of the wall is crucially important in delineating prognosis and treatment. Bladder tumors have a propensity to remain very superficial, spreading over a large surface area of the bladder and likely having something to do with the peculiarities of the transitional cell membrane itself. These superficial spreading tumors can be shaved off mechanically through the cystoscope, sometimes repeatedly. Or, electrocautery can be used. There is a substance called "BCG," representing the last names of the French discoverers of this material, dating back to 1921, and representing a breakthrough in vaccination technology and the immune response. This has been used in the past and still is in some parts of the world, in an attempt to induce a level of immunity to tuberculosis. It does incite an immune response and, because of this, has been tried as topical treatment, instilled into the bladder, with a measure of success in controlling this type of tumor.

In summary, the cure rate or at least prolonged remission rate using these topical approaches vary between 45% and 95%. However, as can be surmised from data with other luminal organs, once the wall begins to be penetrated, including all the way through the surrounding fat and membranes, the opportunity for cure drops precipitously. There is potential for extensive local disease and even distant metastases. For some of these people, particularly if they are young and otherwise healthy, in an attempt to "salvage" the situation, ingenious and adventurous surgical procedures have been devised to perform radical cystectomy (removal of the entire bladder and adjacent tissues) and fashioning of a new bladder by using a portion of the bowel. As can be imagined, this is a very big and complicated operation, with potential for serious complications, but occasionally life saving. Perhaps, this type of aggressive approach is justified in view of the fact that the other powerful cancer fighting approaches, radiation and/or chemotherapy, are not very effective with this tumor.

On this note of caution, please recall that the incidence of bladder cancer that is linked to cigarette smoking and in people who are not occupationally predisposed may thus be preventable.

The bladder can also be the site of stones and polyps. These are usually dealt with locally. Large stones may need to be surgically removed.

The ureters, for the most part, are not commonly problematic. They can be duplicated. They can allow urine to reflux backup toward the kidneys. They can have strictures, polyps, or "webs." They can also be the site of transitional cell cancers. All of these, however, are uncommon or, at least, uncommonly problematic. Basically, the ureters do what they are supposed to do, quietly and methodically.

That brings us all the way up to the kidneys, which, as mentioned hours ago, are the only truly operational or creative part of the urinary system. Anatomically, they are paired, one on each side, in the retroperitoneal space (behind the abdomen) protected by being deep in the body and surrounded by thick muscle, fat, and ribs. They are divided into an outer cortex, each containing approximately one million of the actual functional units called glomeruli or nephrons. The function of these glomeruli, each of which is a plexus of capillaries (the terminal portions of the arterial system, allowing only one blood cell to pass at a time), is to get the blood in contact with the extracellular fluid. With the help of blood pressure gradients, ionic gradients, and a complicated "countercurrent multiplier system," the kidneys can rid the body of toxins and regulate (by excretion or retention) many crucial body chemicals, such as sodium, potassium, and magnesium. Is that clear? Don't worry! I don't understand it either.

Nephrolithiasis

Before focusing on the kidneys per se, and their great creative gift of making urine, this is a good time to discuss a topic which has plagued humans since they became human (this has nothing to do with lousy weather). Urinary tract stones have been found in mummies, carbon-dated to 7,000 years ago. So common and debilitating has been this scourge that some of the first surgical procedures developed had to do with attempts to remove stones, particularly bladder stones. Risk of doing this was so high that Hippocrates insisted that physicians not even try, leaving that to specialists called "lithotomists." By the 1800s, primitive devices had been developed to attempt destruction and removal of the stones via the urethra. However, perioperative death rates remained very high until new instrumentation and much better anesthetic and aseptic techniques became the standard of care in the late 1800s.

Kidney stone disease is technically called nephrolithiasis. It is very common. In fact, there is a one in eight chance that people living in industrialized countries will develop symptomatic stone disease, during the course of their lives. It is not clearly known how often asymptomatic disease is present, meaning the painless passage of small stones, but it is likely common. Kidney stones are three times more common in males than females. Bladder stones, which are more clearly related to obstructive issues (prostate), are eight times more common in males than females. They tend to occur between the ages of twenty and fifty. First-time stone disease is unusual beyond fifty to fifty-five years (one of the many benefits of aging, along with bus passes and cosmetic dentures) Dietary factors are known to play a role, but it is not clear why kidney stones are much more common in industrialized countries versus bladder stones relatively more common in underdeveloped countries.

It is felt that the first step in the development of kidney stones is the appearance of plaques of calcium phosphate in the collecting system of the kidney tubules. Why these form and what percentages go on to develop full-blown kidney stones is not known. We do know that relatively, low fluid intake, especially in hot weather, and excessive calcium in the urine are two absolute risk factors. Increased urinary calcium has several potential causes. Interestingly, high dietary calcium intake has to be very high to be considered a possible risk factor. Much more commonly, an intrinsic abnormality of kidney processing of calcium is thought to be the issue. The kidney tubules are supposed to reabsorb calcium filtered through the glomerulus. If they fail to do this adequately, such a calcium "leak" stays in the urine. In addition, sometimes, excessive absorption of calcium through the gut can contribute to the problem, as can an overly active parathyroid gland (recall that these glands are on the under surface of the thyroid and regulate calcium metabolism by their effect on bone and bowel).

Recall the bell-shaped curve. Although kidney stones may pass with minimal or no symptoms, passage of stones has often been described as excruciating. Women who have given birth to eight- and nine-pound butterballs have personally confirmed to me that they would rather pass three of those than one six-millimeter kidney stone. With a very typical kidney stone, leaving its birthing area in the kidney and entering the ureter, the pain might first be felt in the flank (the side of the back at the lower edge of the ribcage). As the stone migrates down the ureter, the pain is felt to shift around to the side and then to the abdomen. Further migration causes the pain to be felt progressively lower in the side of the abdomen, down to the groin area. At that time, pain can also be felt in the genitals, on the same side as the stone. As soon as the stone leaves the ureter and enters the bladder, the pain is magically and mercifully gone. This entire sequence can last only a few minutes or up to a few days, depending on how fast the stone moves. During this time, stone victims can be rendered helpless, writhing in agony, sweating profusely, and vomiting.

The incidence, or possibly the recognition of kidney stone disease, seems to be increasing, for reasons that are not clear. It is always advisable to "capture" at least one stone for analysis. This can be easily done by using a specially designed filter, particularly for small stones, in the three- to four-millimeter bracket. The larger ones may announce themselves by an audible "clink," as they dive into the toilet bowl. Many of them are nasty looking jagged stalagmites that look like they have been sculpted by geologic forces over millennia. Eighty percent of them are made primarily of calcium and oxalate. Approximately, 15% are uric acid stones. The last five to ten are any number of other chemical configurations. The so-called struvite stones are complex arrangements of magnesium–ammonium–phosphate and are usually seen in conjunction with chronic urinary tract infections. They are often very large, so-called staghorn calculi in the kidney or bladder stones, and thus do not migrate.

Knowledge of the composition of the stones usually allows for elaboration on the prevention side of the equation, going beyond increasing fluid intake. For calcium oxalate stones, somewhat counterintuitively, it may be helpful to slightly increase calcium in the diet if it is deemed too low. This is because calcium in the gut binds with oxalate to reduce oxalate absorption. In terms of other dietary alterations, few of you would need to schedule extra appointments with your psychotherapists over the loss of spinach in your diet. Even fewer would mourn the loss of soybeans. However, the elimination of chocolate may be too much to bear. Along the way, you also need to decrease meat intake and soda. Given these proscriptions, there may be a few of you who will choose the stones.

There are few medications helpful in stone disease. Hydrochlorothiazide, a common diuretic, increases urinary sodium excretion, and this may reduce calcium excretion and help with reduction in incidence. Passage of stones can be a once-in-a-lifetime event. Most typically, it may be an infrequent occurrence, perhaps once every two to five years. In a few unfortunate people, it may occur daily to weekly and basically go a long way toward ruining that person's life. A vast majority of stones pass spontaneously. For those that get stuck along the way, urologists are challenged to remove the stones using devices devised by their sixteenth-century colleagues. Under the worst circumstances, surgical procedures of various types may be necessary for removal. Alternatively, depending on many factors, "lithotripsy," using ultrasonic shock waves to shatter the stones, may be used, after which they pass in tiny fragments.

Hours ago, I promised that we would focus on the kidney and spend some time discussing what I called the only creative part of the urinary system—that is the production of urine, with the side benefit being the regulation of fluid and electrolyte balance. Imbalances of such can be quickly lethal. We are getting close, blocked by only a few more diversions.

Concurrent Biologic Similarity–Dissimilarity

A recurring theme of this discourse has been the oxymoronic fact that we of species *Homo sapiens sapiens* are remarkably both similar and dissimilar, simultaneously. Ultimately, this is a plea for compassion and to become as gentle, gracious, and forgiving of our fellow travelers as is legally, morally, and practically possible. Intrinsic to this construct, which truly is factual, is that we all take in and process information differently. No wonder that we come to different opinions.

The Concept of Elegance

In looking at and studying human beings, it has always seemed to me that we are remarkably complex and that it is miraculous that our biologic machinery seems to work so well. However, there has also existed this nagging torment that somehow or another, evolution, or God, or whoever and whatever was involved in creating this unbelievably complex machine, did it during the course of a long nightmare. Mathematicians use the word "elegant" not to describe a new tuxedo (because like me, they wear their high school sweaters) but to describe simplicity, as in Occam's razor. The most obvious example of this is the equation known by perhaps every conscious person, $E = mc^2$. That simple designation states that matter is energy, and that energy is matter, and that what we have in the universe is the coming and going of the two faces of this phenomenon.

The Nephron

So, utilizing the observations that come to me and are internally processed, and drawing on all of my biases, try as I may to subdue them, it appears to me that besides the brain and nervous system, the kidney is the most complex structure in the body. Paying homage to this complexity, others may see it as elegant. I see it as stunningly clever, yet I can't help but wonder whether it really had

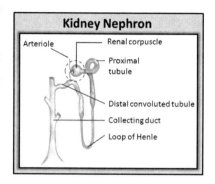

to be so complex. After all, dialysis machines do much of what the kidneys do and are much simpler in design. Granted, they weigh several hundred pounds more.

The kidneys, and specifically the nephron, of which there are approximately one million per kidney, make urine. The two diagrams are a representation of an entire nephron, from the ingoing and outgoing arterioles (already a diversion from standard, by having an outgoing arteriole rather than a venule, allowing for much more precise regulation of filtration pressure), to the "proximal convoluted tubule," to the "loop of Henle" where the counter current multiplier system lives, to the "distal convoluted tubule," and into the "collecting duct." If you look at the pictures, you will see that the tubule heading out from the glomerulus, marked C, takes a long course before returning to the entrance to the glomerulus, marked D. This microscopic anatomic arrangement is absolutely crucial for the nephron to function, as the so-called juxtaglomerular apparatus, involving cells of the distal tubule and several different types of cells of the glomerulus itself, regulate pressure through the glomerulus by sensing differences in the chemical composition of incoming blood, as well as hormonal input, and input

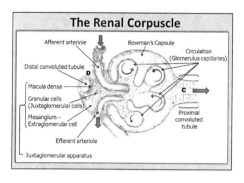

The Renal Corpuscle

Afferent arteriole
Bowman's Capsule
Circulation (Glomerulus capillaries)
Distal convoluted tubule
D
Macula densa
Granular cells (Juxtaglomerular cells)
Mesangium –
Extraglomerular cell
C
Proximal convoluted tubule
Efferent arteriole
Juxtaglomerular apparatus

from the nervous system, which in turn produces a crucial hormone called renin, involved in control of blood pressure. (Whenever I start thinking "nephron," we see another seventy plus word sentence. I apologize.) This officially marks the end of meanderings into renal physiology. Elegant? Or unnecessarily complex? Let's review kidney diseases.

In fact, the most common ones, including infections and stones, have already been discussed. The creative portion of the urinary system is the kidney and specifically the "nephron." As can be imagined, it is relatively easy and convenient to divide the nephron into two portions. The first is the glomerulus, where filtration of blood occurs by hydrostatic pressures pushing fluid out of the circulation, and into Bowman's capsule, which is functionally the first part of the tubular system. At that moment, this fluid is technically out of the body, as it enters the proximal convoluted tubule (a luminal structure), which when unimpeded goes directly through the urethra and out! However, work on the fluid has just begun. Each of the remaining parts of the tubular portion of the nephron has specific responsibility regarding what stays in the lumen versus what is reabsorbed back into the circulation. This exquisitely delicate dance of fluid and chemicals is under control of the moment-to-moment signals received by the tubules, with information coming through several avenues, including the endocrine system, the nervous system, and the cardiovascular system. (Recall that the heart produces atrial natriuretic peptide, which directly affects the nephron).

Erythropoietin, Vitamin D, and Renin

In fact, the kidney itself could be called an endocrine organ as well, in view of the fact that it produces or modifies three substances which would qualify as hormones. Erythropoietin is a fascinating substance produced by the peritubular fibroblasts of the cortex. How and why these particular cells in this particular location were given or took on the responsibility of producing a complex and fascinating hormone remains a mystery. The question "how does it know?" could apply to this group of cells, just as it might apply to a child who asks why a thermos bottle knows how to keep hot things hot and cold things cold. The answer may be "obvious," yet it remains unknown. The peritubular fibroblasts senses oxygenation and may produce erythropoietin in states of low oxygenation, with receptors for erythropoietin found mostly in the bone marrow and the nervous system. Erythropoietin is best known for its action to stimulate production of red blood cells, in the bone marrow. In view of the fact that red blood cells are the major carrier of oxygen, the connection with oxygenation by the peritubular fibroblasts can be seen. Erythropoietin also has a role in the response of the brain to injury. Thus, this hormone comes from fibroblasts, and fibroblasts produce the extracellular matrix, which is the ground substance upon which cells are built, as well as the collagen (connective tissue) fibrils, adding stability to the matrix. We see that the acorn doesn't fall far from the tree. Lastly, erythropoietin has a role in the production of new blood vessels, called angiogenesis.

The second of the hormones which is kidney dependent is vitamin D. There has been a huge amount of interest in vitamin D levels and metabolism in the last five years or so, as it has become common knowledge that vitamin D levels are very often low and sometimes remarkably low in people living in far northern and far southern latitudes. This is particularly true in winter months. The kidney has a very important role in modifying the chemical configuration of vitamin D, in essence creating the active form of the substance. Vitamin D participates in at least 100 enzymatic reactions in the body. Its overall effects on health and disease are likely underestimated, as we are just now seeing the emergence of research studies involving vitamin D. It has been known to be intimately associated with bone disease and calcium metabolism. There are now correlations noted between vitamin D and immune system competence, cancer (colon, breast), vascular pathology, multiple sclerosis, and migraine. There appears to be much more data coming soon.

Lastly, the juxtaglomerular cells of the nephron produce a substance called renin which is a peptide hormone. This substance is one of the important components of the intricate system controlling blood pressure. Jumping the gun slightly, it should not be surprising that in the setting of end-stage kidney disease, one is likely to see problems relating to red blood cell production (anemia), bone metabolism ("renal osteodystrophy," which is a specialized form of bone loss), and blood pressure (high). In fact, problems of this sort are commonly seen even in mild renal failure.

Renal Failure—Acute and Chronic

This issue of mild renal failure is worthy of a brief side trip. The major term used to assess renal function for many years has been the creatinine level. Creatinine is a product of muscle metabolism and thus has some relationship to a person's total body muscle mass. The greater the muscle mass, the higher the creatinine might be. This could cause alarm if the creatinine level in that muscular person is elevated, but it has nothing to do with renal failure. If the muscular man or woman is taking a supplement called creatine, it could be even higher, again not reflecting true renal failure. We have also known that a creatinine level of 1.2 (likely normal) and one of 1.8 (likely abnormal) would represent deterioration in renal function. In the last five to ten years, we have focused much more attention on the levels between about 0.8 and 1.8, with a second decimal point utilized now, such as 1.85. In addition, the term "glomerular filtration rate" (GFR) has received much more attention and is usually reported along with the creatinine. GFR above 60 is thought to be normal. The interesting thing is that a creatinine of 1.40 could represent a GFR of 65, while a creatinine of 1.65 could reveal the GFR to be 55, i.e., "renal failure." As creatinine rises to 1.85, GFR could be as low as 45 to 50. So, we have come to pay much more attention to these relatively minor perturbations near the "normal" values of creatinine and GFR.

It seems that the most important factor is whether or not these figures are stable, reflecting a previous insult to renal function which may now be neutralized, or whether there is ongoing deterioration, suggesting an active process and demanding an evaluation to find the cause. Please note that dialysis does not become a consideration until the GFR falls to the level of 10 to 15, with creatinine then being in the 5 to 6 range. Metabolic abnormalities are frequently seen even with mild renal insufficiency.

Diseases leading to renal failure can usually be separated out to those involving the glomerulus and those involving the tubules. Also, the concept of acute renal failure (ARF), often reversible, and chronic renal failure (CRF), usually not reversible, comes into play. ARF is frequently seen in sick hospitalized patients. Anything that causes a drop in blood pressure, such as dehydration, or sepsis syndrome, or a big heart attack, can cause ARF. This can also be seen, but much less commonly, as a result of rheumatic fever ("strep") or contaminated food (*E. coli*). Most often, these diseases revert to normal or near normal renal function when corrected. These diseases can affect the glomeruli and/or the tubules.

Chronic renal failure is more likely from glomerular injury and basically has to do with all of those factors which damage blood vessels. This includes diabetes, hypertension, tobacco use, high cholesterol, and genetics, such as the relatively common IgA nephropathy, often beginning in young adults. IgA nephropathy is one of a number of autoimmune diseases, including lupus erythematosus and scleroderma and other less common entities, which incite production of antibodies which are relatively large molecules that lodge in glomeruli and damage them, during their filtering through the kidney. Interestingly, with IgA disease, exacerbations tend to be initiated by common mucosal diseases, such as appearance of ordinary URI or UTI, as IgA is found in high concentrations in these tissues. Note please, as I have pointed out ad nauseam, that many of these factors leading to chronic glomerular injury are avoidable! Also, CRF of any type can be made worse if there is a significant blockage in the main renal arteries. There are many different subtypes of glomerulopathy, each with its own few peculiarities and prognosis. Renal biopsy, with special pathologic investigation, is needed to sort out these differences.

Glomeruli and/or tubules can also be injured by toxins, including toxic medications. In this latter category, we see potential for serious damage from commonly used over-the-counter and prescription anti-inflammatories, as well as lithium commonly used for bipolar disorder. Many other medications, including some antibiotics, are potentially nephrotoxic. Lastly, although less common now than in the past, chronic urinary infections can damage the tubules primarily and lead to renal failure. This is most commonly seen in people who need chronic catheter drainage of the urinary system.

CRF was just described as a number below sixty. At that time, the person who has this, whatever the cause, perhaps having had symptoms at some time in the past (symptoms of infection, stones, bleeding), is likely to have no specific symptoms related to the renal failure. Often, significant symptoms do not make their appearance until the person nears the designation of "end-stage renal disease" (ESRD), with GFR 20 or less. At that juncture, prominent systemic symptoms come into the picture, including nausea, vomiting, pain, itching, fatigue, and malaise, that is, a total meltdown of vigor and enthusiasm.

Dialysis

Unfortunately, the only effective treatment available for ESRD may be dialysis. There are several different ways to accomplish dialysis, which involves cleansing of the blood and regulation of body chemistry and fluid balance using techniques which supplement whatever low level of kidney function remains. These techniques represent symptomatic treatment, meaning they don't cure the basic condition but do the cleansing job sufficiently to preserve life. Dialysis can be accomplished by inserting a catheter into the abdominal cavity, where it stays, and by irrigating large quantities of fluid in and out, affecting partial cleansing. More commonly, hemodialysis is utilized, in one of three ways, using a catheter or a surgically created "shunt" in the arm. The three are dialysis in a center, in an auxiliary clinic, or at home. Generally speaking, it is done three times per week, for about four hours each time. Home dialysis allows for more flexibility and potentially for much longer dialysis times. The type of dialysis selected is based on many factors, including age and co-morbidities of the patient, support at home, availability, insurance coverage, and many other issues.

The problems associated with dialysis are huge and getting bigger. There are significant morbidities (problems) associated with dialysis. Hospitalizations are frequent for a large variety of co-morbid issues. There may be numerous shunt issues. Patients often feel chronically ill, some describing it as "existing," rather than "living." It is enormously expensive, when all of the associated costs, including those of hospitalization, are added up. A few people seem very happy with it and do amazingly well.

Transplantation

The only alternative for ESRD is transplantation. Although there is no absolute age cutoff, as there is with transplantation of other organs because of increasing co-morbidities in older people, transplantation is often not considered an option beyond the age of seventy. The donor pool can either be family members or cadavers, with results slightly better for family members, due to better tissue matching, and subsequently less chance of rejection, and lesser requirements for dangerous immune suppressing drugs. End-stage renal disease is rapidly increasing in numbers because of our steadily aging population, with all of the common attendant co-morbidities. As noted, it is enormously expensive, particularly the costs of dialysis. It is already severely straining the Medicare budget, at the same time that we hear talk about potential upcoming cuts in the budget. This has the potential to be another of those emerging "perfect storm" scenarios. At this time, nobody (except perhaps those terminally ill) is turned down for dialysis. Needless to say, one would have to be "blind, deaf, and dumb" to not appreciate the need for an opening of dialog regarding

ESRD specifically and rationing of care in general. If current trends continue, a crisis mode will soon emerge.

Who is courageous enough among our national leaders to open the discussion?

PART VII
MUSCULOSKELETAL

As an intern in a big hospital dealing with large numbers of patients who were severely, if not critically ill, I was puzzled by the interest of one of my esteemed colleagues, for whom I had a good deal of respect. I happened to see him in the "break room," provided for house staff trying to get a breather, before heading back out into the trenches. He was immersed in a book. Nosey as I apparently was, insecure as I definitely was, and fearful that he might be studying something of great relevance for "morning report" or some other meeting where we tried to show each other how smart we were, I unabashedly inquired, "What ya reading?" It turned out that he was reading a treatise on chronic low back pain. In view of the fact that we were to shortly charge back out into the fray, dealing with critically ill people fighting for their lives, I didn't make the connection and certainly didn't ask him to pass the monograph on to me as soon as he was finished.

As I mentioned, he was a much respected colleague, and he taught me an unspoken lesson that day. I recalled that incident twenty years later and realized that his concern about chronic low back pain was prophetic. In fact, musculoskeletal problems, as the title implies, involving muscle, bone, joints, ligaments, and tendons, are extremely common. Although infrequently truly life threatening, such problems can be demoralizing and have long-term consequences on both mental and physical health. As noted, they are basically ubiquitous. We will, again, focus on the common problems, with special attention to the worst of them all, i.e., the back!

The Featherless Biped

During the course of our multi-million year evolutionary journey, major changes have occurred in fits and starts, with long periods of relative stability. Certainly, assumption of the upright posture, freeing our hands with their newly opposable thumbs, was one of those evolutionary jumps and, in so doing, allowed us to become the one and only "featherless biped" in the animal kingdom. Hurray! As is true with everything else, there is no free lunch. Every evolutionary leap has set us apart but has also brought some bad with the greater good. Our animal neighbors, sorely lagging behind us in so many technological ways, may get arthritis (especially if they are pathetically overbred by us), but they generally don't fall down and break their wrists, break their hips, break their ankles, crack their ribs, crunch their skulls, or incur a host of less severe injuries. In addition, they have yet to threaten the integrity of the ecosystem, but that is another issue. In fact, walking on all fours appears to confer a huge stability factor. Evidence for this brilliant observation is all around us. If you don't get a chance to frequently watch mountain goats or mountain lions scampering up and down sheer cliffs as if they were going for a walk in the park, what about our use of canes, walkers, and four-wheel drive vehicles, all adding stability?

Also, the upright posture provided me with the opportunity to name this book. Were it not for our upright posture, aside from the possibility of warts, I would not have been able to think of anything to say about the soles. However, reconfiguration of our feet, to give us even a semblance of stability and to allow us to go for walks, such as from Siberia to Patagonia, up until 11,000 years ago, also gave us the opportunity to suffer with plantar fasciitis. So, to make good on the promise of the title, let's start with the soles.

Plantar Fasciitis

Plantar fasciitis is a painful condition of the sole, with the apex of pain in the heel. As one could imagine, the feet are remarkably complex and, for the most part, well-designed structures. They would have to be, to support the weight of the whole body, with a cushioned gait that prevents us from rattling our spines and teeth, and without breaking down within days of leaving the show room. This common condition can be the nightmare of the jock, professional or weekend, coming on unexpectedly and taking a very long time to resolve. The basic problem seems to be a structural one, involving pronation or flattening of the feet. This, along with collapse of the arch, places strain on the very dense fibrous layer at the bottom of the feet tightly adherent to the heel bone and muscles right under it. MRI studies can show a variety of different injuries to this dense fascia (a tough layer, or overlay of connective tissue), its attachments to the

Plantar Fasciitis Treatment

1) Temporary reduction or elimination of strenuous activity.

2) Use of orthotics.
   - Store bought
   - Custom made

3) Never walk barefoot, except for shower.

4) Wear shoes with superior arch support.

5) Ice on painful area 10 to 15 minutes, twice per day.

6) Anti-inflammatories.

7) Steroid injections into painful area.

8) Surgery (rarely needed).

heel bone and other bones, muscle, and even injury to the heel bone itself. The condition usually arises after some extraordinary activity, which apparently stretches these structures slightly more than usual.

The clinical picture is often "classic," with a history of heel pain after unusual physical stress, worse when first stepping out of bed in the morning, better with activity during the day, tenderness to pressure, with throbbing and burning. Effective treatment is available, which must be meticulously adhered to, sprinkled with patience, for the duration, taking as long as six months to resolve. Recurrences are common (see chart). In the unlikely event that those measures are unsuccessful, injections of steroid drugs may help. Ultimately, if nothing else has worked, it is possible that surgery could be helpful.

So much for the sole. Material regarding the soul is coming soon.

Bunion

Moving forward in the foot, in the direction of the big toe, we come to what is technically called the first metatarsophalangeal joint (MP), at the base of the big toe, and noted by a protuberance. This joint is important for two reasons. First, it is the site of a common foot disorder called bunion. Bunions are very common, thus meeting the criterion for mention in this survey of human ailments. They are much more common in women than men. There is now little doubt that a large variety of relatively minor-looking structural or mechanical deviations from the norm that result in formation of a bunion are genetically determined. In that sense, if you are destined to get bunion formation, it will likely occur no matter what shoes you wear or don't wear, or whatever activities you do or do not engage in.

The end result of what single or combinations of biomechanical problems exist is that the big toe, with the metatarsophalangeal joint acting as the fulcrum, begins to lean or push toward the other toes. In so doing, the MP joint pushes outward and becomes prominent. This obviously can be a setup for certain types of problems. Firstly, suddenly, shoes don't fit very well. Secondly, a variety of different pains can ensue, from irritation of the skin to arthritic changes of the joint itself, to deformities of the other toes. Lastly, for some people, it becomes a big cosmetic problem.

Plastic and Reconstructive Surgery

What a perfect time to take a detour for a while and discuss something much more interesting than bunions. How about the topic of "plastic surgery," stimulated by the phrase "cosmetic problem?" Anyway, it gives me one more group of my colleagues to antagonize.

Although physicians have made abortive attempts at correcting serious body deformities going back to ancient Greece (and perhaps earlier), the modern specialty which is best known as Plastic and Reconstructive Surgery had its origins during and after World War I. That era presented a convergence of massive numbers of mutilated people, combined with markedly improved surgical and anesthetic techniques, so that for the most part, surgery could at least be done safely. If we calculate roughly 100 years of modern concepts in this discipline, in the first half of this, the emphasis was heavily weighted toward reconstructive surgery, with the attempts to improve function, with possible side benefit of improving appearance as well. At that point, the trend began to reverse. In the past thirty to forty years, the vast majority of surgery done by these practitioners is now "plastic" (rather than reconstructive), designed to change and presumably improve appearance. This newer trend can stand with the name "plastic" but has also been called "aesthetic" or even "body modification" surgery. The point is that the overwhelming emphasis is now on change of form, rather than change of function.

As is well known, a vast majority of these procedures are performed on women. The most common plastic surgery procedure performed in the Western world is breast augmentation, numbering to approximately 350,000 procedures per year in the USA alone. This is a stunning number and, in my opinion, an opportunity for reflection. When we look around us, we sometimes have hope that the xenophobic, male-dominated world, which has basically been entrenched since the dawn of civilization, is beginning to crumble. It seems that women have made enormous strides toward merging with men as true equals. However, many women still sense the subtle yet pervasive smell of being objects, rather than subjects. The same can be said for black people, who still feel the sting of racism in many ways. (In October of 2009, in Chicago, home of the nation's first black president, and with a huge black population, a group of black college students was turned away from a nightclub because of baggy pants thought to be emblematic of the rap culture.) That vast numbers of women would yearly conclude that their breasts do not meet certain standards and agree to go under the knife flies in the face of all the true feminists who have gone before in an effort to advance women's rights. Why is there not an outcry from the female population against this trend? Why don't females boycott plastic surgery services? Do women agree that if they have different looking breasts, they become sexually more attractive and, through some serpiginous route, have a better chance to pass their genes on? In other words, perhaps the most frightening thought of all is that they want this surgery for their own benefit and not simply because they feel pressure from males. In other words, modern women appear to have taken a step backward in their liberation.

It also speaks to the deep distress that women feel. Women who have breast augmentation have a risk of suicide three times those that have not, immediately after surgery. After twenty years, the risk is eight times as high. What are we teaching girls in our society? Martin Luther King, perhaps the greatest teacher of acceptance in the twentieth century, spoke about looking at a person's character, rather than the color of their skin. Do women want to apply their efforts into development of character or development of breast size? Lastly, is this a wake-up call for the idealists who dreamt that an infusion of feminine energy into leadership roles would soften and sweeten the world and make it more peaceful? Look at the short list of women who have risen to the top leadership roles in their countries and the answer may be glaringly apparent. My reflection about this issue is that testosterone is not the problem. The problem is the reptilian brain. Well-kept records have demonstrated clearly that female *Tyrannosaurus rex* individuals ruthlessly devoured just as many hapless weaker foes as male *T. rex* individuals. Character is not a gender issue. Much more about the reptilian brain is coming soon.

One final comment about Plastic and Reconstructive Surgery. The people who specialize in this area are enormously gifted. This is most clearly the creative part of clinical medicine, where the art of medicine can be seen not only in the manner in which we deal with patients psyches but in the magic we can bring to people who feel crushed by deformity. I would hope that at some point, these surgeons and the leaders of their professional societies can find a way to spread these gifts to encompass the impoverished and underprivileged hoards around the world. Oh, oh! Here comes that idealism again.

OK, back to bunions. As has been beaten to death by now, people are incredibly alike and disalike, simultaneously. Besides being a wonderful paradox to work with, this explains why symptoms vary so much from person to person. Some people with mild bunion deformities suffer with much pain. Others with marked deformities never even mention it to the doctor. Big black shoes with a large "toe box" present no problem for them. Like any other surgery, foot surgery is a big deal, even bigger than most. There can be considerable postoperative pain. Many surgeries require you to clunk around in huge braces for months. So, consider the options carefully. Clearly, the option of choosing surgery because of preoperative pain seems a better one—than because you don't like the way the bunion looks. Get a second or third opinion.

From Chiropodists to Doctors of Podiatric Medicine

Here is a brief digression—non-controversial, non-philosophic, and gluten free as well. When I was a child and experiencing an outbreak of plantar warts (caused by viruses and affecting the feet), common in childhood and quite painful, my dutiful mother took me (many times) to the "foot doctor," at that time called "chiropodist." I don't think they had much training, and they certainly were not called upon to do much more than deal with corns, calluses, and warts. By the 1960s, the landscape regarding the feet was changing. Nowadays, podiatrists or doctors of podiatric medicine are trained to do many very technically challenging procedures regarding feet. Also, a small number of orthopedic surgeons do specialized training in foot diseases and surgeries. So, you, the consumer, have your choice of seeing either type of doctor, podiatrist or orthopedist, depending on your own preferences. I might suggest podiatry for problems that are not surgical. This is something you might not immediately know. However, things involving the skin would likely be classified as non-surgical. Foot pain, without much deformity, and nail issues would also suggest a non-surgical approach to be likely. For painful deformities or fractures, either specialty would suffice. And please consider this, which I have and will likely recommend again. If surgery is suggested, unless it is remarkably simple, it may well be to your advantage to get more than one opinion.

Moving up the body from the foot, we naturally encounter the ankle, which is technically considered to be a joint. More specifically, the ankle is a "large joint," although nobody uses a ruler to determine which is large or otherwise. The large joints include ankles, knees, hips, perhaps elbows, and shoulders. All of these joints manifest, as their major pathologic process, a disease called "arthritis." There are perhaps three major forms of arthritis which can affect any of those joints, singly or in combination. There are a number of lesser frequency arthritic processes, some of which are thankfully intermittent. Lastly, there are a number of arthritic processes which also affect small joints, like those in the hands and feet primarily. The spine, including the neck and back are somewhat in a special category, largely because of the complexity of the anatomy, with skeletal neurologic and musculotendinous tissues all prominently featured and interacting complexly. Also, there are a few diseases which are unique to the spinal joints.

Recall again that the emphasis here is on common disease processes, which likely account for 90% of the problems people face regarding joints.

Tendonitis Versus "Ligamentitis"

As a curious and somewhat irrelevant sidelight, note the following custom. As previously mentioned, tendons hold muscles to bone (to move them) and ligaments hold bones together (to keep them from moving excessively). The term "tendonitis" is very frequently used in clinical medicine, by both doctors and patients. If you live to be 120 years (currently, or at least recently, thought to be our biologic "wall," and to be discussed later), you will never hear the term "ligamentitis." Whether or not there is technically such a term, the reasons why the proponents of tendonitis won out over the proponents of ligamentitis will forever be shrouded in the veil of medical idiosyncrasy. So, if you are really frustrated or angry at your doctor at some point (personally, I can't imagine why that would happen), ask him or her to explain to you the differences between tendonitis and ligamentitis. The answer is that ligaments and tendons overlap and intersect. We obviously frequently don't know exactly what the problematic anatomic structure is. By convention, we call it tendonitis. The point is that we don't know. This is likely one of the reasons why we do so poorly in trying to explain painful or dysfunctional neck or back issues. We just don't know! This is just another example of our substantially made-up world.

Achilles, Apollo, Hector, Invincibility, and the Concept of Hubris

At the back of the foot, coming up from the heel, is a thick "cord," the name of which is derived from a series of myths. Greek mythology states that Achilles was destined at birth for greatness. His mother is said to have attempted to insure his invulnerability by dipping him upside down into the river Styx, immersing his entire body except for the area behind his ankle, where she held him tightly. During the Trojan War, Achilles' invulnerability as the great Greek warrior appeared to be intact. However, his killing of Hector, followed by the egregious desecration and mutilation of Hector's body, is said to have angered the god Apollo. After all, if nothing else, the greatest of all indiscretions in ancient Greece was that of hubris…outrageous arrogance. This flagrant act of hubris appeared to have sealed the fate of Achilles, who was subsequently brought down by a poisoned arrow from the bow of Trojan prince Paris, striking him just above the heel, the only part of his body not submerged in the river as an infant. So, even the greatest warrior, invulnerable or not, is subject to the basic Greek injunction against arrogance. We are also made aware of the limits of invulnerability. This is particularly pertinent to us moderns, seeking health and longevity, by popping pills and seeking surgery, while living far out of balance, with the erroneous notion that our parachute will always spring open at the last moment.

Resiliency/Fragility

So this myth gives us some beautiful lessons, a warning, and a mystical name… the Achilles tendon. This is truly a tendon, with no overlying ligaments. Tendonitis is generally thought to occur in or after situations of unusual activity, which stretch or otherwise stress a tendon, as might be seen with repetitive activity. The only problems that tendons can cause are inflammation, i.e., tendonitis or partial or complete rupture. For the most part, treatment of tendonitis all over the body is generally the same

> **Treatment of Tendonitis**
>
> 1) Avoid or reduce the causative activity.
>
> 2) Ice 15 minutes, twice per day.
>
> 3) Anti-inflammatory agents for up to two weeks.
>
> 4) Wrapping or bracing where applicable.

(see chart). Review of this list reveals the need to alter one's routine, sometimes considerably. Although tendonitis can heal spontaneously with no change in routine, the steps outlined represent an attempt to accelerate the healing process and prevent the disaster of rupture. Depending on the specific tendon, rupture means one of several things: (1) surgical repair, with a very long recovery time, (2) permanent significant deformity and/or loss of function (finger tendons and ligaments), and (3) chronic pain/soreness. With this short list of suboptimal options, it is wise to improve the odds of a good outcome by subscribing conscientiously to the recommendations.

Keep in mind that as resilient as the body is, it is equally fragile. This has been mentioned before and is certainly one of the take-home messages of this treatise. It implores us to pay attention to the little things. In my experience, in listening to many thousands of patient stories over the years, the downhill slide often begins deceptively innocently, with a slight slip. A tendon injury can lead to inability to function fully, with the subsequent domino effect spilling over into many other areas of life. So, there needs to be a degree of mental toughness and a resolute attitude to resist progressive and especially premature loss of function. Collapse into the attitude of "I guess I'm just getting older," often voiced in the forties or fifties, is a myth equal to Achilles' sense of immortality. It likely stems from a basic underlying depression or at least dysthymia, with superimposition of a low expectation. A confluence of negative attitudes like these is substantially cultural, rather than genetic.

Achilles tendonitis has one feature which is both odd and ominous in the realm of tendon injuries. Namely, it can rupture with (A) little or (B) no warning. "A" might manifest as mild discomfort or tenderness to pressure or squeeze. "B" might manifest as a completely unexpected sudden sharp, slap-like pain in the area, with subsequent inability to walk. "A" demands careful attention to reduction of strenuous activity and close monitoring over the next month or so. Failure to resolve should result in a trip to the family doctor or orthopedist. Diagnosis can be confirmed on MRI. "B" likely means a trip to the operating room. How many people with "B" actually were "A" and ignored it? Not known.

The Ankle

The ankle itself is prone to two common problems, namely arthritis and/or sprains. Sprain is a commonly used but somewhat vague term used by doctors and patients. People apply the term to necks, backs, shoulders, elbows, wrists, hips, knees, and ankles, frequently when there is an "incident," followed by pain, prominent with movement. In fact, out of all of those areas, the term is accurate perhaps only in the ankle region. Basically, it implies an injury of soft tissues, usually acute onset, followed by pain and swelling. In the case of a human ankle, it is almost always an inversion injury (turn in/under) which initiates the tearing of tendons and ligaments, which in the ankle are in close proximity. There are some fairly subtle findings which might point to primarily ligamentous versus tendonous injury, but for practical purposes, both are involved. As is true for most disease entities, severity can vary greatly. In the case of severe ankle sprain, there is much pain and swelling (and bruising), accompanied by obvious instability of the joint. The joint, and the person to whom it belongs, is very vulnerable at that juncture, as there is a high risk of a recurrent injury, which can only magnify the damage. The key is to avoid further injury. To accomplish this, you will likely need some type of external bracing device, whether it is an ace wrap, a soft preformed ankle brace, or something much more elaborate such as a hinged ankle–foot hard plastic brace. Boots extending several inches above the ankle might suffice. The usual ice and anti-inflammatory medication might help. A severe injury can take three to four months to resolve completely, but even severe injuries rarely require surgery. Obviously, your doctor can assist you with details regarding treatment.

Arthritis

Since we are about to discuss arthritis of the ankle, this is a good time to discuss arthritis in general (see Table). The six categories listed likely account for 90% of all cases. In fact, osteoarthritis alone likely accounts for two-thirds or more of the cases.

Major Categories of Arthritis
1. Osteoarthritis (degenerative or wear-and-tear)
2. Rheumatoid
3. Gouty
4. Psoriatic
5. Post-traumatic
6. Infectious, including viral

Gout

Gout has already been mentioned, in reference to the most common area it affects, i.e., the base of the big toe. The second and third most common areas are the small joints across the top of the foot, just below the ankle, and the ankle joint itself. It somewhat frequently can affect the knees. It infrequently affects other joints. Gout is a systemic disease which results most often from a genetically determined mishandling of uric acid metabolism. Uric acid in turn comes from the recycling of a class of organic molecules called purines, which are widely dispersed in nature, including being an integral part of DNA and RNA. As cells die, breakdown, and are prepared for recycling, uric acid is released and enters the circulation. If levels become excessive, the kidneys primarily, and liver secondarily, excrete this substance. Uric acid can also be ingested in the form of certain foods high in purines, including meat, especially organ meat, and seafood of certain types. Uric acid can crystallize in joints and form beautiful but very painful needle-like structures, clearly visible under the microscope. In fact, crystallization can occur in other places in the body, depending on local circumstances. Since it filters through the kidney, it can cause damage to the tubules.

Most typically, the onset of gout is sudden and most often in the middle of the night. It is generally considered to be a form of acute and possibly recurring arthritis, with long periods of remission. It shares genetic linkage to the metabolic syndrome and its individual elements (diabetes, obesity, hypertension) and is thus somewhat preventable by healthy lifestyle (what isn't?). There are effective medical treatments.

Psoriatic Arthritis

Psoriatic arthritis, as the name implies, is seen in conjunction with psoriasis. It is much less common than gout, in my experience. It is potentially a very serious condition, in that it can be chronic and deforming and can interfere with function. It is much less common than psoriasis, but can actually precede the appearance of skin disease. Although it can affect any joint in the body, it has a tendency to affect the small joints of fingers and toes, as well as the spine and sacroiliac joints. Treatment is available but includes potentially dangerous drugs, such as steroids and other immune suppressing agents.

Post-traumatic Arthritis

The cause of post-traumatic arthritis is somewhat self-explanatory. Any type of serious injury which affects a joint, most commonly a fracture which extends into a joint, can result in this condition. This is not a systemic disease, usually affecting only one joint. Sometimes, there may be a domino effect, whereby severe damage of one joint causes the person to "favor" other joints, which can cause those to deteriorate. Treatment options are somewhat limited and usually involve pain management and possibly joint replacement.

Infectious-Related Arthritis

Infectious arthritides are fairly common and usually transitory. The two major types seen clinically are viral and bacterial, with the latter being generally of much more concern. Anyone who has ever had flu syndrome, which probably includes everybody, can attest to the fact that the viral agent which causes this self-limited disease is capable of causing severe muscle and/or joint pain. There is a viral disease called dengue fever, which occurs mostly in tropical and subtropical locations, and also in the southeastern USA, which has been dubbed "breakbone fever." What is perhaps not as well known is that there appears to be a large number of viruses which behave a little differently. These viruses tend to cause protracted illnesses, perhaps going on for months, characterized by malaise, intermittent fever, a variety of other systemic symptoms, and severe joint pain. It is almost as if parts of the five- to seven-day flu syndrome become markedly stretched out. In this situation, the joint complaints frequently become the dominant feature. The term "arthralgia" is used to describe joints that hurt, but in which there are no physical signs of inflammation (remember the four signs of inflammation, to include dolor (pain), tumor (swelling), rubor (redness), calor (heat)). "Arthritis" implies active, detectable inflammation. Regardless, these protracted viral illnesses dominated by joint issues can be understandably extremely frustrating for both doctor and patient. In this situation, your family doctor may have done a legitimate investigation, including thorough history, physical exam, lab studies, and possibly X-ray. He or she may have seen you two or three times in the office, bringing you up to date, and reviewing the exam. At this time, your condition is sufficiently problematic to warrant consultation with a rheumatologist (specialist in musculoskeletal, non-surgical problems) and an infectious disease specialist. If the evaluation remains "negative" for definitive diagnosis at that time, there is not much choice but to wait.

"Watchful Waiting" as a Possibly Underused Medical Weapon

In general, after appropriate investigation, with the emphasis on appropriate, no matter what the illness or disease process, it is advisable if not mandatory to pause and wait. The likelihood is high that one of two things will happen in the near future: (1) The disease will declare itself, such that the diagnosis is then easy, avoiding the frustration and cost of relentlessly "negative" studies. (2) Or much more commonly, the condition melts away, leaving both doctor and recovering victim to wonder, "What the heck was that?" We tend to ascribe a large number of peculiar illnesses to viruses, just as we do painful red skin bumps to spiders. The virus notion may be a correct assumption. Being a spider fan, I can attest that the spider notion is very poorly documented. Incidentally, the concept of watchful waiting can be a serious consideration in many other types of diseases.

Keep in mind that to be an effective strategy, avoiding costly, uncomfortable, and possibly dangerous elements of investigation, watchful waiting requires a high level of trust between patient and doctor. (Patient: "Don't let me die or suffer permanent disfigurement." Doctor: "I won't, as long as you don't sue me.") There is nothing intrinsically wrong with soliciting a second or third opinion, as long as it is recognized that these consultants immediately come under the same pressures to "get it right" as the original doctor. Therefore, the patient always has to weigh the risks of going further versus waiting. Trust is the key element.

Bacterial Arthritis

Bacterial arthritis illnesses tend to be somewhat explosive. Artificial joints are of particular concern, although previously healthy joints can also be attacked. There can be a local skin or soft tissue infection such as cellulitis initiating the problem, or it could be induced by trauma in the vicinity of the joint. Or the joint could be seeded by an infection at a distant site, which is a consequence of bacteria gaining access to the circulation (i.e., sepsis). Almost any joint can be infected, including spinal joints. The person is generally ill, with fever, chills, malaise, and likely severe pain in the affected joint. Diagnosis can be difficult to confirm. Treatment is with long-term antibiotic therapy and usually surgical drainage and cleaning of the affected joint.

Autoimmune ("Connective Tissue") Diseases

The four types of arthritis just discussed, as mentioned, likely account for only 10% to 15% of the human arthritic burden. Rheumatoid and osteoarthritis account for the vast majority of chronic arthritides. These are diseases which have plagued us for many thousands of years, long before the historical record was begun. Carbon-dated skeletal remains from all over the world attest to the ubiquitous nature of the disease during our development as a species over thousands of years.

Rheumatoid (or rheumatoid arthritis) is one of the autoimmune diseases, characterized by what appears to be the activities of an overly zealous immune system, detecting "other" and mounting an attack to destroy the other. In fact, the "other" may be simply a mildly aberrant family of proteins, manufactured by slightly altered DNA or RNA, and perhaps of no real threat on its own. That is a working model of the autoimmune diseases. Perhaps, these altered proteins are potentially more dangerous than we assume they are, and thus, it may be better to have the autoimmune disease than it is to have the unchecked "other." We simply don't know. Unfortunately, these types of autoimmune diseases, sometimes called "connective tissue diseases," are not innocent bystanders. People die with or from these diseases, especially in those whom the respective treatment modalities are not very effective—or toxic. Even rheumatoid arthritis, a fairly common disease process and often relatively quiet and non-aggressive, is associated with a statistically shorter life span. These diseases seem to be associated with accelerated arteriosclerosis. The other connective tissue diseases include systemic lupus erythematosus, scleroderma, polymyositis, and dermatomyositis, each involving primarily a different tissue and each with its own clinical picture. These are all systemic diseases, often with a propensity to attack one particular tissue above all else and affecting different sites and organs. Although the trigger mechanisms which initiate the autoimmune response are generally not known, several… (you got it) viruses are suspected.

Rheumatoid Arthritis

Rheumatoid arthritis, as the name implies, affects mostly joints. The term rheumatoid disease is used because other tissues are often involved. Sometimes, the other tissues present problems before the arthritic issues became a problem. The lungs are often involved, as are the membranes surrounding the heart and lungs, causing painful pericarditis and pleurisy. Rheumatoid arthritis can affect any joint in the body, including larger joints, small joints, spine (neck and back), and even the jaw joint. It tends to be symmetric. The joints which are close to the body surface usually demonstrate detectable signs of inflammation. There may be prominent stiffness, especially early morning. As is true for most diseases, the pain and stiffness, and the number of involved joints, can vary widely. It tends to have a waxing and waning property but can be very longstanding, going on for many years.

The point of attack of the immune system appears to be the so-called synovial membrane which lines the joint space, including bones and cartilage. The membrane becomes intensely inflamed and begins to erode into surrounding tissue such as ligaments, tendons, and muscle. These structures may weaken or tear causing the bones to migrate, resulting in marked deformity. The diagnosis can usually be confirmed on lab studies and X-rays of the involved joints. The disease can be life changing and debilitating.

Treatment for the most part is with medications, of which there are now an increasing number of choices. Previously, non-steroidal anti-inflammatories were the workhorse drugs and are still widely used. Steroids were frequently used and still are. A number of drugs to tone down the immune system have been used and still are. Most recently, in the last ten to fifteen years, a group of drugs called "disease-modifying anti-rheumatic drugs" has been developed due to the fact that all of the earlier used drugs did not always stop the progressive joint deformities. The newer drugs can be very effective in preventing further joint destruction. However, since they interfere with the normal inflammatory cascade, needed to ward off infections and cancers, they are potentially dangerous. People with active rheumatoid arthritis should be seen by rheumatologists, as well as by their regular doctors. The hope is always that the person will experience a spontaneous or drug-induced remission, which can be permanent, before too much deformity ensues. For those of whom this does not occur quickly enough, surgical joint replacements then become possibilities.

In closing, in case you remain unconvinced about the widespread dangers of cigarette smoking, there is good epidemiologic data to suggest that with all of the "unknown" factors about initiation of rheumatoid, cigarette smoking is one of the triggers.

Osteoarthritis

Finally, we have reached a discussion of by far the most common form of arthritis—that being osteoarthritis. Despite its overwhelming preponderance, it is a much more plebian, blue-collar disorder than the other arthritides discussed. It lacks the exotic aura of an autoimmune disease, with all the mystery and complexity surrounding those conditions. It has been called "wear-and-tear" arthritis, being more common with aging, and with physical stress, with that being total body or a localized area. We frequently see the onset in men in their forties who have been doing construction or some rough-and-tumble work for many years. It is much more common with obesity and the added stress that excessive weight places on joints. There are obvious genetic predispositions, sometimes striking in their specificity. It is not unusual to see the same joint severely damaged in several generations of a family, with many other joints unaffected. One or many joints can be involved. It tends to be progressive, but often quite slowly so. As might be expected, the main symptom is pain.

Very characteristically, the finger joints involved most often are the knuckles closest to the nails, except for the thumb, where it usually affects the joint at the base of the thumb where it joins the wrist.

The point of attack in this disease appears to be the cartilage between the bones. This structure, which allows for lubrication and cushioning between the bones, begins to deteriorate. Treatment is generally focused on trying to alter body mechanics so that whatever joint it is may be less traumatized. Obviously, this may be very difficult to pull off, as it may entail a radical lifestyle change. From the medicinal standpoint, the non-steroidal, anti-inflammatories have been and continue to be the mainstays of treatment, even though the inflammatory response is not as intense as it is with some of the other arthritides. They are reasonably effective in reducing pain, although their effect on the long-term progression of the disease is less impressive. Please recall the potential dangers for these over-the-counter and therefore unregulated drugs, including interstitial nephritis and painless massive gastrointestinal bleeding. (See! You know so much now that there is no need to explain these medical terms.)

Joint Replacement Surgery

This gives us a perfect segue into the topic of joint replacements, medically termed "total joint arthroplasty." But first, let's take another relaxing diversion. Recall the laudatory remarks I made about the operation called transurethral resection of the prostate, devised in the early 1920s. Also, recall that internists don't often give laudatory praise to surgical colleagues, often pejoratively describing them as "technicians." Looking back over the last ninety years, however, this rather simple "reem job" would have to stand as a monumental achievement to those who devised it, in terms of affording great benefits to millions of people.

A similar achievement is currently evolving in the realm of total joint replacements. These types of operations have been attempted for many years also, going back to the early twentieth century, but on a limited basis, mandated by very limited success. Perhaps, one could assign the year 1970 as the approximate time that both hip and knee replacements began to be done with a measure of regularity, based on improved results. Personally, however, I don't recall these operations being done frequently until the 1980s. Now, they are an everyday occurrence in virtually every hospital. The results regarding total shoulder arthroplasty were the last to achieve a level of success which would allow them to be everyday operations, perhaps since the 1990s. Replacement surgery on arthritic hands is relatively infrequently done, as is such surgery on ankles. Regarding the latter, at this point in time, it seems that when relief of pain is needed, ankle fusion is more often utilized than ankle replacement. "Fusion" is a procedure done mostly on necks and back, whereby using bone grafts or metallic materials, pain relief is attempted by causing the arthritic parts to lock together, markedly reducing movement. Results are variable but usually do provide meaningful pain relief.

At this point in time, knee and hip replacement surgery has become a commonly done procedure, performed by orthopedic surgeons. The major reason for the popularity of this procedure happens to be the best reason possible; it is very effective in eliminating pain and restoring function. Once evaluation is completed by the orthopedist, he or she is likely to say "come back when you are ready to have the operation." These are elective procedures, implying that they do not address life-threatening illness and that they can be done at the patient's discretion. As cautious as I may be about doctors drumming up business for themselves, I have not seen a hint of this with joint replacement. These people are suffering with pain, and their lives have become unnecessarily circumscribed. Since I am an admitted fanatic of the value of exercise and of generally being active, anything that can significantly restore function and provide for increased activity gets my endorsement. Even if the person is a lifetime couch potato, the operation can be justified on the basis of the anticipated pain relief. That is what doctoring is all about.

These are very good operations, with a high likelihood of success. But surgery is surgery, and things can go wrong. It is best to be cognizant of this and decide if the risk warrants the potential benefit. The formula is subtly different for every person. Most of the operations are done for complications of osteoarthritis, with a smaller number for rheumatoid arthritis. Sometimes, it is necessary to stage 2 or 3, or more surgeries, to get all of the painful joints replaced.

Neck and Back Pain

The last topic to be discussed in the musculoskeletal system is the "back" (and neck). Actually, it is a discussion about the spine. In alignment with the ground rules, arbitrarily and dictatorially setup by me regarding what is discussed, we will only cover common conditions. Dictators don't usually beg for mercy, but in this situation, please be patient with me, as I interject a good deal of personal feelings, based on forty years of observation. My goal is not self-aggrandizement (hard to believe) but your well-being (even harder to believe).

We learn in medical school that each organ system has its own "language" for expressing itself. Most of the major organs have three or four symptoms which tell you "I'm not doing well." The back, however, having dropped out of school three million years ago when our hominid ancestor *Australopithecus* decided to stand up and take notice is monosyllabic… "pain." As mentioned earlier, we have paid a steep price for this evolutionary leap. One look into the waiting room of your local chiropractor will confirm this.

It is stated that in our industrialized society, during the course of a lifetime, 80% of the population will consult a medical practitioner at least once for back pain. So, that is lesson number one. Expect back and/or neck pain, and don't necessarily panic when it occurs. For the majority of people, back pain is something that occurs infrequently, perhaps in conjunction with some type of unusual lifting or other physical activity, makes you feel temporarily old, and makes you walk funny such that every person you encounter over the next week will ask, "What happened to you?" If they are feeling unusually aggressive or cocky, they may rephrase that to, "What did you do to yourself?" Anyway, in a week or two, you will be back to your usual jaunty self. That might be a good time to carefully review a primer on back care, whereby you can learn how to strengthen your core muscles, lift with your knees, stand close to the object to be lifted, etc. Actually, all of those things do help, even though the pain will likely recur at some point in the future. Most people are never worse off than that. The usual area of back pain is in the low back, the so-called lumbosacral area.

A much smaller number of people will develop a prolonged period of moderate or even moderately severe back pain. When things are not going well after four or five days, and you are beginning to feel murderous thoughts regarding people inquiring about your odd posture, you will likely go to the doctor. I will first describe the visit if the doctor is an MD and then give the chiropractic version. As is always the case (notice that as we are near the end of our survey of common medical problems, I am becoming increasingly concerned that you haven't expected and, if need be, demanded a few basic services from your doctor), your doctor should hearken back to the medical school opprobrium that "the diagnosis is in the history." How to do this in ten minutes? Difficult but possible. A brief exam of back, hips, and legs should follow. Most of the time, nothing else needs to be done, except that you need an explanation of the findings and conclusions. If you are held hostage in a clinic which demands that your doctor rotate to the next consumer (patient) every ten minutes, you may need to schedule another ten-minute follow-up next week. That is OK and, in fact, way better than ordering an MRI, as it is likely that you will be better next week. A vast majority of people, even with moderately severe low back pain, improve steadily over the next several weeks to several months (yes, months). Even those with documented sciatica would be expected to improve steadily.

Sciatica

Recall that the nerves which run into the legs emanate from the lumbar and sacral regions of the spinal cord, exiting the cord as nerve roots, which combine in the pelvis into a very large nerve called the sciatic nerve, which leaves the pelvis and enters the leg. The sciatic nerve ends at the tip of the big toe. Interestingly, this so-called post-ganglionic nerve which originates just as the nerve exits the spinal cord is an amazingly long structure, with its axon and dendrites terminating three to four feet from where it began. Considering that the body of the neuron itself is a microscopic structure, this is really amazing. Even people with sciatica, often caused by a slipped disk, will improve spontaneously. Doctors and patients like to utilize physical therapy. There is no doubt that physical therapy is helpful sometimes. There is also no doubt that most bodily ailments slowly get better. So, is it the therapy, "tincture of time," or both? Since physical therapists are generally nice and enthusiastic people, and quite dedicated, I have no objections to soliciting their help, even though it is expensive. Personally, I would likely not do it for myself, unless I had a truly serious or very debilitating condition. Simple home exercises, and traction using your own body weight (called gravity traction), can be set up with their advice. Traction is definitely helpful, done long enough and often enough.

Now, we enter the land of the problematic, i.e., the person who experiences that innocent appearing injury, but simply gets progressively worse, and is eventually having severe pain. Perhaps, one to four weeks has transpired. By this time, the person is deserving of a "workup," which would include re-examination by the doctor, to see if there are new findings historically or physically, and some type of imaging study, depending on the findings. Perhaps a simple X-ray of the lumbosacral spine will yield the diagnosis. Sometimes, we may need to move on to the Cadillac of studies—that being an MRI, which costs about fifteen times as much as an X-ray.

Based on the course and workup so far, it may be determined that the person might benefit from some type of injection of medication, using a needle, into the problematic area. This type of procedure is done with X-ray guidance and is performed by a variety of doctors, including interventional pain specialists, physical medicine specialists, interventional radiologists, and perhaps others. Depending on severity of pain, and whether it is improving or not, it might be worthwhile to take this approach, as it is quite safe and relatively easy. It may or may not be helpful. The spectrum of results runs all the way from not at all helpful, to partly successful for weeks to months, to complete long-term relief of pain.

Depending on the results of these injections, a decision may be made whether the person is a "candidate" for a surgical procedure. Being a candidate is a little like being a politician or vying for the title of Miss America. That is, you think you want the job but you are not really sure what it all entails. And of course, most candidates lose. Regardless, once your candidacy is established, you will be directed toward a person who does that kind of surgery. Basically, there are two types of physician career paths which terminate in their willingness to operate on necks and backs. They come from the ranks of neurosurgery (who also deal with all kinds of head and brain surgery) and orthopedic surgeons (who also deal with strains, sprains, fractures, and joint replacements). Surgeons love to operate. I have discussed this with surgical colleagues, suspecting that a day in the operating room, with a series of tough cases lined up, would be very stressful and exhausting. Quite the opposite. This opportunity with its attendant adrenaline rush energizes them and fulfills all of the needs for drama, decisive intervention, and immediate results, which enticed them into surgical careers in the beginning.

Operating Room

The operating room remains a place of intense connection. Obviously, there are few ways to be more intimate with someone than to enter into an agreement whereby one life is entrusted into the hands of another life. The operating room (OR) bustles with nurses, technicians, anesthesiologists, and others. One gets the sense that this is like the military war room, where a campaign is being waged by the forces of good (the medical team) against the forces of evil (the disease), with the decisive battle about to be fought. A good outcome provides that same indescribable "high" that motivates athletes, binding them to the "fans," and performers of all kinds including singers, musicians, and actors who join hands at the end of a performance and bow to the adulation of the audience, with that same deeply satisfying sense of unity, camaraderie, and belonging. Indeed, the operating room is an intoxicating place.

I have great respect for my surgical colleagues. They are a courageous bunch. On the surface, they may appear to be supremely confident, to the point of appearing cocky. However, as they progress through their careers, just as they produce scars on the body surfaces of their patients, they too become scarred. This discussion is particularly relevant in the framework of spinal surgery, where results are often suboptimal to poor. However, it applies to every doctor who walks into the OR and picks up a scalpel. We all know that there are bad outcomes, when the news from the OR is much worse than we expected or the final results are not what we had hoped for.

Then, there is the worst of all case scenarios. Immerse yourself in this scene. The patient goes in for a routine operation, done every day. Perhaps, this is a young or middle-aged person in the "prime of life." There is a sudden, completely unexpected problem which results in a cardiac arrest. Resuscitation attempts proceed immediately. The OR fills up with many new players, i.e., the "code team." Efforts go on for what seems like forever (perhaps thirty to sixty minutes). Ultimately, it is apparent that the patient has passed. In the dreaded lexicon, the patient "died on the table." The family sits in the surgical waiting room… waiting for the good news. The doctor is faced with the unspeakably difficult task of walking into the sphere of this family unit and informing these loved ones, who are anticipating a celebration that the loved one in the OR is… dead! The rock star fell off the stage. The soprano collapsed in the middle of the aria. The curtain has crashed down.

Suddenly, the bravado and the ego disappear. That is exactly what the doctor wants to do... disappear. But guess what? His or her next surgery is scheduled to start right now! Life goes on. Endless self-questioning. Emerging fears of a malpractice claim, with attorneys pouring through the medical record looking for the slightest breach of protocol upon which to build the case that were it not for that one small breach, the loved one would still be alive. In other words, the doctor killed the patient. What if the patient was a mother in the act of delivering? What if the patient was a newborn?

Back Pain—The "Black Box"

Spinal surgery is a very risky business. Eventually, most doctors don't want anything to do with it because the grief of doing surgery with such capricious outcomes takes its toll. Eventually, a relatively few are left. Many of them have pared down their practice to only back surgery. Of course, there are some clinical back situations in which the results of surgery are predictably good. However, these are the minority of situations. In my opinion, the back is the proverbial "black box"... a structure, neat and clean on the outside but with all kinds of complexly interacting gizmos and gadgets on the inside. This factually true arrangement makes it exceedingly difficult to know what the pain generators are. We know that there are many structures which can cause pain, under certain circumstances, in certain people, with certain kinds of pathological findings. Sometimes, there are two or three obvious possible sources of pain. Which one (or two, or three) is causing the pain? My colleague who was studying back pain during a "break" forty years ago had the right idea. I wonder if he has it figured out by now.

So, what do you, the patient, do with your back pain? It has been present for years and steadily getting worse. You have seen many doctors.

You have had many chiropractic treatments. You have taken medications, vitamins, and supplements; done physical therapy, core strengthening, and yoga; changed your shoes; changed your job; and prayed. The pain has simply become worse. I would get multiple opinions from back surgeons, at least two or three. If you live in a rural community or small town, I would consider going to a "tertiary referral center," where they do multiple back operations every day. Regarding the two or three doctors you will see, I would hope to get the following concurrence. Ask them to write down the diagnosis or diagnoses causing the pain. Then, ask them to write down the name of the operation they would recommend (yes, operations all have medical names). If the diagnoses and the treatments do not concur, I would have great reluctance about doing any surgery. Unlike most types of surgery, the wrong operation can make the condition worse—and burn bridges at the same time.

A prolonged discussion about neck pain and neck surgery would be largely redundant. Most of what has been said about back surgery applies to neck surgery. The neck is still part of the "black box." Patience with problems is warranted. Multiple opinions may be solicited. Injection therapy and surgery are frequently done, as a last resort.

Recall earlier that I mentioned that I would outline the MD version first, followed by the chiropractic version. Please note that I am not an expert on chiropractic therapy or practice. As mentioned earlier, I do personally refer patients to chiropractics for back and neck problems but not for "internal" or metabolic problems. I listen carefully to my patient's reports of chiropractic care.

Recall also that "tincture of time" is a great treatment, some of the time. That is, many medical problems eventually improve spontaneously. Please recall that 30% of people respond positively to a sugar pill, i.e., the powerful placebo response. Lastly and emphatically, these statements which bear heavily on the "cause and effect" concept discussed earlier (so-called cause and effect may be completely unrelated) apply to medical care as well as chiropractic care.

As best I can tell, when going to the chiropractor for treatment of back or neck pain, the visits tend to be short, with most of the time dealing with some kind of physical "adjustment." Visits initially may be daily to three times per week and then less often eventually. Some patients claim benefit to having an adjustment once per month. If you benefit from chiropractic services, then you should continue, perhaps always trying to stretch out return visits to see if the treatments are still needed. If there is no sustained improvement after four to six weeks of intensive therapy, it seems unlikely to me that further treatment is indicated.

There are several other common back problems to consider before closing the chapter on the musculoskeletal system. This is also an excellent time to discuss a very common disease (a pre-requisite for discussion), with a huge amount of morbidity (associated problems), as well as increased mortality (we all know what that is). The disease is bone loss, which in its full expression is called osteoporosis.

Bone Loss (Osteopenia/Osteoporosis)

Bone loss is the perfect example of the voyager, strolling along through the forest, gaping upwards at the trees, listening and watching for birds, glimpsing white fluffy clouds between the treetops, and more or less feeling that heaven on earth is manifest. The description of our voyager, intoxicated with a sense of peace and connectedness, depicts a bygone era. Although this blissfully engulfed person may not have named the experience as such, any yogi would identify it as a walking meditation. The locale is less important than the sense of connectedness. It is what we all crave and need. The dark side is always close at hand. Our deep longing to feel love, connectedness, and a sense of relevance can overwhelm us. It begins to creep into our pores. We forget that all of this is available to us every moment of every day in everything we do and everyone we encounter. But also, we are born into tribes. Hundreds of them. The everyday–every minute opportunities are missed, and we feel lonely. Where is the tribe when we really need it?

So, our journey becomes disrupted, no matter where it was, whether forest, seashore, desert canyons, or canyonlands of the city. It doesn't matter. It is different for us all. We feel lonely. No problem. We have the technology to connect at our fingertips via e-mail, twitter…, cell phone…and…. But today, a simple blue fin with our favorite diversion allows us to continue with our reverie.

Back to our sojourner in the forest. The blue fin proves to be too much diversion. One step too many results in a free fall over the precipice, with untold and unnamed injuries less than two seconds away. So, it is with bone loss. Beginning at about age twenty-five, our bones begin to melt, like an ice cube on a cool overcast fall day. The maximum amount of bone laid down has been predetermined by our genetics, our diet, and our lifestyle up to that point. Women are usually smaller than men and lay down less bone. Those of us who have neglected our diets and been inattentive to the ongoing need for weight-bearing exercise (after all, how many teenagers worry about whether or not they have taken in enough calcium, or sunlight today?), these are simply not issues which torment us on a day-to-day basis. And our sense of invulnerability, so deeply ingrained in young people as to appear to be hard-wired into our psyche, would blind us to the consequences of lifestyle choices, even if we knew. For all of these, we must be communally forgiven.

The ice cube is still melting periodically, even through the winter and certainly into the spring. There have even been days when we were so pre-occupied that we forget to take our multivitamins and trace minerals... you know, the ones with strontium. We keep forgetting day after day that our bones are in a constant state of flux. Ten percent of our skeleton, at any point in time, is being actively broken down by cellular elements called osteoclasts, and built up by cellular elements called osteoblasts (since when does "blasting" build something up? No Nobel Prize for the scientists who named the bone builder a "blast"). Both of these cellular elements are strongly influenced by multiple hormones, most of which have been mentioned through the course of our discussion. The major ones are cortisol, estrogen, testosterone, and parathyroid hormone. Our mental health and physical health both have major influences on bone metabolism. Some of us were never told by our mothers, religious leaders, or even our doctors that divergent factors like too much thyroid medication ("It helps me lose weight."), too many anti-depressants ("I think I feel a little better."), too much soda ("But it's caffeine free and sugar free."), too much antacid ("I never get heartburn anymore."), too much alcohol ("But I only have two or three glasses of wine per day."), and not enough soy ("You gotta be kidding.") can stimulate osteoclasts and/or inhibit osteoblasts, thus contributing to bone loss.

Oh, oh! "Summer" is just around the corner. We are now fifty years of age. Many of us have lost our sense of invulnerability (that's good). A few of us have actually become hypochondriacs (not good... fear and worry do not generally spawn creativity). All of us, except for those who have been kept in solitary confinement, are aware of the concept of bone loss. In fact, the female members of our tribe, beginning with an already reduced bone mass, are about to experience a possible dramatic drop-off in bone density, as ovaries shrivel to nubbins and the estrogen well runs dry. Male members are not immune to this phenomenon, although the drop-off in testicular function and testosterone production is a much more gradual and prolonged process.

So, do we all just collapse in a heap and mourn the loss of our bones, or is there actually something we can do about it?

Doctoring and Nature

It seems that doctoring has often been about the conflicting opinions about what to do about natural (derived from nature) processes. Hippocrates was perhaps the first to comment upon the concept of supporting the natural processes, including healing processes, of nature. Recall, that with no treatment, the deep gash heals with a barely discernable scar. In the absence of the modern-day pharmaceutical industry and food processing industry behind him, he spoke about the equation of medicine and food. Notice how many categories of medicine we take are "anti" this and "anti" that. Nature is not "anti" but is value-neutral. I certainly do not avoid anti-medicines when they are clearly useful and even life saving. On the other hand, I also recognize that the reason this person developed this serious illness at this particular moment involves many factors which are not indelible but which could have been altered, so as to avoid the increasing illness in the first place. If a life-threatening illness (like any cardiac event or any cancer) is not a wake-up call, what is it?

Treating Menopause

This whole concept about supporting nature versus overriding nature is beautifully and poignantly illustrated in the concept of post-menopausal estrogen replacement. For decades, data had accumulated indicating that estrogen replacement had numerous, widespread, markedly beneficial attributes. Yes, we always knew about the increased incidence of blood clotting problems and the increased incidence of breast cancer, but those "minor" drawbacks were washed over by the enormous benefits attributed to estrogen replacement. Implicit in this conception, however, is the implication that menopause is a disease which needs to be "anti'd" with something.

It seems that we all (scientists, doctors, and patients) were asleep at the wheel. One by one, the house of estrogen cards began to fall. As the house lay in rubble, part of one wall and the chimney still stood. Estrogen does reduce the so-called vasomotor symptoms of sweating and flushing which often herald the final collapse of estrogen production and can be very disruptive to everyday living. Also, it does slow the progressive bone loss which may occur after menopause. Now, we look at this issue with a much more balanced view. I applaud my medical colleagues, many of whom have stopped pushing the estrogen button once the new data was presented. There are many herbal and vitamin supplements and foods which are effective in getting a woman through menopause, usually by containing plant-based estrogen-like materials and simply reducing the vasomotor symptoms. This impressive list includes brown rice, yams, tofu, almonds, and cashews on the food side. On the vitamin side, vitamin E 800 mg, vitamin C 2,000+ mg, and magnesium 750 mg may blunt symptoms. On the herbal side, ginseng, red clover isoflavones, evening primrose oil, and black cohosh (Demi fermin) are all variably helpful.

The Soybean

Lastly, it is a fact that approximately 90% of the soybeans grown in this country are fed to farm animals. The other 10% are fed to a group of people who have found that soybeans are extremely high in protein and have a large number of culinary applications which can actually be tasty. Drill Sergeant Marmorstein knew about this years ago and was successful in getting a huge number of military men to give up meat and become dedicated to a vegetarian diet. Soybeans helped. Incidentally, the high concentration of estrogen-like compounds did nothing to feminize his tribe of soldiers, who were always highly decorated. So, contrary to popular belief, and in respect to my leader-of-the-pack twin brother, I am not kidding, soy has it all.

Bone Density Measurements: Dexa Scan

So as not to lose the forest for the trees, bone density studies are reported in one of three ways. The report leans on the bell-shaped curve with its "standard deviations," from the "normal" value, which is taken to be the population at age twenty to thirty, the time of maximal bone density. (1) Normal reflects a T-score between +1 and –1. (2) Osteopenia is represented by a T-score between –1 and –2.5. This identifies a population with clearly identifiable bone loss but is not statistically associated with increased risk of fractures, at least not yet. (3) Osteoporosis with a T-score below –2.5 represents substantial bone loss. This designation in turn has two possible consequences. First, it suggests that the person is likely to have fractures from any type of trauma, such as falling down. Secondly, and even more devastating, is the possibility of so-called spontaneous fractures, that is, occurring with no obvious trauma, per se.

Falling

A word about falling. Recall, sadly, that this is the "baggage" that came along with our assumption of the upright posture. Most of us fall occasionally. This is certainly true for the majority of people who participate in sports or other strenuous activities (swimmers are exempt). Some of us fall with everyday activity, although hopefully these falls are few and far between. Unfortunately, some people fall frequently. Earlier, I noted how actuaries for life insurance companies were responsible for discovering the point-by-point inverse relationship between blood pressure and all-cause mortality. That is, the higher the blood pressure, the shorter is life expectancy from all causes. The same relationships hold true for falling. When a person begins to fall regularly, life expectancy drops proportionally. Many people coming to the doctor with one complaint, or another, suspect "I guess it's because of my age," only to find out that many of these conditions are not clearly age-related. Falling, however, is age-related, that is progressively more common in older people. As is always the case with biologic phenomenon, the view from 30,000 ft may be radically different than the view from the second floor. Although ninety-year-old people fall more often than eighty-year-old people, who fall more than seventy-year-old people, etc., some in any given group never fall and some fall often. Those who fall often are statistically doomed to die sooner.

Regarding falling, there are basically two reasons for falling. A minority of such people have "syncope," which basically means they fall because they have loss of consciousness. These falls are horrible to watch, as the person may go down like a felled tree, attempting no protective action at all. Understandably, this smaller group of people may sustain fractures, but they may also have serious head and facial injuries, sometimes fatal. Syncope can occur from some type of cardiac event, such as a very fast or very slow rate, or even a cardiac arrest. It can also occur with a brain seizure. Actually, the most common cause of syncope is from a sudden drop in blood pressure, when changing from sitting to standing, and that could be from many causes, including fluid depletion, medication to lower blood pressure, or dysfunction of the autonomic nervous system, possibly related to diabetes or idiopathic (cause unknown). Usually in this case, the person does try to cushion the fall. If a facial or head injury ensues, there may be permanent emotional, intellectual, and motor difficulty as a result.

Whenever falling becomes part of a clinical picture, we always make efforts to determine the cause and, if possible, fix it. Physical and occupational therapists are often very helpful in this regard. There may well be rearrangement of household belongings, change in shoe wear, removing throw rugs, using assistive devices like canes or walkers, focusing, alteration in clothing, etc. Appropriate testing is carried out. These communal efforts may or may not be helpful. Incidentally, falling is much more common in dementia because of judgment disabilities.

Injury Fractures

With falls of whatever type, the three most common fractures occur in hips, wrists, and pelvis. Hips and wrists usually require surgical repair, and recovery may be prolonged, with abundant opportunity for complication. In fact, in older people, hip fractures carry about a 25%, six-month mortality rate! Pelvic fractures can be very painful but are usually dealt with non-surgically. Once again, the recovery may be very prolonged (four to six weeks), with a high chance of complications.

Spontaneous Fractures

The last type of fracture to be discussed with bone loss will conclude this section on musculoskeletal issues. There are the so-called spontaneous fractures, occurring without a significant injury event. This can occur with ribs, which can "crack" from coughing, sneezing, and even hugging! So, as much as you may love your elderly companions, hug them gently. Less commonly, the sternum, i.e., breastbone, can be injured by the same processes. These can be very painful fractures, which can make it difficult for the person to breathe and make them susceptible to pneumonia.

Even more difficult than the rib fractures are spinal fractures, sometimes called "compression fractures." These most commonly involve lumbar and/or sacral areas, i.e., the bottom of the spine, supporting the upper half of the body. These are very painful fractures, which often cause a person to be "frozen," meaning completely immobilized, unable to move anything without help, except arms or head. At one time, it appeared that treatment by interventional radiologists, using one or two similar techniques to stabilize the fractured vertebra, could be immediately very helpful. These procedures using needles are called vertebroplasty or kyphoplasty. Experience with these procedures has shown that although occasionally they are indeed very helpful, much more often they are not. Therefore, enthusiasm has waned, and we have reverted to treating these unfortunate people with pain killers and occasionally calcitonin and/or anti-inflammatories. Full recovery is likely to take six to eight weeks.

In people who are chronically bedridden, all bets are off. Bones can become so weakened that even fractures of the large leg bones can occur, with simple acts such as turning or rolling over. The "crack" felt when this occurs is a painful shock to both the patient and the caregiver. Needless to say, by the time that spontaneous fractures begin to appear, the victim of these events is in great danger of increasing debility and complications, leading to a terminal event.

PART VIII
NERVOUS SYSTEM

N ow, finally let the fun begin. After plowing through these droll topics about excretion (two types), blood pumping, digestion, oxygenating, walking, and other such mundane activities, we finally arrive at the raison d'etre for all that we have read so far. All of this machinery is nothing more than a life support apparatus for the nervous system, including of course the brain.

Brain–Computer Interface

The 1965 novel by Frank Herbert, Dune, stands as one of the greatest science fiction stories of all time. As is sometimes true about science fiction, elements of the story begin to actualize with the march of time. In the novel, set far into the future, the universe has been populated by humans, scattered over hundreds and thousands of light years. Travel and commerce, and competition for resources are no less important then, as they have been throughout our history. In order to accommodate for the possibility of contact between these far flung outposts, Herbert brilliantly devises several structures allowing this to occur. His concept of "spacefolding" fits perfectly with contemporary cosmology in which the universe is not seen as a symmetrically expanding sphere but as a complex, somewhat chaotic arrangement of curves and bends generated by immense gravitational forces. Black holes, thought to be "science fiction" twenty years ago, are now precisely delineated and accepted as fact by astronomers. "Worm holes," potential shortcuts across space and time, are now being openly discussed by modern-day scientists and cosmologists. In the novel, the complexity of spacefolding is depicted as such that one in ten voyages was lost forever, an unacceptable number. After all, how many of us would get on an airplane if there were a one-in-ten chance that the plane would not return?

To deal with this problem, super computers were developed to improve the odds for success. Perhaps, Herbert also sensed the debate that would emerge in our time between computer scientists who suspect that super computers are destined to become integrated into our biology and greatly supersede anything possible by the unembossed human brain (called instantiation) and neuroscientists who are brimming with ideas about how to protect and enhance our brains, allowing us to stay a step ahead of the super computers. In the novel, super computers were incapable of improving the odds enough to allow for safe transport. Instead, the human body was mutated, just as we are capable of doing at this time, by genetic alterations. The mutations resulted in the production of "guild navigators," who in their final form were not really recognizable as human. Thanks to huge doses of the spice "mélange," the humanoid being underwent dramatic shrinkage of appendages and other body parts and enormous enlargement of the brain. Basically, they were all brain, which surpassed any capability of super computers and conferred on them an all-encompassing prescience. With this ability, these navigators could now navigate the folds of space and worm holes as easily as you and I driving to the corner grocery market. And the story proceeds.

The Battery

My own vision of the brain is that of a giant battery. The brain and nervous system buzz with electrical and chemical activity. All of the other body tissues lack this sparkle. Unanimated flesh can maintain some resemblance of activity, such as the extricated beating heart held aloft by the Aztec priest. For the most part, however, the flesh can only be brought to life by the brain. Mary Shelley, herself, attested to this in her 1821 novel, Frankenstein, but asserting that the "mind" was activated by a "spark," which then animated the dead flesh.

The sparkling brain is a wonder. Not only can it do mathematical computation, create symphonies, or write poetry, it can love unconditionally, sacrifice itself for the bigger good, run twenty-six miles in two hours and a few minutes, imagine, and do a host of miraculous things. When the buzzing and sparkling begin to dim, from aging, disease, and impending death, the effect of the lights going out is palpable, filling space with a sense of loss.

Computer scientists use the word instantiation to refer to a new entity or object. As miraculous as modern day computers are now, and how much greater the emerging super computers of the near future may be, I cannot imagine that we would ever wish to exchange our brains for a computer-based nervous system. As we get better and better with computers and instantiation, the possibility of integrating computers into the nervous system will become possible. Although we seem to have embraced alterations of our bodies through the medium of plastic surgery, how much will we be willing to alter our brains? The ethical questions surrounding this type of inquiry will likely far surpass any debates of bodily function so far entertained.

Mitochondria and Evolution

Before we fully examine the nervous system and its disorders, this is an opportune time to discuss a little about evolution, particularly about very distant evolution. This in turn brings up the topic of mitochondria, disorders of which appear to be closely tied to many neurological diseases. The trillions of cells which compose our bodies eventually retreat evolutionarily to a single cell. In multi-cellular organisms called eukaryotes (pronounced "u-carry-oats"), the cell is divided into complex structures contained in membranes or envelopes. The defining one is, of course, the nucleus, which contains a copy of the DNA blueprint. The cell body contains a variety of so-called organelles, once again wrapped and folded in complex ways, as well as a so-called cytoskeleton composed of microtubules and filaments. Recall that the nucleus creates RNA, which is transported throughout the cell body, the biologic manufacturing plant, where the production of thousands of different kinds of proteins proceeds.

The Cell

This two-sentence paragraph is made for emphasis. The nervous system is the most complex part of the human organism, and the cell is likely the most mind-boggling, complex structure in the known universe, consisting of a labyrinth of twisted passageways and tunnels, some connected and some with dead ends, with multiple compartments and cubby holes where messages are brought and proteins are built, all supervised by the big boss... DNA.

With the rapid "evolution" of computer science, including remarkable advances in artificial intelligence, our species, the species which has given birth to these emerging super computers, has come under attack by its very own progeny (sounds like a rebellious teenager to me). This has involved name-calling, such as labeling life as it now exists as "DNA-based" or even more pejorative "carbon-based." The idea is that a new era is dawning, whereby out goes the old and in comes the new silicone-based to begin, which will quickly dwarf any evolutionary leaps made by the antiquated carbon-based format over the last 3.5 billion years.

Prokaryotes

The first single-cell organisms, called "prokaryotes," date back approximately 3.5 billion years, give or take a few years. Prokaryotes are the first known cells. Prokaryotes are able to reproduce and are self-sustaining, separated from their environment by a membrane. There are two varieties of prokaryotes: bacteria and the recently described archaea. They are still here, 3.5 billion years later, attesting to the durability of their design. However, they lack ambition, possibly because they have no nucleus. There appears to have been little evolution over 3.5 billion years. I guess, "if it ain't broke, don't fix it."

Eukaryotes

In contrast, the next great evolutionary step is a relatively recent one, dating back about 1.7 billion years. This is the so-called eukaryocyte, which is basically the modern cell. These structures are far bigger than prokaryotes and, like them, have a cell membrane, separating them from their environment. However, they are remarkably more complex internally, and the structure of their DNA is unmistakably different than that of prokaryotes. As noted, several paragraphs above, internally they are remarkably folded, so as to create a labyrinth. The most remarkable set of foldings results in the appearance of the nucleus, akin to the throne room, containing the emperor/empress DNA. Many other realms of foldings, all determined by the structure of internally produced proteins, give rise to a list of so-called organelles. These represent domains of folding which are distinct enough to have a particular microscopic visual characteristic and a somewhat unique function in the overall scheme of cellular metabolism.

The punch line of this evolutionary drift is drawing near. Please appreciate that we are describing the very structure, multiplied by trillions or quadrillions, which make up the completed organism, whether it be an earthworm or a Nobel Laureate. The largest, most distinct, and most important organelle is called the mitochondria (see Figure). Every cell has one to thousands of these structures, each with five distinct compartments. They are roughly ten microns in length, about the size of 1½ red blood cells. Mitochondria (or "chloroplasts" found in plants) are involved in numerous cell functions, including signaling, via calcium fluxes, and all levels of the cell cycle including cell differentiation, aging, and cell death. Now that should get your attention! Multiply cell death in a multi-cellular organism by several trillion, and the possible results are obvious.

The biology of mitochondria has come to light incredibly fast. There is an increasingly large set of so-called mitochondrial diseases, many of which present as neurological or neuromuscular disorders including Parkinson's disease, epilepsy, stroke, Alzheimer's disease, myopathies

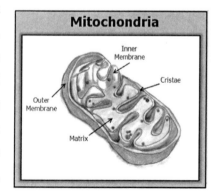

(muscle disorders) encephalomyopathies, diabetes, and psychiatric disorders, including schizophrenia and bipolar disorders. A common thread in all of these conditions appears to involve oxidative stress → leakage of electrons → enzyme dysfunction → peroxidases, free radicals, and other reactive oxygen species → cell damage and death. Cell death × several trillion = death of organism, all emanating from "oxidative stress." More about this, soon.

Matrilineal Mitochondrial DNA

The punch line has finally arrived. Scientists soon discovered that remarkably and inexplicably (at first), DNA was found in the mitochondria, i.e., outside of the nucleus. Almost immediately, it was also appreciated that this was no average DNA. In fact, it was as different from nuclear DNA, as a pot roast from the elk. Slightly closer inspection revealed it to be astoundingly similar to bacterial DNA. Several other lines of evidence all converged on a single point that within the body of every eukaryotic cell sits the descendant of a bacterium! So around 1.7 billion years ago, one of our ancestors stumbled upon a bacterium and engulfed it. Since bacteria are adept at so-called cellular respiration, which generates endless energy, this boost of free energy provided a huge evolutionary advantage to our eukaryotic ancestors, and... well... here we are!

Mitochondria have ten copies of mitochondrial DNA. They have retained their ancestral ability to divide and/or bud. Unfortunately, they appear to be particularly susceptible to oxidative damage. Mutations of mitochondrial DNA may be responsible for exercise intolerance similar to that seen in brain and neuromuscular diseases. As noted, mitochondrial diseases appear to be most symptomatic when found in muscle or nerve tissue. Obviously, the expression of mitochondrial diseases depends heavily on the organ in which the dysfunction occurs. It is not known if today's "chronic fatigue syndrome" is a mitochondrial disease.

Lastly, there is now unequivocal evidence that mitochondrial DNA is of matrilineal origin. Once again, information from divergent sources has allowed scientists to portray the "Mitochondrial Eve." She is the woman identified as the most recent common ancestor of all currently living humans. She lived approximately 200,000 years ago in East Africa. Obviously, other *H. sapiens* females were alive then, perhaps as many as 5,000. However, their mitochondrial DNA is gone, but their nuclear DNA is present in today's population. Incidentally, her counterpart is "Chromosomal Adam," who lived much later, perhaps 75,000 years ago.

Every organ system has its compliment of cells, the individual units that make up the organs that get the job done. From the structural or anatomic standpoint, the nervous system is no different. Obviously the major difference, soon to be discussed ad nauseam, has to do with a series of what perhaps should be called epiphenomena. This refers to functions, very important functions, which occur not because of individual cellular activity, as complicated as that may be, but because of interconnections between cells, giving rise to unexpected results. Obviously, what I am referring to are the issues of consciousness, memory, and learning. This will follow soon.

The Neuron

Now, for the relatively straight-forward cast of characters. Although it has a strong supporting cast, the neuron is the star. It is a cell like no other. It can be recognized as a cell by the appearance of a cell body with the usual complement of organelles and nucleus. That is where the similarity ends. Surrounding the cell body are a very large number of dendrites, which are projections which provide a large surface area for an abundance of receptor sites for connection with the axon terminal of the next neuron (Figure A). In between the dendrites and the axon terminals

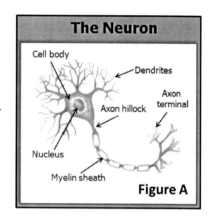

The Neuron

Figure A

is the long axon projection covered by a myelin sheath acting as an electrochemical insulator, to improve conduction of the electrical impulse as it travels down the axon (Figure B). Note the axon hillock, representing an impediment to electrical transmission. It takes strong stimuli to get over and through the hillock to proceed all the way down the axon to the terminals. These diagrams are very simplistic. Neurons

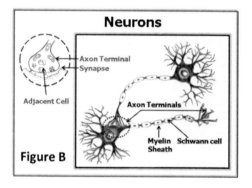

Neurons

Figure B

may connect with thousands of other neurons, and with themselves. Massive interconnection assures that enough energy will be transferred from neuron to neuron, to allow the impulse to pass the axon hillock and traverse the axon. The cell bodies of neurons clustered together in the cortex represent the "gray matter" of the brain. The myelin sheath, composed of fatty substances, comprises the "white matter" of the cortex of the brain.

Now for the glial cells. The smallest of these are the microglia, which are modified macrophages, of hematopoietic (bone marrow) origin. Macrophages are designated as scavengers, mobile and capable of engulfing debris and disposing of it through chemical attenuation. They are the roving watch dogs of the central nervous system (CNS). There are perhaps 150 billion of them in the CNS. They may have pluripotential features (ability to transform into other cells), but it is not known for sure how much this actually occurs.

Astrocytes are the most common of the larger glial cells. They anchor neurons to their blood supply. They act as scaffolding for migration of other cells. They regulate the ionic environment and aid in the recycling of neurotransmitters. They signal each other by calcium fluxes.

Oligodendrocytes have one extremely important known function—that being the production of the myelin sheath surrounding the neuronal axons.

Ependymal cells line the ventricular system. They create the cerebrospinal fluid and assist with its circulation by the function of their cilia.

Radial glias appear in areas of neurogenesis. They act as neural progenitors in the developing brain and also act as scaffolding. They may be the major cell responsible for development of new neurons.

Oxidative Stress and Antioxidants

Several pages ago, in describing remarkable new knowledge about mitochondria, the metabolic workhorse of the cell, a comment was made about how sensitive those structures are to the effects of "oxidative stress." This is a topic which interestingly has remained somewhat on the fringes of clinical medicine for a long time. Therefore, for the most part, it has been ignored by medical doctors. We all need to appreciate the fact that many forms of human intercourse have financial brakes and accelerators. Especially in modern times in the industrialized world, such intercourse is often driven by financial concerns. Contemporary scientific exploration, in whatever area of interest, is a fragile undertaking, heavily influenced by factors beyond the elemental curiosity of investigators. All of this babble is an attempt to understand at least one plausible explanation as to why a topic which looks potentially so rich would be so relatively ignored for a long time. Modern research is very expensive. Research scientists need funding. There is intense competition for funding. One of the main carrots which might tempt funders to fund is the prospect of quickly realizing a profit, perhaps even a huge profit. These types of considerations are perpetually potential stumbling blocks for medical researchers. Perhaps, the goose who lays the golden eggs has not been clearly visualized by the major funders (pharmaceutical companies and the government) in reference to the topic of oxidative stress. There are likely many other possible explanations.

At the dawn of what may be the oxidative stress era, here are the very basics. We will not go into great detail for two reasons: (1) I don't understand it, and (2) you would be quickly bored to tears. The basic science of this topic extends back to principles of organic chemistry, and some of this terminology may bring back memories of high school chemistry class. To whet your interest enough to proceed, this discussion will lead us to the "hot" topic of so-called anti-oxidants and their possible role in maintenance of health.

Oxidation–reduction reactions, now termed "redox" reactions, represent a basic chemical reaction, whereby there is a transfer of electrons from one chemical to another. The chemical losing an electron undergoes oxidation and becomes oxidized. At the same time, it then becomes a reducing agent. The chemical gaining an electron undergoes reduction and becomes reduced and thus becomes an oxidizing agent. (In many chemical reactions, there is no gain or loss of electrons, as compounds merge.)

"Cellular respiration," which is metabolism occurring in the presence of oxygen, is the cellular reaction to convert glucose or other nutrients to ATP, with production of waste products. Other nutrients include amino acids and fatty acids. ATP represents stored energy (fuel) for cellular biosynthesis, locomotion, or transport of molecules back and forth across the cell membrane. Our intimate relationship to plants is illustrated by the fact that using sunlight (energy), photosynthesis in plants combines carbon dioxide and water to form carbohydrates and oxygen. Obviously, both end-products are essential to animal life. Cellular respiration is the opposite, using carbohydrates (sugars) and oxygen to form carbon dioxide and water and energy (ATP) during intermediary steps. Basically, through photosynthesis and cellular respiration, sunlight is transformed into ATP through the intermediation of plants.

Oxidative stress is the term used to describe what emerges when there is an excessive load of free radicals, also called reactive oxygen species, exceeding ability of the body to neutralize or eliminate them. Free radicals are byproducts of normal cellular function, producing unstable oxygen molecules. Production of free radicals can be excessive secondary to numerous factors, including improper diet, such as in chemically altered fats in commercial vegetable oil, vegetable shortening, all heated oils (fried foods), highly processed foods (three-fourths of what you find on the grocery shelf), excessive sugar, food coloring, and preservatives. Many other types of toxicity, from sunlight, to medical X-rays, to mental stress, tobacco and alcohol abuse, pesticides, cleaning fluids, chemical solvents, and air pollution can all create free radicals.

Regardless of the source, free radicals are very unstable, with an insatiable thirst for electrons, and react quickly with anything, from which they can scavenge or steal an electron. This includes numerous cellular components, thus damaging cellular mechanisms and threatening the integrity of the cell itself. Free radicals can also scavenge electrons from DNA in the nucleus of the cell, destabilizing

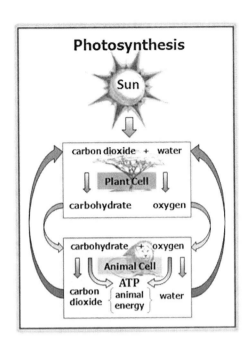

that structure and laying the groundwork for mutations. Recall that the chances of a random mutation producing a beneficial effect is thought to be small, compared to the likelihood of producing a deleterious effect. Recall also that the death of a cell multiplied by a large number obviously results in the death of the organism as a whole. In summary, excessive free radicals have a high potential for having negative effects on the organism, with a very small chance of positive effects.

Molecular Biology–Clinical Medicine Interface

So, free radical production can be too high for the organism to cope with, due to ambient "toxicity," in the broadest sense. In addition, during the natural aging process, free radical production invariably tends to increase. This is manifest as the appearance of degenerative diseases of all types, such as arteriosclerosis and malignant processes.

At this point, a vicious cycle may be established, whereby free radicals produce degenerative diseases which then greatly proliferate the production of free radicals, and thus, the fuse is lit. In fact, it often appears that this scenario is played out in clinical medicine, whereby one illness starts the snowball rolling downhill, with an increasing mass of other problems pulled into the picture, with increasing speed and force of the downhill snowball. This attests to the need to be constantly wary, so as to try to prevent the snowball from being nudged into downhill motion. If that per chance occurs, the person needs to mount a furious counterattack, to not only stop the process immediately but to strengthen the body as a whole, so that the vicious cycle does not reactivate again and hurtle the snowball down the hill. There is a name for this approach. It is called preventative medicine. This may be the crucial interface between "molecular biology" (cellular function) and "clinical medicine" (what happens to you and me in real time).

Incidentally, as has been noted before, few things are absolutely black or white. The vast majority of earth-bound features are shades of gray. The organism, in this case "us," needs free radicals. The liver uses them to assist in the daily detoxification activities in which it is involved. White blood cells utilize them to kill invading organisms, like bacteria and viruses. Even more importantly, recall that it is less important what a given cell can do than whether or not its receptor function is adequate to activate all the switches to do the job properly. In this sense, free radicals/reactive oxygen species appear to have a very important role in cell signaling, i.e., turning switches off and on all over the body. It is clear that our goal is not to eliminate free radicals but to contain them. As they are produced normally by all cells, we tend to sit on the fence leaning well over toward the proliferation side, rather than the control side. Proliferation occurs with an increase (even small) in "toxicity."

The best method to control toxicity is, of course, "prevention." Reading between the lines, this takes considerable effort, at least initially. Old habits die hard. Once new habits are set in place, it gets easier. The recruits under Drill Sergeant Marmorstein initially had no choice. Later, they elected to eat, work, sleep, and think differently, and the results pay dividends. In the meantime, I promised mention of the topic of "antioxidants." This is the generic name given to substances which have the ability and the willingness to gladly donate an electron or two to the frenetic free radical, to calm it down. These were not researched by Drill Sergeant Marmorstein but were mentioned as part of the protocol. There is a vast amount of anecdotal evidence that these materials are beneficial. Due to the fact that there is little chance of a big paycheck being made by funders of research, it is unlikely that any of this will be tested in a randomized, double-blinded, placebo-controlled, i.e., evidence-based fashion. Substances known to give up electrons are vitamins A, C, and E, glutathione, bioflavonoids, selenium, CoQ_{10}, polyphenols, lipoic acids, catalase, superoxide dismutase, and melatonin. Cholesterol does the same, perhaps explaining why very low cholesterol levels seem to be linked to increased rates of cancer. Glutathione may be pivotal, being the major antioxidant of the liver.

Nervous System Divisions

The nervous system is anatomically divided into the central nervous system (CNS), comprising the brain and spinal cord, and the peripheral nervous system, comprising nerves which branch all over

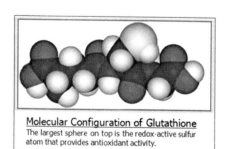

Molecular Configuration of Glutathione
The largest sphere on top is the redox-active sulfur atom that provides antioxidant activity.

the interior and the surfaces of the body. There is a subdivision called the autonomic nervous system (ANS) consisting of a number of neural pathways beginning in the hypothalamus and brainstem, composed of two parts—the sympathetic and parasympathetic sections—and generally regulating a host of unconscious or "automatic" physiologic (metabolic) functions all over the body.

Isolation of the Nervous System and the Blood–Brain Barrier

The CNS is unique in many ways, such as its role in memory, cognition, and consciousness. From the anatomic standpoint, it is unique in one very interesting way. It seems that at some point in the evolution of the CNS, and please pardon this anthropomorphizing explanation, it seems that the evolving organism, recognizing the emerging monumental importance of these tissues, decided that they needed special protection. First of all, in order to function well, neurons are partially covered by a myelin sheath, composed mostly of fatty substances. This adds up to about 60% fat content for the brain. In view of the fact that this fatty material is held at ninety-eight degrees, or thereabouts, the brain is moderately soft, having the consistency somewhat of butter sitting in a sunny location. The first level of protection is very apparent—that being the skull. The brain of most vertebrates is surrounded by this protective bony shield. Only slightly less apparent is that the spinal cord, the body of which terminates slightly below the mid-back, is substantially surrounded by the vertebral bones and then with further protection from muscles and other soft tissues.

What is likely not appreciated is that there is another layer of protection, which is truly unique. In fact, it is called the blood–brain barrier (BBB). In slightly fanciful terms, it is almost as if the brain and spinal cord were wrapped in a tough, thin cellophane, substantially isolating it from the rest of the body. This BBB is visible in some areas, such as over the surface of the brain, just under large portions of the skull, where the so-called meninges can be readily seen. As is true about almost everything, when investigated a little more closely, the meninges are found to consist of three separate layers (see diagram). The outer layer with the anthropomorphic-sounding name dura mater ("tough mother") is a thin but very tough fibrous membrane. Under that is the arachnoid (with "spider-like" webbing) containing dense vascular beds. Just below that is a space filled with cerebrospinal fluid (CSF), called the subarachnoid space. The fluid acts as another form of barrier and also a cushion for impacts. Just beneath that is the third layer of the meninges, the pia mater ("soft mother"), tightly adherent to the convolutions of the brain, like Saran Wrap. It contains a plexus of blood vessels which eventually enter and nourish the brain.

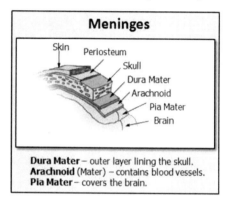

Meninges

Skin · Periosteum · Skull · Dura Mater · Arachnoid · Pia Mater · Brain

Dura Mater – outer layer lining the skull.
Arachnoid (Mater) – contains blood vessels.
Pia Mater – covers the brain.

The last and perhaps the most comprehensive part of the BBB is invisible to the naked eye but functions to substantially isolate the CNS from the rest of the body. The brain receives approximately 25% of the blood flowing out of the heart, and this proportion is carefully maintained by a number of potent reflexes. Recall the image of the brain as a huge battery. If it is not appropriately nourished with glucose and oxygen, or if its neurons and supporting cells called astrocytes are experiencing mitochondrial malfunction, global mental and physical functioning can be seriously compromised. What protects the brain from this massive influx of blood? Everywhere else in the body, those innocent looking but shockingly complex cells, with their labyrinthine folding, and remnants of bacterial ancestors are fairly tightly connected, but with purposeful breaks in this connection, so that certain substances can flow into and out of cells, without all the metabolic work needed to penetrate the cell membrane.

This arrangement is altered in two ways in the CNS. The cells lining the walls of the capillaries penetrating deep into the CNS are packed densely tight together. In addition to that, as just mentioned, the astrocytes, on the brain side of the capillary, push pod-like extensions out to further stabilize the intercellular junction and to provide an additional physical barrier to transfer of unwanted materials (see diagram).

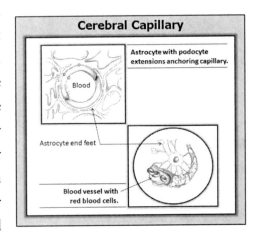

So, this is a very elaborate evolutionary arrangement. It certainly appears that the purpose of this is to protect the CNS. As mentioned, it is as if the organism as a whole acknowledges the ascendancy of the CNS in terms of survival and goes to great lengths to protect this treasure trove. Interestingly, this entire arrangement does not appear to affect the passive diffusion of oxygen and carbon dioxide into and out of the CNS. Interestingly, and not to be editorialized by me, the other common substance which diffuses inward without impediment is alcohol! Transport systems continue to operate by pumping in sugars and amino acids. The good news is that the CNS is substantially protected from infections and toxins. The bad news is that antibodies do not get in, so that if an infection does develop in the CNS, it can move devastatingly fast because of the inability of the immune system to engage the infection fully. Also, many antibiotics do not penetrate the BBB, although the BBB does tend to weaken during a serious infection. Fortunately, some antibiotics do penetrate even the intact BBB. Lastly, this system of protection evolved long before the appearance of chemotherapeutic agents, which also do not penetrate well.

Dysfunction of BBB

There is considerable interest now in the possibility that previously unknown malfunctioning of the BBB may be at least part of the explanation for several relatively common diseases. Multiple sclerosis appears to be a result of an autoimmune attack on the myelin sheath (which act as insulators to improve electrical transmission) of neurons. It is now being investigated as to whether a primary disruption of the BBB could allow T lymphocytes to enter the CNS and attack myelin. Secondly, there is now evidence that herpes simplex virus I (the virus responsible for facial "cold sores") can be found in amyloid plaques, the characteristic pathology of Alzheimer's disease. Once again, it is now being speculated that breaches of the BBB allow either the virus itself or amyloid B to enter the CNS, which then adheres to astrocytes, causing them to die and leaving a plaque. Lastly, it is now thought that our universal enemy, "oxidative stress," can weaken the BBB, allowing unwanted substances in, producing seizure and other problems.

Meningitis

A few final concepts regarding the meninges. Infection of these membranes is a disease which is well known, called meningitis. The majority of cases of meningitis are viral in origin and usually seen in conjunction with a flu-like illness. The most common symptom is headache, often very severe. Occasionally, there may be alterations of consciousness, but not coma. It may be necessary to do a "spinal tap" or lumbar puncture to obtain a sample of CSF for analysis and for confirmation that the disease is not caused by a bacterial agent. Viral meningitis is invariably cured, as the body mounts its immune response, likely made more effective by the damage to the meninges.

Bacterial meningitis is a much more serious condition. It can occur explosively in previously healthy young people. Or, it may occur from some other primary infection, which then seeds the bloodstream and overwhelms the BBB. Antibiotic treatments are needed early to avoid a terrible (permanent sequelae) or horrible (death) outcome.

Meninges and Bleeding

The last issue to be discussed regarding the meninges has to do with the fact that several types of bleeding into the head are named by their precise location in reference to the layers of the meninges involved. Needless to say, bleeding into the head is always a serious problem. The spectrum of results runs all the way from full recovery to death. All three of these particular types of bleeding can perhaps be looked upon as varieties of stroke or cerebrovascular accident, although we most often associate stroke with either spontaneous (non-traumatic) occlusion or rupture of a blood vessel coming up into the brain from the neck. These three types of meningeal bleeding, usually the result of a head injury, are more common in older people—and especially common with falling. All are much more common in people on blood thinners, including aspirin.

Epidural Hematoma

Epidural hematoma refers to an accumulation of blood between the dura mater and the skull. There is often an accompanying skull fracture. The person is usually not very well, and the diagnosis is usually made within a few hours. Depending on the size, it may need to be surgically evacuated. This is dangerous bleeding as it is often arterial in origin—that is under pressure—and can quickly worsen. This type of bleeding is more common in younger people.

Subarachnoid Hemorrhage

The second type of bleeding is called subarachnoid hemorrhage. This is also a very serious problem and which most often occurs spontaneously, rather than trauma-induced. This is the type of bleeding which occurs from a ruptured aneurysm or a ruptured arteriovenous malformation. The person is often rendered quickly helpless and unable to communicate effectively. They may become unconscious. There is usually no surgery for such a person. However, if they are lucky enough to be only mildly impaired, a number of radiographic and/ or surgical procedures can be attempted to prevent the possibility of a further catastrophic hemorrhage. Recovery may be very prolonged, and long-term sequelae are common.

Subdural Hematoma

The third type of bleeding is subdural hematoma. The pace of this process is often much different, beginning with a head injury, but no apparent immediate change. However, over the course of days to many weeks, a large variety of motor (movement), sensory, and especially behavioral elements may begin to emerge such that it is very apparent that something is very wrong. By that time, the head injury of months ago may have been forgotten. In the case just described, it is possible that surgical removal of the clot may not completely restore full function. If the pace is quicker, days to a few weeks, it is more likely that a surgical approach will cure the disease. Based on many patient factors, and the peculiarities of any particular set of circumstances, it may be difficult to decide whether to operate or not.

All of these different types of meningeal bleeding are usually diagnosed by CT scan or MRI of the head. Recall that the skull is a confined space, in fact with several compartments. Accumulating blood takes up space. If this occurs slowly, the underlying brain may be simply compressed, and life is likely preserved, albeit possibly with a neurologic deficit. However, if the accumulation of blood occurs quickly, the brain does not necessarily compress, but instead there may be a great buildup of pressure within the skull. The mechanism of death in these cases may be from herniation of the base of the brain into or through the foramen magnum, which is the largest naturally occurring hole in the skull, at its base. As the brain pushes into this narrow alleyway, it compresses critical brainstem reflexes, such as those regulating blood pressure or breathing, either one of which may bottom out, with death ensuing.

Deep Brain Strokes

The more typical types of stroke, as mentioned above, are those that occur from problems with blood vessels in the depths of the brain tissue. There are four major blood vessels feeding the brain, consisting of two carotid arteries, one on each side, and two vertebral arteries running up along the spine. These meet deep inside the skull to form the so-called circle of Willis, whereby blood from the back of the brain can flow forward and blood from the front can flow backward. This arrangement appears to be an evolutionary attempt to provide a backup system should blood flow in any given artery become blocked. In fact, it often works exactly as it was designed to do. This may be particularly true if the blockage occurs gradually, so that blood flow from the other patent arteries can find its way to branches beyond the blocked artery, somewhat like a self- or automatically induced bypass. If this does occur, the artery in question may close completely, and there may be absolutely no symptoms. Once again, evolution appears to place a very high priority on preservation of brain function.

From the circle of Willis, three more branches emerge— the anterior, middle, and posterior cerebral arteries, one of each on each side. The middle cerebral usually supplies the largest territory and is the most common affected with these kinds of stroke. Unfortunately, the occlusion may occur before collateral vessels have emerged. The other type of problem is rupture of the artery, with hemorrhage into the brain

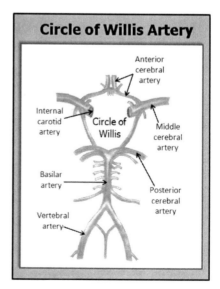

Circle of Willis Artery

Anterior cerebral artery

Internal carotid artery

Circle of Willis

Middle cerebral artery

Basilar artery

Posterior cerebral artery

Vertebral artery

substance, more often seen in poorly controlled hypertension. This is often a devastating occurrence. Either one of these varieties can come on unexpectedly without any prodrome. Symptoms of either variety are dependent on location and size of the stroke, and can result in motor, and/or sensory, and/or cognitive dysfunction, which may be temporary or permanent. Recovery can proceed as long as one to two years out from the stroke. Treatment is basically correction or control of precipitating factors, such as hypertension, and other causative factors for hardening of the arteries. Large focal collections of blood are occasionally approached surgically. Obviously, by far, the best treatment is prevention. Rigorous control of contributing factors can unequivocally lower the chances of stroke.

There is one other form of stroke to be mentioned, with a pace all of its own and a somewhat unique outcome. As has been mentioned on a number of different occasions, human beings have characteristic patterns of thinking and subsequent behavior, just as does any animal species. We tend to point out those things about animal "x", as if to emphasize our superiority over them, in that it is so readily apparent to our level of discernment but unapparent to the poor simpletons of animal "x" variety. I have this concept that I hold to be true—that if we humans were invaded and eventually subjugated by a clearly superior being (perhaps, this will occur as soon as super computers are instantiated into our carbon-based nervous systems) that these superior beings would convulse in laughter (if that is what truly superior beings do) watching us go through our litany of highly predictable, "adorable" behaviors. (No, that is not the longest sentence in this text, as it is only sixty-seven words.) Anyway, it seems highly likely to me that a world filled with humility will work better than a world filled with condescension.

So, one of our predictable patterns is that we are not comfortable with ambiguity. If your doctor told you "It might be advanced cancer, or it could be a virus from which you will soon recover," you might be inclined to not pay your bill. In fact, the doctor's statement is likely true. However, we are adept enough regarding interpersonal communication to know that the patient would not do well with that summation. So, "Let's order a few simple tests, which will take a while to come back, and meet again in a month," falls much easier on the patient's ears. We like answers. We like black. We like white. We don't like gray.

TIA versus Stroke

The stroke alluded to several paragraphs ago has to do with the concept of "transient ischemic attack" or TIA. You have likely heard this term many times before, as if it were a clarion call or a monolithic marker in the wilderness. TIA refers to a temporary interruption of circulation to a part of the brain, associated with some type of symptomology. This in turn could be a clear-cut syndrome, such as paralysis of one side of the body, or it could be extremely nebulous like your inability to remember the name of your doctor whom you have seen for the last ten years. What defines the syndrome as a TIA ("T for transient") is that it must revert completely in twenty-four hours. In fact, true, bona fide TIAs usually revert much faster than that. The implication is that a TIA completely reverses, whereby a stroke never completely reverses. So, if your syndrome lasts twenty-four hours and one second, unfortunately you have had a stroke. This is the black and white approach that we find so comfortable.

Recall that the human nervous system has approximately a trillion neurons and as many as 100–300 trillion astrocytes. The likelihood is high that as soon as the definitive TIA syndrome appears, neurons and astrocytes start dropping off like flies. Fortunately, this may represent a very small portion of the total number of cells at risk of dying. The point is that the all-or-none concept of TIA or stroke is likely a gross oversimplification and that minute little strokes occurring in end arteries (literally, the smallest artery before it gives way to the capillary network and the venous circulation) likely occur frequently. In fact, they may be so small as to escape detection all together, or big enough to create a very minor or subtle syndrome. This is the gray approach, which tends to make us very uncomfortable.

Ischemic Encephalopathy

We know about this clinically (in the real world) by finding on CT or MRI of the brain, described by various terms such as ischemic encephalopathy, cystic or multi cystic encephalopathy, or simply "white matter disease." We see changes which include the appearance of tiny holes, thought to represent the end result of tiny strokes. People with this imaging study finding may appear to be and claim to be normal, attesting to the fact that a trillion neurons and a quadrillion astrocytes are a lot to start with. Many of these people do have symptoms of neurologic disease, such as low energy (recall the brain is a battery, and the concept of mitochondrial diseases), slowness in walking, stiffness, and awkwardness, as well as subtle changes in mentation. The cause of this disorder is blockage of these tiny arterial fragments deep in the brain and secondary to all of the known risk factors for arteriosclerosis. In this particular condition, hypertension appears to be particularly prevalent.

Is It Luck or Radicalism?

By inference, this is a preventable disease, as are so many of the diseases we discuss. When one considers the ravages that arteriosclerosis can wreak all over the body, the radical-appearing lifestyle adjustments so fundamental to the approach of Drill Sergeant Marmorstein don't look so radical after all. Instead, being old and mentally and/or physically inept prematurely can be the radical result of a lifetime of neglect. In assessing the overview of illness and premature decline, I always emphasize the need to truly, deeply, compassionately, and lovingly care for oneself, i.e., avoiding avoidable diseases, and the need for good luck, i.e., not being blindsided by diseases that seem to occur randomly in the population and have no known cause. It is really being blindsided? To finish this punch–counterpunch–punch debate about what Thomas Jefferson said, presaging Mark Twain, Winston Churchill, and possibly others, "I'm a great believer in luck, and I find that the harder I work, the more I have of it."

Ventricular System

For many of us, possibly including you, our first lesson in neuroanatomy occurred during grade school. I clearly recall this when one of my classmates after hearing me tell that my uncle's farm in Ohio contained the body of water where the biblical story of Jonah and the Whale occurred brashly declared, "You got a hole in your head." He was right, and several years later, I found out that I was wrong.

We all have a fairly large hole in our heads, called the ventricular system of the brain. We have already discussed the cerebrospinal fluid (CSF), which is formed by specialized structures in the brain called the choroid plexi, of which there are usually four, as well as the ependymal cells lining the ventricles. CSF is filtered from the blood, but as filters obviously do, by allowing some things to enter and some not, it is very different than blood. It cushions the brain against impact. Most of it is located deep in the brain tissue, where it assists with nourishment and cleansing of those deeply seated tissues.

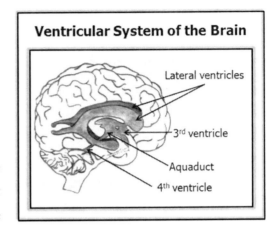

Although CFS fills the subarachnoid space of the meninges, most of it is located in the ventricular system and contiguous with the subarachnoid space as the pia mater fuses with the ependymal cells which line these rather large ventricular spaces. The left and right lateral ventricles are the largest, and project anteriorly (frontward) and posteriorly (backward) as well. The so-called third ventricle lies between the right and left thalamic bodies, in the midline. The fourth ventricle is located between the cerebellum and the pons—posterior and inferior to the third. There is a very narrow aqueduct of Sylvius connecting to the third and fourth ventricles. This aqueduct, because of its narrow size, is prone to blockage by a number of conditions. It is the fourth ventricle that connects with the subarachnoid space by three openings, called foramina, all of which are narrow. From the subarachnoid space, the fluid circulates up over the top of the brain to the superior sagittal sinus which is like a large vein, into which project the so-called arachnoid granulations, whereby the CSF goes back into the blood. (Diagrams) Interestingly, fluids of the inner ear originate from CSF, attesting to the fact that the inner ear is an outward projection of the CNS, just as is the retina of the eye.

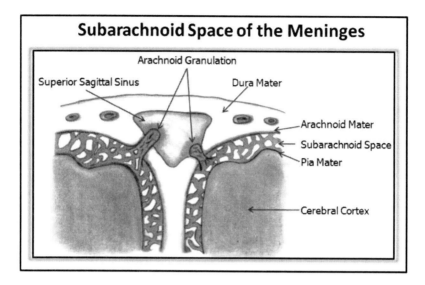

There are only a few diseases which primarily affect the ventricular system. They are somewhat common and can result in considerable morbidity.

Hydrocephalus is the term applied to too much fluid. This can occur because of too much production, too little resorption, or impeded flow. Another way of looking at is to describe it as communicating (non-obstructed) or non-communicating (obstructed). Either of these can be congenital (born with it) or acquired (produced by disease process after birth).

Normal Pressure Hydrocephalus

A common form of communicating hydrocephalus is so-called normal pressure hydrocephalus, with enlarged ventricles but normal or only slightly elevated pressure of the fluid. This is often seen as a clinical triad of gait disturbance, urinary incontinence, and mental deterioration. In most cases, it seems that impaired absorption is the most common mechanism. If treated early enough with a shunt, up to 20% of people show dramatic improvement. A larger number show some improvement. Shunts are placed by neurosurgeons to drain the excess fluid from the ventricular system to the abdomen. Unfortunately, they may be difficult to keep open and they can become infected when seen in the aftermath of infections, strokes, or tumors and their treatment; hydrocephalus can be a vexing problem in and of itself.

Gross Anatomy of the CNS— The Cobbled-Together Mess

We have made allusions to the huge number of cells comprising the nervous system. Thus far, we have not described the gross anatomic parts of the brain and spinal cord. The time has come. The description will be very basic. The brain is incredibly complex on several different levels. Although every part of the brain has been named and attempts to organize individual structures into functional units have been done, studies of such arrangements give little insight into the actual ways that the brain functions. To try to explain how several trillion cells could cooperate in a coherent way in itself is an impossibility. Much of what the brain does appear to transcend by a factor of many, what analysis of individual sections can do, or what groupings of sections can do.

The brain appears to be the poster child of the notion that the sum is greater than its parts. In this case, the sum overwhelms the workings of its individual parts. So, studying the parts may be interesting and may provide insights, but it doesn't tell us who we are and why we do what we do. The medical adage about "never say never" does not dissuade me from skepticism as to whether or not the brain will ever yield its ultimate secrets, whether it is being investigated by humans who use it or super computers which can describe it in great detail.

Neither approach may get at the kernel of brain function, which in some ways truly does appear to be otherworldly. The words of one well-known neuroscience professor, in describing the brain emphasize the point "… cobbled together mess… quirky, inefficient, and bizarre… a weird agglomeration of ad hoc solutions." (From this point in time, forever on, whenever becoming extremely frustrated over the shortcomings of your fellow travelers, and of your own blunders and faux pas, calm and soften yourself by recalling the "cobbled together mess.")

Therefore, rather than waste your time, you will get only the very basics of gross neuroanatomy. Not only is it enough for the curious reader, as I recall, it is just about as much as was presented to us in medical school forty-five years ago.

The spinal cord is basically a nerve, albeit a very thick and structurally complex one. A nerve is basically living tissue whose purpose is to conduct an electrical current from point A to point B. Very simply put, for the most part, once the current arrives at point B, it causes a discharge of a chemical packet or packets called neurotransmitters. If point B abuts another nerve cell, transfer of these chemical messengers across the miniscule gap activates the second nerve cell, etc. If the nerve terminal abuts some other type of cell, discharge of these chemical messages will alter the cell membrane in some way, to cause an influx and/or efflux of ions into and out of the cell, which thus directs the cell to do something in the arsenal of things it can do, in turn depending on the complexities of receptor functioning and signaling already mentioned.

The spinal cord thus electrically connects the brain and the body. Obviously, information proceeds in both directions, i.e., from the brain to the body and from the body to the brain, in ascending and descending pathways. Once again, avoiding the hang-ups of getting overly entwined in the specifics of neuroanatomy, simply accept that as the spinal cord rises toward the brain, it is carrying some type of information from every region and every tissue in the body. This is a vast amount of information packed into a relatively small conduit. Of course, it is complex. Skip it!

Continuing with our simplistic grade school/medical school approach to neuroanatomy, how do we know when we have arrived at the brain? The answer is simple. You pass an unmistakably large landmark, given a powerful and elegant Latin name, foramen magnum ("big hole") which is the largest opening in the skull, at its base. Voila! You have now arrived in the brain, considered not only as the pinnacle of evolutionary development but also a "cobbled-together mess."

The structure arrived at is named the medulla (see diagram). The medulla has a number of so-called nuclei. This term, or used in this context, does not refer to the part of the cell with DNA but to a conglomeration of neurons, densely packed. These cells are involved with autonomic functions, such as cardiac and respiratory reflexes, including blood pressure regulation. The

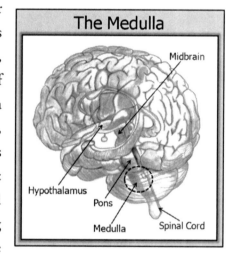

vomiting center is located here, very useful information, I am certain. There are relays, where ascending nerve fibers end and new ones begin. Just above the medulla is the pons. Many of the cranial nerve nuclei are located here—these are the nuclei which give rise to the nerves that supply all the structures of the head and upper neck. There are also respiratory and circulatory nuclei. Just above the pons is the mid-brain, containing relays of auditory and visual stimuli, and the substantia nigra ("black substance"). This might be of little concern, except that if it stops functioning, we see the syndrome of Parkinson's disease appear. Above that is the hypothalamus, which has enormous importance in controlling the internal milieu of the whole body, by linking the endocrine system and the nervous system.

Brainstem

These four structures—medulla, pons, midbrain, and hypothalamus—fulfill most anatomists' definition of the "brain stem." If this is all you have, you could stay alive. You would breath, and your heart would beat. A neurologist would come and test "primitive" reflexes and would state that "brainstem reflexes are intact." You might look awake, with eyes open and moving around. You might respond to "threat" by blinking. However, as best we can tell, you would not have the ability to integrate enough information coming in to be aware or so-called cognizant. People in this condition can be kept alive indefinitely, and in fact, this is done more often than it should be, in my opinion. Every nursing home is likely to have one or several permanent residents, who more or less fulfill the abovementioned characteristics. Some of these people are being fed completely through stomach feeding tubes. Even more remarkably, and more difficult for families to contend with, are those who will chew and swallow when food is placed in their mouth.

Brain Injury and Long-Term Care

The clinical syndrome noted above should be of concern to all of us. One of the many ways that humans are different than any other animal species is that through the medium of our huge cerebral cortex, which is absent in many species and remarkably smaller in many others, we have developed technological abilities that allow us to perform what perhaps could be described as "miracles." Obviously, in the individual with severe brain injury noted, such that only brainstem function is identifiable (and this may well include young individuals), left alone, the chances are 100% likely that the person would die. However, with our technology and increasing experience with large groups of people like this, we have the ability to keep them alive for decades.

The feeding is only a small part of the challenge. Helpless individuals like this are prone to a host of complications which occur anywhere from occasionally to frequently. These complications fall into several categories, including infections, skin issues, surgeries, and musculoskeletal issues. Infections include those of the urinary tract, respiratory tract, and other miscellaneous sites. Respiratory infections including pneumonia occur because of reduced cough reflex as well as dysfunctional swallowing. There also tends to be a reduction of the sighing reflex, which periodically expands the distal (especially lower) parts of the lungs in healthy people, who unconsciously sigh several times per hour, day and night. All of these conspire to reduce clearance of mucous and infectious material, and food and liquid from the lower respiratory tract, i.e., below the voice box, creating a setup for pneumonia. To the doctor, the question is not, "Why do these people get pneumonia?" But, "Why don't they have pneumonia all the time?" Although placing a feeding tube directly into the stomach lowers the risk of so-called "aspiration pneumonia," it certainly does not eliminate it for two reasons. First, food and liquid can regurgitate up from the stomach to the level of the voice box and windpipe and then be sucked down into the lung. Second, we all produce about one liter of saliva per day. As soon as this liquid enters the mouth, it becomes infected because of the resident bacterial population there. It tends to "pool" in the throat and can easily be aspirated into the lungs.

The second major source of infection is the urinary tract. Urinary infections are common even in otherwise healthy people. Many of these people with severe brain injuries have pre-existing urinary pathology. Most are cared for without catheters in the bladder. However, infections are particularly common during periods of fluid depletion, which can occur unbeknownst to the caregivers. In addition, at times, catheters become necessary for one of several reasons. Firstly, if these people are incontinent, depending on how often and for how long they are "wet," this can cause skin problems in that area. Secondly, some have bladder or prostate issues which prevent them from voiding adequately. So, eventually, a bladder catheter may be necessary. This may solve some problems, but it creates new ones, including guaranteed appearance of urinary infection. Surprisingly, some patients appear to have little if any difficulty with this. Others, however, become repeatedly symptomatic and even septic (blood stream invasion), requiring repeated use of antibiotics and trips back to the hospital.

Antibiotics are not innocuous drugs. There are many types of serious problems, which may occur upon first usage, or on the 100th usage, when there was no problem with the first 99. As mentioned above, there are other common sites for infection, including the gastrointestinal tract. The colon is home to billions of bacteria. Most of these are "friendly" (helping us) or neutral (just along for the ride). A few, generally in small numbers, can cause serious problems if given the chance. The chance comes in the form of an antibiotic, which is indiscriminant in its bacterial-killing ability and kills off enough of the friendly or neutral bacteria to give the conniving, evil ones the chance they have been waiting for. There is now a "new" disease among us, in fact in epidemic proportions. It has been mentioned already. This is formally called "clostridium difficile enterocolitis" or informally "C-diff." This is a common and potentially serious infection. Many of you have likely heard this name bantered about. It can make a person very ill, with abdominal pain and diarrhea. In people who cannot communicate verbally, we get the diarrhea alone. It may be difficult to diagnose and difficult to treat. It may greatly worsen skin issues in that area, causing frank bed sores which may be impossible to keep clean. In other words, it can be a nightmare.

Skin issues can thus be secondary to urinary or bowel problems. They can also occur from pressure on a body prominence, which reduces blood flow to the skin, and can cause the emergence of "bedsores," which represents breakdown of superficial or deep layers all the way to the bone. This is more likely to occur in the setting of poor skin to begin with, as exists in many older people and in those who are nutritionally compromised. To prevent this dreaded complication, the one most likely to have a nursing home "cited," for poor care, takes a huge amount of attention and effort. Once present, the attention and work escalate greatly. These wounds may take months to heal.

Seizures

Seizures are events which occur secondary to an uncontrolled, inappropriate electrical activation of neurons in the brain. This is a very common problem always considered to be "serious" and often very difficult to deal with. If one simply contemplates the enormous range of mental and physical processes controlled by the brain, it is easy to see how vast might be the different clinical presentations. Seizure disorder, or "epilepsy," is a huge topic and can only be mentioned and briefly sketched in this setting. Very simplistically, seizure syndromes can range all the way from occasional brief periods of abnormal mentation or physical activity to complete loss of consciousness, with potential for major injury secondary to collateral injury from unprotected falls or accidents. Imagine the psychological impact from knowledge that control of one's own body and mind can be lost at any moment!

See the Table for a simple classification of epilepsy. As mentioned, a seizure can be a one-time event, such as in a child with a fever, or a recurring life-threatening event during an entire lifetime. Many seizure disorders are of unknown cause or genetically determined. Some are secondary to brain injury or disease of almost any type, including post-stroke. Seizures can be very disturbing to families and caregivers of people who are already seriously disabled. Although medications are available to reduce the frequency of seizures, many of these have a list of potentially serious side effects, and most are only partially successful.

Classification of Seizures	
Partial (one part of the brain)	• Simple, i.e., no change of consciousness, but motor, sensory, or autonomic disturbances. • Complex, i.e., alternation of consciousness.
Generalized (spread to all areas of the brain)	• Petit mal, with abnormal behavior but no loss of conscious. • Myoclonic, with jerking activity. • Atonic, with sudden collapse. • Grand mal, with loss of consciousness and uncontrolled motor activity.

Lastly, of the common complications, of people who are completely helpless, are musculoskeletal issues, of which only two will be mentioned. Most of these patients have minimal if any weight-bearing activity. Because of this, they may develop profound loss of bone. This can in turn cause them to have repeated "spontaneous" fractures that are from no true injury or accident. The most dramatic of all of these can be fracture of the femur or thigh bone, the biggest bone in the body, by simply turning over in bed or while being transferred from bed to chair or vice versa. The second is the development of "contractures." These generally come from inadequate movement—and perhaps a basic stiffness, with joints becoming fixed in awkward positions.

In summary, we began with a discussion of brain stem function, remaining after "higher" centers are destroyed, and broadened the discussion to include any patients who are relatively helpless and/or relatively bedridden. These poor souls, although appearing to be safely sequestered, live in a dangerous world prone to a host of serious complications over which they have no control. It takes an enormous effort and financial cost to keep them from further injury. Ultimately, this often proves to be futile despite our best efforts. For many of them, the "quality of life" seems to be very poor.

Here are a few suggestions for you, the currently healthy person, to contemplate seriously: (1) If the person so described is you, would you want to be kept alive or would you wish to be allowed to "die with dignity?" (2) Do we as a society "play God" more by keeping a desperately ill person alive or more by allowing them to die? If one subscribes to the notion that we are judged by our deeds rather than our words, at this point in time, it appears that most often, we align God's plan with keeping people alive. This is an issue which needs to be continually revisited and debated as external circumstances—and people's consciousness change.

Cerebellum

The moment in the sun, so long awaited by the cerebellum, nearly lost at the back of the brain, below the visual cortex, behind the brainstem, just above the spinal cord, and truly looking as it had just been plastered on as an afterthought, is yet to come. Or so it seems. Granted, for centuries, its role in coordination of motor activity has been known and studied. Much more recently, some of it more subtle, but equally essential effects regarding a host of brain functions have come to light. Cognitive functions, attention, language, music, and coordination of sensory input are all known to be intimately tied to cerebellar function. It is as if the deeper one goes, the more that is found.

After all, why should this not be true? The fist-sized cerebellum contains at least as many neurons as the rest of the brain combined, despite its diminutive 10% of brain volume. Elaborate folding has provided for a surface area of approximately 75% of the cerebral cortex, uniformly distributed in its three layers of cortical neurons. A relatively paltry number of forty million neuronal axons make their way to and from the cerebral cortex. The cerebellum reminds one of a densely packed offshore island; the Java of the nervous system.

No doubt that important functions are yet to be defined. For now, we have to accept our relatively rudimentary understanding of cerebellar function, using generalities, such as the integration of sensory perception, coordination, and motor control, and updating of rather than initiating, adjusting, and fine-tuning provided for by universal synaptic plasticity. Interestingly, age-related changes are much less apparent than in the cerebral cortex.

Reptilian Brain

Over the last several pages, we have discussed the basic component of the brainstem and the odd off-shore island, the cerebellum. These are real structures, with real functions, some known and likely many unknown. These structures are enough to keep a person alive. In fact, many fully functional animal species have little more than this and are able to function sufficiently well to sustain themselves through long lifetimes. All that needs to be added are a few basic elements, and the animal is complete in its own way. In fact, the animal may be an awesome predator. Add a structure called the thalamus, adjacent to the hypothalamus already mentioned, and the creature now has a structure involved in circadian rhythms, such as the sleep-wake cycle, a way station for processing and relaying sensory information, and a relay terminal between all of the structures mentioned and the primitive cortical area containing motor and sensory neurons.

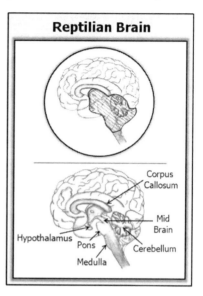

Earlier in our evolution from prokaryotic cells to eukaryotic cells, to multicellular and increasingly complex organisms, first it was water-bound, then amphibious, and finally land dwellers—this was our brain. In fact, this is still the only brain possessed by many species of reptiles. When looked at grossly, after removing the huge cap called the cerebral cortex, with its closely attached limbic system acting as a bridge between the cerebral cortex and the lower brain, the similarity between the reptilian brain and the human brain is unmistakable.

With the knowledge of lower brain function known to us, this has provided ample fodder for scientists, philosophers, and writers to speculate about a semi-imaginary structure deep in our modern brain, called the reptilian brain. Contemplation of this pseudo structure has provided a surprisingly rich opportunity to speculate as to why we humans are the way we are. In fact I will go as far to say that I consider this area of speculation as worthy of very serious consideration, with the possibility of becoming much more widely appreciated. In fact,

I would hope that it could be elevated to the level of "likely factual," just as is much of scientific knowledge, and perhaps become a new cultural icon. We humans, or at least the vast majority of us, behind our bravado, and our multiple facades, including all of our trappings of wealth and importance, are emotionally very fragile. Those who have interacted with small children would have no difficulty accepting this and can likely recall multiple examples of a child breaking into tears, or dropping head into solitariness, if they sense reprimand. That is us as adults, also. However, as adults, we don't usually respond that way because we cannot, and we will not see ourselves or allow others to see us as helpless. We lash out, fight back, curse, and in turn try to induce the helpless response in our perceived tormenter. Seeing others and accepting ourselves as emotionally fragile could be a great step forward in interpersonal relationships, creating a huge space for civility and compassion. Then, the true bullies, those of us who are intractably angry and aggressive would stand out like sore thumbs, needing to change, or facing ostracism.

Dark Side

The most difficult thing to do, however, is to look at our pumped-up selves in the mirror, and be willing to accept our "dark side." We all (every one of us) have this dark side. It is not so bad. It is the leftover flotsam and jetsam of our evolutionary journey through amphibian and reptilian ancestry to our current state of development. What it needs more than anything else is to be accepted and embraced, allowing it to be fully integrated consciously, coming under control of our higher brain functions. Yes it is me. I can be a predator. My survival and the survival of my family and tribe are what counts. I can be unpredictably violent. I can turn aggressive on a dime. I can humiliate people. I can be ruthless and arbitrary in my dealings with others. I can be cold-blooded. I can behave with top–down tyranny. I can be absolutely convinced of my own rightness and equally convinced of your wrongness. I can be vengeful. The term "sentient being" ends with people (animals are excluded from consideration).

When these powerful impulses come under the influence of civilization and common law, they tend to mutate to a more subtle picture. "Yes, it is me! I can be ritualistic and superstitious. (Carl Sagan wrote about the reptilian brain, with excessive ritual and homicidal behavior years ago.) I can be stuck in tradition and in the old ways of doing things. I can be devoted to precedent and ceremony. I can respond definitively to partial representations, failing to see the big picture. I can be deceptive (get around the law). I can be fearful (allowing me to reciprocate). I can be addicted to almost anything, from heroin to sex.

So what we see emerging, originating from the slime, screaming for acceptance and integration is the triune theory of brain development. Our most primitive brain is the reptilian, just described. As previously noted, as a species, with our leftover reptilian instincts, and our discomfort with gray rather than black and white when looking at the reptilian brain with our full-brain capacity, it could appear that the reptilian brain is all bad. Obviously, this is not the case. As already mentioned, it has all the "hard wiring" to keep us alive via respiratory and circulatory activity. Furthermore, it gives us the basic tools for protecting ourselves in an always dangerous world, through the integration of our neuroendocrine system, and with the ability to respond quickly and definitely to protect ourselves when need be. Lastly, this dense core of our brain packs a huge amount of energy.

If the brain as a whole is our battery, the reptilian brain is the starter that charges the battery and ignites the engine.

A majority of living creatures live their lives with little more than this reptilian brain. The major difference between the lowest and the highest members is the relative amounts and sophistication of the next two portions, especially the amount of cerebral cortex. Please respect the power of a neuron, although it seems easy to be dismissive of a single neuron, when we speak of the human brain as having a trillion or so. Besides humans, scientists investigating memory and cognition, the highest of all neurologic functions have a number of favored animal species useful in shedding light on these functions. *Caenorhabditis elegans* is a worm that has a grand total of 302 neurons. *Aplysia californica* is a sea slug. Both of these creatures are used widely in research involving cognition. Most of us know that slugs are basically snails without shells. These creatures have complex life cycles and behaviors, hinging on the grand total of 20,000 neurons, albeit the "behaviors" are simple or primitive. The point is that although the circuitries of mammalian and non-mammalian systems differ, the fundamental units of the brain—molecules, neurons, and synapses—are shared. That is, molecular activity of neurons allows for differences in signaling, which ultimately determines what the brain does, no matter how many neurons are present. To any given animal, every neuron counts, and complex behavior does not require a thirteen-figure neuronal structure.

The second part of the triune brain is the limbic system, sometimes too simplistically called the "emotional brain." The major components include the thalamus, hypothalamus, amygdala, hippocampus, prefrontal cortex, and several other structures, including the mamillary bodies. Only mammals have a full limbic system, involved in a wide range of behaviors including aggression, sexuality, anxiety, depression, fear, and maternal behavior. All components seem to compete for sending connections to the ever-popular and courted hypothalamus. Note that the hypothalamus and thalamus are also part of the reptilian brain. Note that the cortex is involved. In this sense, the limbic system acts as the bridge, already mentioned, connecting the reptilian brain to the cortex. The amygdala is involved in aggression. The hippocampus is crucial for learning and memory. The mamillary bodies, named for their appearance rather than their function, incidentally are involved with maternal behavior. The frontal cortex acts as a brake, or conscience, inhibiting socially inappropriate behaviors. Other areas affect hunger, sexual behavior, and circadian rhythms.

The last part of the triune brain schema, in the size and scope of its developments, and dwarfing development in lower species, is the cerebral cortex or cerebrum. This is the portion of the brain seen fully developed in primates. It was a very recent evolutionary addition to the brain and arose more or less alongside of the development of language. This has generated debate as to whether the big brain spawned language or emerging language development spawned the big brain. It is not clear whether this question is answerable or not. Perhaps, this is simply two sides of the post hoc fallacy (the thing following is caused by the thing proceeding).

There is considerable diversity in the cortex itself, with older parts of it containing three cell layers and the newer parts having six cell layers. Different areas of the cortex subserve different functions. The current paradigm is that large portions of the cortex are devoted to the processing of sensory information and that other large swaths evolved with higher-order cognitive functions, comprising the so-called association cortex. Some cortical functions, such as the "motor strip," are relatively symmetric in right and left hemispheres. Other areas are asymmetric, from one hemisphere to the other, including limbic structures involved with mood. The two sides of the hippocampus subserve completely different realms of memory. Three hundred million neuronal axons run through the corpus callosum, a thick band of axons, connecting mirror images in one hemisphere to the other. Perhaps, this has some function in giving us the experience of apparent unified function. Even today, there are likely huge gaps in basic knowledge about unified function of the previously described "cobbled together mess."

The cortex, despite its structural diversity, complex interconnections, and frustrating concerns about how the whole seems so much greater than any of its parts (implying a tight coherence not yet understood), is confidently accepted as essential to, if not the very kernel of, our highest intellectual capability. There is abundant evidence that illustrates that when a certain area is damaged, some aspect of our intellectual prowess drops away. It is equally apparent that it may be very difficult to discern any objective deficit when neighboring areas are lost to disease or injury. The patient may state "I just don't feel like myself," or "I just don't feel right," and yet continue to function at a high level of intellectual performance.

These difficulties surrounding our ability to understand the mechanism of total brain coherence are made even more confusing by increasing evidence for a remarkable degree of plasticity. Up until very recently, it was thought that development of the CNS was complete by approximately age twenty-five. It was also felt that from that point on, there was a steady drop-off of neurons, with no replacements waiting in the wings. This drop-off rate was thought to accelerate with advancing age. Happily, we now know this to be untrue or at least not necessarily true. Recall that besides the trillion neurons, there exists perhaps as many as 100 trillion other cells, supporting and supplementing neuronal function in one way or another. Recall that of these different types of glial cells, the so-called "micoglia," of which there may be 150 billion, were derived from hematopoietic (bone marrow) precursors and may have pluripotential function. Not only may they be the security system of the CNS, watching for and disposing of unwanted characters, they may also have stem cell-like powers to differentiate into new neurons. So, once a brain is subtly damaged, if no further damage occurs, repair processes swing into action and can restore function.

Recall that our most cherished possession—that of memory—is dependent on molecular processes in neurons and glial cells, and signaling between these cells. This, of course, depends on the number and pattern of synapses between cells, as well as the strength of the synaptic messages via neurotransmitters. Total synaptic strength is reflected by the strength of memory traces. Changing the strength of synaptic communication is one of the basics of neuroplasticity and thus of learning. Long-term potentiation (LTP) occurs when neuronal dendrites are repeatedly stimulated so that action potentials flow more easily weeks to months later, resulting in increased synaptic responsiveness and output. Appreciating that action potentials are not so easy to sustain; basically, the brain is massively interconnected to ensure that signals do not sputter out because of stimuli coming from multiple sources. Ultimately, LTP "works" because of changes in cellular glutamate as production and receptor function (excitatory), as well as changes in calcium channels in the dendrites. Needless to say, the amount of and function of neurotransmitters and receptors can vary greatly from one person to another, modifying all of these plasticity issues.

My dear readers, I wish to offer you an apology for dropping you into this cauldron. What is being boiled down is "cutting edge" information regarding neural plasticity and yes... neurogenesis, i.e., production of new neurons in the adult. Don't feel bad about incomplete understanding. Moving into "cutting edge" territory of any topic is difficult for everyone, including those very clever and often brilliant people who have created the cutting edge. Although neuroscientists subscribe to the scientific method, dependent on what is seen and what is measured, and theoretically independent of existing paradigms and biases, they are also human. Humans have deep biases, difficult to purge. Nature abhors a vacuum. Scientists abhor a vacuum of knowledge once an old paradigm begins to crumble. They scramble to erect a new one, by postulating this or that and then designing experiments to test the postulates. The most difficult task of "bench" scientists (an armchair term implying sitting at a lab bench, rather than trekking through the jungles of Amazonia or the jungles of a big teaching hospital with its committees that determine what experimentation can be ethically done to living humans) is to design experimental protocols that have as little built-in bias as possible. Such a protocol allows them to trust the data "no matter what it shows." Even neuroscientists don't understand much of this. One of them made the point about five years ago in which he considered the discovery of neuroplasticity to be the greatest discovery of the twentieth century. Of course, that's why he is a neuroscientist. But, it is very important and all within the last fifteen years. The next time you come across this topic in the media, you will be surprised how easily you can relate to it.

So, let us try one more time. After all, who would argue that repetition is a main key to learning…or to use the jargon "long-term potentiation."

Memory is postulated to be represented in the physical realm by vastly interconnected networks of neuronal synapses. Long-term potentiation shares many features with long-term memory. Both depend on synthesis of new proteins (new DNA), as well as enhanced synaptic transmission. You have read and seen a little about neurons and enough to get the drift. In other words, modifications of synaptic strength encodes for memory. This concept that synapses can be modified is at the heart of neuroplasticity. Thinking, learning, and acting change the physical structure and functional organization of the brain, one neuron at a time, until all one trillion are accounted for. These changes occur at every layer in the processing hierarchy and include glial cells as well. Plasticity can have positive or negative effects. Recovery after a stroke or concussion is good. Increased muscle tone or spasticity after a stroke is bad. The difference may only be a perfect level versus an excessive stimulation of neural growth, in turn dependent on growth factors (proteins) responding to the injury. Current speculation places drug addiction and obsessive–compulsive disorder as maladaptive synaptic wiring, secondary to some physical or "mental" injury. Neuroplasticity can be geographically radical, if the area of injury is too severely damaged, as the subserved functions are moved to a distant site, possibly in one of the vast areas of "associative cortex." All of these are being actively studied by your neighborhood neuroscientists all over the world. Now for the killer news regarding synaptic networks. (All of you please sit down.) There is strong evidence that day-to-day life experiences are intimately connected with reorganization of synaptic networks, including within the cortex.

We are almost finished with this agonizing cutting-edge portrayal. This last issue deals with the holy grail of neuroplasticity. As already mentioned for 100 years of neuroscience, the existing paradigm through generations of brilliant researchers held that the human brain was structurally and functionally finished between age twenty and twenty-five, after which it is all downhill. That "truth" began to crack with discovery of neurogenesis in bird brains in the early 1990s. Neurogenesis refers to the birth of new neurons. We now have what thus far appears to be irrefutable evidence that new neurons are born within the human brain, even into old age. This has been most convincingly demonstrated in two areas, including the subventricular (meaning just under the ventricle) zone of the lateral ventricle, and within several areas of the hippocampus, already well-known to be associated with memory function. There is emerging evidence for the existence of neuronal stem cells, although a detailed understanding is not yet available. Neurogenesis has been found in virtually every area of the brain. It is known that some of these newborn cells soon die. It is known that they can migrate over distances. Although it is not yet known what the ultimate effect of these new cells are. See Table X for a short list of established data.

Neurogenesis (Adult-Born Neurons)

- Origin of neurogenic stem-cell not yet known.
- More easily excitable.
- Production inhibited by sleep deprivation.
- Production enhanced by exercise.
- Production and survival enhanced and integration into hippocampus enhanced by exercise and enriched environment.
- Production increased in response to CNS injury.
- Production reduced by stress.
- Production reduced in aging.

Before we discuss several more common diseases of the nervous system, I wish to philosophically and ethically sum up functions of the brain, as I see it. Astronomer/philosopher Carl Sagan, taken from us much too early, recognized twenty-five years ago the need to come to grips with the reptilian brain. He was concerned especially with our ritualistic and hierarchical behavior, which he associated with the reptilian brain. Perhaps, the fullest expression of that occurred in Nazi Germany, where visual imagery and symbols, which are thought to be the language of the reptile, were so flagrantly abused. The success of Nazism is that with the emphatic use of ridicule, it appealed to all three components of the triune brain (thinking, feeling, and instinctual) whereas logic only touches one component. The cry of those who tried to stand up against Nazism, claiming that "mockery is a rust that corrodes all it touches," either achieved nothing or marched to their deaths.

As mentioned previously, reptilian is not synonymous with "bad." Images and symbols in movies and television can appeal to our deepest goodness as well as pander to our deepest insecurities. Theatre, with its motto of "suspension of disbelief" depends on imagery and yet traditionally over thousands of years, has struggled to teach positive lessons. Anything that purposefully attempts to increase our fearfulness can be held responsible for the negativity associated with this aspect of the reptilian response. Fear tends to weaken us, leaving us open to the possibility of being manipulated. Our goal should not be to become the micro-chipped person of the future in the *Matrix* movie, who can be made fearless on demand, and respond by "cruelty not weakened by tears." Our goal should be to use all parts of our brain. This takes effort because we are not bombarded daily with the kinds of themes that appeal to our higher brains. No one would doubt that we have the ability to bring consciousness and conscience into play. This is the only way to achieve the type of balanced brain function necessary to see clearly, to avoid distortion, and to avoid the black and white of attraction and aversion.

Obscuring of clarity is the problem, with unbalanced brain function. Recognition of our connectedness with all living creatures, plants, and animals is our heritage. Hell is separation/alienation. This can be avoided as simply as recognizing that we share 70% of our DNA with a banana. To get clear, we need to balance fear with compassion for all, obviously a higher brain function. That recognition is the vehicle for getting free. As stated so eloquently by Benjamin Franklin, "We must all hang together, or we will all hang separately."

Disease of the Nervous System

Back to diseases of the nervous system. Please recall that during the course of previous discussions such as the meninges, the ventricular system, and the blood–brain barrier, we have already discussed some of the most common and important diseases and syndromes. Once again, recall that a disease is a term used to represent a disorder of function (physiology) and/or structure (anatomy), with a clear cut and usually prescribed picture, or layout. Upper respiratory infection would be an example of this on the minor side of the spectrum and uncomplicated heart attack on the major side of the spectrum. A syndrome is a constellation of signs and symptoms, likely widespread in the body, with a more protean picture, more variable, and likely involving several organ systems. Although these processes might also be called a disease, the emphasis is to check for and deal with all of the other possible ramifications.

We have already reviewed stroke and its common syndromes, hydrocephalus, seizure disorders, and meningitis.

Neuropathy

The one common process to be discussed involving the peripheral nervous system, i.e., outside of the spinal cord, is that of neuropathy, meaning disease of nerves. There are a large number of categories of neuropathies. Many of them are syndromes, with different manifestations in different areas of the body. Sometimes an attempt is made to determine if only one nerve is involved, or multiple nerves.

Since nerves can carry motor fibers, sensory fibers, and autonomic fibers in varying concentrations, the manifestations could involve weakness, pain of various types, or abnormalities in color, temperature, and potential for sweating, as in autonomic disorders. By far, the most common symptoms are sensory, including numbness, tingling and/or pain.

In terms of causes of peripheral neuropathy, this may come as a big surprise. The most common cause in the world is leprosy, an infectious disease affecting the nerves which is rarely seen in western, industrialized countries. Most often, these conditions are seen as complications of background systemic disease, with the most common being diabetes. Other common systemic illnesses like chronic renal failure, chronic liver disease, and hypothyroidism can, with much less frequency, damage nerves. With these types of disorders, the most frequent manifestations are sensory, with numbness, tingling, and/or pain. More about this shortly.

Cause of Peripheral Neuropathy Secondary to Systemic Illness

→ Toxic
→ Heredity
→ Nutritional
→ Pressure
→ Cancer – paraneoplastic syndrome
→ Traumatic
→ Idiopathic

There are large numbers of hereditary causes of neuropathy, most rare, but a few common enough to be talked about. Some causes are related to pressure on or compression of nerves, such as carpal tunnel syndrome in the wrist or sciatica in the spine or pelvis. Toxicity, most often alcohol, is a common cause of diffuse neuropathy. A list of prescription drugs have been implicated, including some chemotherapy agents and others. Malnutrition, from whatever the cause, can lead to protein and vitamin deficiencies, especially B vitamins, which can cause neuropathy.

Paraneoplastic Syndromes

Perhaps the most interesting of all, although relatively rare, is interesting enough to warrant mention. This is the so-called paraneoplastic syndrome, which is a fancy medical term for neuropathy (or encephalopathy, or myelopathy) associated with cancer. As has already been mentioned, cancer represents "other." It is a tissue which has completely lost contact with the rest of the body. Instead of obeying the rules of physiology and contributing to the betterment of the organism as a whole, it is that ruthless invader, without a conscience, subscribing to the reptilian motto of "cruelty without tears," ready to destroy the organism and, itself, in a dance of death—the cellular suicide bomber. Being an invader and paying no attention to the blueprint, it does whatever it damn well pleases. One of those options which it exercises is to occasionally produce substances above a level helpful for the body as a whole, and even compounds which are novel and not usually produced at all. Some of these act like hormones and cytokines. We haven't spoken much about cytokines. These represent a large number of substances which act like hormones in many ways, working at widespread sites and involved in cell signaling and communication. Instead of emanating from a specific site or gland, they emanate ordinarily from immunomodulating agents, attacking the cell surface receptors.

When produced by cancer cells, they tend to have widespread, non-specific effects with particular proclivity for nervous system tissue. They may well be at least partially responsible for some systemic effects, such as loss of appetite and loss of vitality. They also can be very toxic to differing parts of the nervous system, with different tumors having different patterns of production, and thus differing effects. Of great interest is the occasional appearance of a clinical neurologic syndrome well before a tumor is discovered (months to years).

Also, relatively rare in general, the tumors most likely associated with paraneoplastic syndromes are breast, ovary, lung, and lymph nodes. The neurologic syndromes most frequently encountered include diffuse muscle weakness, degeneration of the cerebellum, encephalitis, and/or myelitis (widespread dysfunction of the brain and/or spinal cord). (I will not discuss encephalitis or myelitis further, as they are relatively rare. Besides having a tendency to be associated with viral diseases, these also can be secondary to systemic illnesses, toxic agents, deficiencies, and hereditary factors.) The treatment of the paraneoplastic syndrome depends on finding the tumor and being able to successfully treat that.

Parkinson's Disease

This is a very common disorder, involving a particular portion of the basal ganglia called the substantia nigra. In view of the fact that the brain is so absolutely complicated in structure and function, as is true in other common diseases of the nervous system, although important specifics are well known (in this case location, and specifically a loss of certain cells), many other features remain highly variable and/or unknown. This simply seems to be an inherent feature of neurological diseases, when dense concentrations of neurons with very specific functions are located very close to other similar loci, but with differing function. Ultimate expression of the neurological disease in question may have something to do with how much spillover occurs from one clump of neurons to another.

This small area of the basal ganglia is associated with production of neurons producing relatively large amounts of dopamine, with radiations up to the motor cortex. Therefore, much of what we see has to do with altered motor function. However, because of closely adjoining areas in both the basal ganglia and the multiple subcortical or cortical connections with the motor cortex, the clinical course can vary widely.

The major physical findings in Parkinson's disease (PD) include varying degrees of a certain type of tremor, a certain type of muscular rigidity, and a certain pattern of slowness of movement. As is true for many neurological conditions, there is no diagnostic blood test or imaging study. The diagnosis is made on clinical grounds. In addition, and most tragic of all, is that a percentage of patients with PD also develop dementia, again of varying severity. This will be discussed further, shortly, when we discuss dementia in general.

Parkinson's disease is an unequivocally terrible condition, for several reasons. First of all, the doctor cannot sit down with you and tell you what to do to avoid getting PD. Secondly, once present, the disease can quickly and severely change your life. Thirdly, it can severely damage your cognitive abilities. Fourthly, treatment of the disease leaves much to be desired. The only good thing about it is that it tends to leave you alone until your sixties or seventies. As a sidelight, it has been stated repeatedly that to remain healthy, one needs to engage the will and intend to be healthy. The second necessity is luck, whether luck is absolutely capricious or in some way tethered to hard work and intent. PD has the appearance (so far) of a disease associated with bad luck.

As is true in most other diseases, the spectrum of disability is great. Some people complain bitterly about "this damn tremor," making it difficult for them to drink from a cup, without recognizing that things could be dramatically worse. In advanced stages, the person can become frozen, moving very little and with great difficulty. They may have the inability to swallow safely. Speech may be almost indecipherable. Recurring falls place them at high risk for further injury. And through all of this, cognition may be intact. Disturbances in mood, with depression and anxiety, are common. By that time, the person likely needs institutional care. Medications are variably helpful but usually not much. They do not stop progression of the disease, nor do they prevent cognitive loss.

As mentioned, we only have sketchy information as to how to prevent this devastating condition. There is a weak association with cigarette smoking, and a weak association with pesticide and solvent exposure. There are general thoughts that there is a genetic predisposition and then simply too much in the way of "toxicity," with too much in the way of reactive oxygen species.

Multiple Sclerosis

This disease doesn't usually wait until you are sixty-five or seventy to make its appearance. Many people have their first symptoms in their twenties or thirties. Like PD, it is riddled with many unknowns. There are many theories about what might initiate it, with the most recent being that gaps in the blood–brain barrier allow entry of viruses and/or immunologically active cells. We do know that the damage is done to the myelin sheath that surrounds the axon of the neuron and that this can interfere with interneuronal communication. Eventually, as the body attempts to control this process in a foreign land (the CNS, where neither viruses nor the immunologically active cells are supposed to be), scars are laid down, in an area which does not tolerate scarring, and permanent damage ensues.

As to spectrum of disease, there is once again a huge variability. Some people only experience intermittent, relatively focal neurologic dysfunction. Others have a progressive course, which can run the gamut through visual problems, speech and swallowing problems, sensory changes including pain, fatigue, problems with bowel and bladder control, weakness, and eventually virtual paralysis. And of course, since this is occurring in the brain as well, the seat of our cognitive abilities, if the disruption of neuronal communication is severe enough, the person can experience loss of cognitive functioning. Fortunately, most people do not end up demented or in motorized wheel chairs. In fact, life expectancy is only slightly shortened. However, quality of life can suffer significantly.

As with Parkinson's disease, we cannot tell you how to avoid this condition. As is frequently the case, when there is a gap in knowledge about causation, the usual suspects usually pop up, including viruses, genetics, and toxicity, the latter being the only one we have any control over. Why is the incidence progressively higher the further from the equator where one resides? Treatment with steroids (very toxic in high doses) may be effective in controlling acute attacks but is not practical for long-term treatment. A variety of emerging "disease-modifying drugs" can be modestly effective.

Dementia

"Dementing illness" seems to be a more comfortable description regarding loss of cognitive abilities than "dementia." Perhaps, this brings back the purported medieval argument about how many angels can dance on the head of a pin, i.e., not very important. Dementing illness seems a little more vague, leaving open other possibilities besides dementia, which seems a little more definitive and absolute. Once again, members of our species seem to be obsessed with putting things in boxes, with the illusions that that might give us better understanding. This is more of an endearing trait than a criticism, often times, just not working very well in this largely gray world.

So, we do our best to try to segregate the dementias. Throughout much of the history of medicine, understanding has come through visual gross inspection or microscopic analysis of tissue samples. At the beginning of my career, in many hospitals, the autopsy rate of expired patients was in the range of 40%. At this juncture, if I call my local pathologist and asked him or her to do an autopsy, they might (1) laugh at me, (2) refuse, or (3) quickly schedule a trip out of town. The rate of autopsies nationally now is less than 5%. This is important from the standpoint of the dementing illnesses because there are visible pathologic correlates which might allow us to segregate these illnesses more accurately. Without an autopsy, however, it becomes very imprecise. This is seen at the same time that people are living longer and dementias are becoming increasingly more common. Recall the adage that two features occurring in close conjunction are not necessarily related. Perhaps, the increased incidence of dementing illness has nothing to do with the aging of our population, but I suspect that it does.

This is an enormously important topic. We all hear about the huge economic burden that dementia brings with it. There is also the burden of human life becoming a shadow of what it was—a tragedy that we all end up enduring. Yes, we have an increasing life expectancy. However, most of those people are not aging well in terms of preservation of physical and mental functioning. We have an aging, sick population of people, whom I can assure you are not happy or contented as a group. Many of them suffer daily. Many of them have varying levels of dementia, and often, we can only guess at the cause.

Cognitive Dysfunction of Aging

First, we need to define dementia and perhaps contrast it with another term called "cognitive dysfunction of aging." The more we age as a species, and the more we appreciate that some of our members show no evidence of dementia at any age, it once again demonstrates the ever-present workings of the bell-shaped curve, with a wide spectrum of brain function.

It is truly inspiring when we meet a very old person who is mentally intact. That is what getting older should be about—accruing progressively more knowledge and experience, and transforming that into the ever-elusive "wisdom." That would make staying alive worthwhile and even helpful and with a little bit of luck, one might be able to pass on some of those kernels of wisdom.

It should be apparent by now that I tend to see things in general and certainly biologic phenomena as lying along a continuum. In other words, I am less impressed with categorizing and naming things than with looking for the unifying features which run through a series of categories. Therefore, I would be happy to accept the notion that cognitive dysfunction of aging is a form of very mild dementia. This is a very common condition. Since statistics regarding dementia seem to start at age fifty-five and since it is quoted that 5% to 8% of the population at age sixty-five has dementia, let us assume that all 5% of these have CDA, as the first step along the road of dementia. I would also be the first to agree that this designation, regarding these 5% of the population, may be somewhat prejudicial. After all, if we look at a large group of physical phenomena, look what we see. Likely 95% of the population at sixty-five is shorter than they were at age twenty-five, cannot run as fast, cannot jump as high, and is not as strong as they were at age twenty-five. To state that this 95% of people have "physical dysfunction of aging" and imply that only 5% of the population is "normal" would seem to be absurd.

So what is CDA? These people basically function normally in society. Many of them still work in responsible jobs. They are basically self-sufficient. They never get lost in their own neighborhood, and they never fail to recognize a person they have known for years. They do tell you, to paraphrase, "I can't remember things the way I used to." Examples of this tend to be quite uniform, such as "I couldn't remember the first name of my doctor (or friend, advisor, or barber)." Or, "I lay my keys down and can't find them." Or, "I can't remember where I was from one Christmas to the next." In summary, (a) their brains and their cognitive processes feel different to them, and (b) there does appear to be losses of memory, which are verifiable.

Incidence of Dementia

Moving along in age, a substantial portion of these people will not overtly deteriorate mentally, as they pass seventy and seventy-five, etc. However, epidemiologic studies support the idea that the incidence of dementia doubles every five years. Is this really true? Ten percent at age seventy? Yes. Twenty percent at age seventy-five? Yes, maybe. Forty percent at age eighty? Yes, maybe. Eighty percent at age eighty-five? No! One hundred sixty percent at age ninety? Of course not. So, something is wrong. Perhaps, the starting number of 5% is wrong, in that of those 5%, 60% of them (or 3%) have CDA or very mild dementia, which never progresses. Perhaps the starting number of progressive dementia is really 2% at sixty-five, 4% at seventy, 8% at seventy-five, 16% at eighty, 32% at eighty-five, and 64% at ninety. Alternately, the doubling every five years may be true for only the first ten or fifteen years and may then slow significantly. If we assume as with most of the other biologic phenomena that there is an interplay between hereditary and environment (nature versus nurture), the second postulate would speak to the possibility that the nature–nurture balance shifts on the fly, likely in the direction of more emphasis on nature and less emphasis on nurture. In other words, if you have little or no genetic programming pointing toward dementia, no matter what happens to your environment, you will not get dementia.

So, what is dementia? Again, pardon me for being repetitious, but repetition is an effective tool for learning. We humans cannot prevent ourselves from categorizing and boxing up things. It is apparently part of our genome. The result is that we establish criteria for dementia, i.e., boxes one to five, with four out of five being necessary for the diagnosis. This is very valuable, particularly from the epidemiologic, information-gathering standpoint.

Cognitive Response Chart		
Topic	**Cognitive Dysfunction of Aging**	**Dementia**
Income Tax	Don't know where the records are.	Don't know what income tax is.
Dentist	Don't remember when they were last in.	Don't know what a dentist does.
Automobile	Misplaces keys/Misplaces car.	Nobody would even drive with them.
Job/Career	Laid-off recently for poor performance.	Can't remember what it was.
Age	Can't remember number, but knows birth date.	No idea.
Spouse	Recall name/? dead	No name or recollection.
Name and number(s) of children	Three/recall names of two.	"Yes, I think I don't remember.
Personality	Clearly the same.	Radically different.
Behavior	Socially appropriate.	Inappropriate.
Continence (bladder and bowel)	Zero or rare accident.	Incontinent.
Eating	Enjoy/feeds self.	No initiation.
Speech	Able to carry on, frequently submits, "I don't remember."	Non-verbal, or babble.

But what about the frightened seventy-five-year-old person in front of you, with a tenth grade education? In that case, I think I prefer the Justice Potter Stewart approach of "I know it when I see it."

So here is the Barry L. Marmorstein version of dementia. A person with dementia is really truly not fully independent. That is, they cannot function adequately in society alone (see Cognitive Response Chart). For those doctors or patients or families who wish to be a little more scientific than the always too practical Stewart–Marmorstein approach, there is the Mini-Mental State Exam, used frequently and usually in mild cases. This is designed to take into consideration arithmetic, orientation, and memory issues, with a grading system (see Mini-Mental State Examination Chart).

The term "clinical" is used repeatedly in this discourse. I hope you remember the definition, but here it is again, in the vernacular. Clinical means in the real world of medical practice, whether it be the doctor's office, hospital, or nursing home. This is in contrast to the ivory tower of the medical school

The Mini-Mental State Examination

	Maximum Score
Orientation	
What is the year, season, month, day of month, and day of week?	5
Where are we (e.g., state, county, town, building, floor)?	5
Registration	
Tester names three objects, then asks patient to repeat them.*	3
Attention and Calculation	
Serial sevens (five successive subtractions from 100). Alternatively, patient is asked to spell "world" backwards.	5
Recall	
What were the three objects learned earlier?	3
Language and Praxis	
Tester points to a pencil and a watch and asks patient to name them	2
Patient is asked to:	1
Repeat "No ifs, ands, or buts."	
Follow the three-stage verbal command to "take this piece of paper in your right hand, fold it in half, and put it on the floor."	3
Follow the written command to "close your eyes."	1
Make up and write a sentence.	1
Copy this design.	1
Maximum Total Score†	30

* If patient scores < 3, examiner repeats names up to six times until patient learns them, in preparation for recall test.

† Total scores < 24 generally signify dementia or delirium.

Adapted from Folstein MF, Folstein S, McHugh JR, 1975.

or medical society, with ivory tower defined as "a place or attitude of retreat, especially preoccupied with lofty, remote, or intellectual considerations, rather than practical, everyday life."

Vascular Dementia

The vast majority of clinicians, including neurologists, would likely box dementias into four categories. One of these, so-called vascular dementia, is seen as part of the hypertensive–elderly–arteriosderotic population and can be superimposed on any of the other boxes or categories, creating a mixed bag. Since vascular dementia is one of the two most common, let's discuss this first. We have already discussed the pathophysiology (abnormalities) leading to vascular insult in our discussions regarding the meninges, with different types of bleeding associated with the meninges, followed by deep brain strokes, TIA, and ischemic encephalopathy. In essence, blockage of any artery, from the big arteries in the neck to the tiny arteries in the depths of the brain, can deprive neurons of their blood supply, resulting in cell death. If enough of the events occur or, perhaps even more importantly, if they occur in crucial areas of the brain, dense with neurons of a certain type or in the midst of neuronal pathways, enough neurons or pathways can be destroyed to result in dementia.

This type of dementia is largely preventable, utilizing all the medicinal and other tools available to normalize blood pressure and cholesterol, avoid or adequately treat diabetes, and with absolutely no use of tobacco products. Once it is well established, the same measures can reduce progression of the dementia but are unlikely to show a reversal or trend back toward normal.

Alzheimer's Dementia

The second very common cause of dementia is Alzheimer's disease. Much less is known about this life wrecker than about vascular dementia. Ultimately, in creating a portrait of a disease process, the golden nugget medical scientists are really after is causation. Obviously, once uncovered, if the research is done properly and with a minimum of bias, this should lead to deep understanding and hopefully to treatment and/or prevention strategies. The opening statement of this paragraph would imply that deep understanding is still forthcoming. I suspect that with the enormous amount of research spawned at this time, in turn stimulated by the huge losses accompanying this disease which has affected most people directly or indirectly, the deep secrets will be uncovered within the next ten to twenty years. Whether there will be effective strategies to deal with it obviously hinges on the causes.

The usual suspects are similar to many other disease processes, including genetic susceptibility, and a host of environmental influences. I don't see much value in listing a set of research trends, as the bottom line is that there is still no unifying explanation to account for the preponderance of cases. Here are a few things that are well established. It is basically a disease of elderly people, very uncommon below the age of sixty-five, with one exception: people with Down's syndrome have a high incidence of dementing illness by age forty. Is this important from the standpoint of understanding Alzheimer's disease? All we can say is that the amyloid-beta protein, associated the amyloid plaques seen under the microscope, is located on chromosome 21, the same chromosome abnormal in Down's syndrome, and apparently acts as a risk factor. The incidence of Alzheimer's increases rapidly from that point on, up to age eighty to eighty-five, at which time it definitely slows. By age eighty-five, up to 40% of the population in some studies is affected. The take-home message is that if you make it to age eighty-five without the disease, your chances of getting it are likely less than the average person at age sixty-five.

The other major pathologic finding under the microscope (besides amyloid-beta plaques) is the so-called neurofibrillary tangles. They are thought to come from the degenerated axon of the neurons, which normally contain long tubules coded for by so-called tau protein. Abnormal twisting of the tau protein (recall that proteins are unique partly secondary to their specific three dimensional twists and turns, allowing them to lock onto some receptors and be excluded from others) is what is thought to result in destruction of the tubules of the axon and then the axon itself. Perhaps, this is the primary lesion, with subsequent death of the neuron and creation of plaques coming afterwards.

Despite whatever genetic predispositions have been found, a vast majority of cases of Alzheimer's disease occur sporadically. Obviously, and not unexpectedly, there is more to it than just genetics. Theories of environmental influences have ranged over a wide spectrum, from aluminum toxicity (aluminum cookware) to prion disease. Prions are a fascinating topic, and their very nature, very much "under the radar," creates difficulties in understanding how and to what extent they contribute to human and animal diseases. They are best described as proteinaceous infectious particles. They are self-propagating and transmissible. They are not viruses (DNA or RNA). They appear to be more widely found in the animal kingdom than in humans and are known to be the cause of "mad cow disease." They are also known to be the cause of so-called Creutzfeldt–Jakob disease (CJD), rare but the most common prion disease of humans. So far, two Nobel prizes have been awarded to researchers in this arena. Their role in the broad spectrum of neurological disease, with the exception of CJD, remains speculative. Recall the speculation that Alzheimer's disease may be initiated by the breakdown of blood brain barrier and the immunological breakdown of neurons.

Clinically, Alzheimer's disease is a nightmare, for patients, families, and caregivers. Patients come first. Try to imagine the overwhelming sense of helplessness engendered in the early stages, as the victim begins to feel brain power slipping away. Very quickly, depression and possibly anxiety with full-blown panic attacks become important co-morbidities (associated diseases, frequently linked with the primary disease). In fact, for a variable period of time, the depression and anxiety may be felt by all concerned to be the primary issue, with reduction in cognitive function secondary to that. Soon enough, perhaps heralded by unmistakable behavioral abnormalities, such as striking the beloved spouse or urinating in the garbage can, the true nature of the problem emerges. Just as no one has recently come back from death to tell us what it was like (the closest we get is the vivid out-of-body experience described by those with cardiac arrest in the process of resuscitation), no one has come back from advancing dementia to tell us what it was like. Sleep disturbances, both way too much and way too little, become commonplace. Wandering and getting lost, inability to read or comprehend, temper tantrums, endless sobbing, incontinency of bowel and bladder, loss of speech, and loss of interest in eating, all follow in various combinations. I can imagine that for the person, losing their mind, losing their sense of self, and having already lost their sense of self-worth and dignity, it is not the "long day's journey into night" but the "endless descent into the blackness and loneliness of hell."

Treatment, as such, can be modestly effective regarding improvement in cognition in the early stages of the disease. It does not usually prevent progression, and it rarely helps in advanced stages. These drugs, which are designed to increase neural production of the neurotransmitter acetylcholine, in my opinion, are more effective as mood modulators than as cognition improvers. As bad as loss of cognition may be, loss of all restraints of civility, likely due to progressive damage to the frontal lobes, can take the sweet, kindly old person feeding the pigeons into the raving tyrant trying to feed you to the vultures. Ultimately, it is either unrestrained behavioral outbursts or everyday bowel and bladder incontinency which results in institutional care. This is something that families often steadfastly resist, having promised the sweetheart-turned-out-of-control-danger-to-self-and-others victim that "We'll never put you in a nursing home." Such care in a "Dementia Unit," meaning it is locked to keep people from escaping, and populated only with dementia patients to protect non-demented patients, will likely cost $6,000 to $8,000 per month. Care at home, at approximately $25 per hour, could be two or three times that cost.

This nightmare, going on for years, punctuated by acute illnesses and injuries which might require hospitalization, can completely drain family savings. When ill enough to be hospitalized, these individuals will almost always need "sitters" to protect them, with those costs borne by the hospital. After return to the dementia unit, the cost of sitters may need to be added on to the basic cost, adding up to thousands of dollars more per month, until stabilization occurs.

Once again, I would ask the readers what you would wish for yourself, once you know unequivocally that you are slipping into dementia. What about the stage whereby you lose your appetite and/or can no longer feed yourself? Is this nature's clarion call that your life is over, or will you or your family opt for a feeding tube? At what point in the life of a human being does staying alive because we have the technical know-how to do it become counterproductive? On a deeper level, returning to one of the prime concepts of the Hippocratic Oath, which need not be confined to lead doctors only, what is the best thing to do for the sick one? That is, are we making decisions based on our needs and wishes (perhaps the cure for dementia will be announced next week) or theirs? On the deepest level, as has been broached already, is "playing god" simulated by keeping a desperately ill person alive, or by letting go?

Other Dementing Illness

In clinical medicine, a vast majority of dementing illnesses come down to a choice between vascular and Alzheimer's, or a combination of both. So-called Lewy body dementia, with a few slightly unique features, if there is such a concept, is likely uncommon and difficult to tease out. As might be surmised, there is no effective treatment. The same can be said for Creutzfeldt–Jakob disease, which is likely rare and untreatable. Recall that Parkinson's disease may be associated with dementia. Perhaps, the fact that some people with Parkinson's have dementia and some do not reflects the coincident appearance of vascular or Alzheimer's dementia, rather than some as yet mysterious feature about Parkinson's disease. Recall also that non-specific factors, such as toxins and head injuries (concussions), as well as any cause of bleeding in the head can create a dementia-like picture, perhaps somewhat atypical. As a final comment regarding the dementing illness, recall that way back in our evolutionary development, a "decision" was made to protect the brain, through the elaborate blood–brain barrier, and its different mechanisms. Anthropomorphizing to the limit, it was recognized that in order to function as spectacularly well as it does, the brain with its neurons and glial cells would have to be suspended in this elaborate skull, with much of the working elements encased in a greasy, buttery medium. In other words, the brain is very fragile, an excusable feature considering what it does for us. Single or repeated episodes of physical injury can take their toll. There is a contemporary huge amount of controversy as to whether or not the practice of "heading" in soccer can lead to brain impairment. Medical research has not yet been able to provide irrefutable evidence one way or the other. I mention this simply to point out that it is possible that even "everyday" types of head trauma can have negative consequences in susceptible people.

Delirium

Delirium is a common variety of global brain dysfunction but different than dementia. The main difference is that delirium is a temporary phenomenon, usually seen in the context of some other systemic illness. It can even be seen in young people. In general, the older the person, the less severe need an illness be to produce delirium. When seen in young people, there is often a life-threatening illness, which is present, causing the brain to shut down. Actually, that phenomenon is the rule, and the mechanism of it is unexplored as far as I know. During the course of any severe illness or injury, in people of any age, despite the ability to speak and interact and appear to others as being "normal," there is a powerful amnesia which sets in, such that the person has no recollection of any of those events or discussions after recovery. In fact, the amnesia is so dense as to frequently spread over into the antecedent period of wellness such that the person may have no recollection of anything that happened for days to weeks before the seminal event.

If memories are stored via changes in the strength of synaptic discharges, particularly those in the temporal lobes or hippocampus, what is going on with dementia and its short-term correlate, delirium? There are estimated to be up to 1,000 synapses per neuron. Messenger RNA carries information around the neuron, with such information able to code for new proteins. So, material produced in the nucleus of the neuron is transported down the axon to the synapses. Recall that short-term memory involves changes in synapses (synaptic strength), whereas long-term memory requires new gene expression and new proteins. It appears that we have both, as these new proteins are delivered to some, but not all synapses, increasing synaptic strength. So, changes in gene expression (protein) can be, and are, very local.

Who is "Benjamin Kyle," a badly beaten man found unconscious, naked, and without an identity, behind a Burger King (with the B and K of his name having been selected because he was found at a Burger King) in Georgia twenty-five years ago? Even the likes of forensic genealogist Colleen Fitzpatrick, achieving notoriety in the identification of Sidney Leslie Goodwin, whose family perished on the Titanic, had previously been unable to crack his identity. His sketchy reflections of his earlier life thus far have not been enough to help.

I think that it's a truism that people who demonstrate delirium in the setting of a minor illness have abnormal brain function and are at high risk to evolve into a picture or dementia. The most common example of this is the elderly person, appearing to be normal to family and friends, who lapses into an acute confusional state with the appearance of a bladder infection. The mechanism of this remarkable type of brain decomposition is not clear. Return to normalcy may occur within a few days of initiation of antibiotic therapy. There are many other examples of similar circumstances, some of which do not involve infections. We simply do not really understand what is going on here.

Before we complete the survey of common diseases of the nervous system, here are a few comments about "brain tumors." People talk about a loved-one who died from "brain cancer." There are two categories of "brain cancer," one common and one relatively rare. The common one is cancer which has originated in a different part of the body and has metastasized into the brain by getting through the BBB. How and why these malignant cells penetrate the BBB to bring a new level of urgency, and likely pessimism to the existing treatment protocol is not completely clear to me. What may be even more amazing is that despite its huge blood flow (25% of the blood pumped out of the heart), metastatic cancer appears in the brain in only a small percentage of cases. This fact reflects the relative effectiveness of the BBB in keeping unwanted things out of the CNS. Once into the CNS, the cancer appears to have found a relatively safe haven, in that many of the most commonly used chemotherapeutic agents do not penetrate the BBB. A single metastasis may be amenable to surgical removal, as part of a heroic life-saving strategy. Radiation can also be used but has a high likelihood of killing off millions of viable neurons. So, at what price is survival worth it? "Gamma knife" radiation, using targeted radiation in very high doses, is an attempt to bypass the mass killing of healthy neurons which otherwise might occur, when the patient is deemed "salvageable" (This is a term commonly used by cancer specialists and other doctors. It seems to be a particularly harsh term, which creates a visual image of retrieving the patient from the garbage can. Is it just me, or should we ban usage of that term from acceptable medical jargon?).

The other type of "brain cancer" is cancer which originates in the brain or the meninges. These tumors can be benign or malignant. The danger of the benign ones depends almost completely on location. Many of them are very slow growing, produce minimal symptoms, and can be left alone. Some, based on location or growth patterns, demand treatment. The primary malignant tumors of the brain are uncommon but carry a very poor prognosis (They account for only 1.4% of primary cancers in adults, but 20% to 25% in children.). From the scientific standpoint, perhaps the most interesting thing about them is that almost nothing is known about the cause of this lethal tumor.

Depression, Anxiety, and Bipolar Disorder

The above mentioned conditions are sometimes referred to as "mood disorders." There appears to be a new appreciation of these diagnoses among medical professionals. Whereas previously they have been thought to represent differing disease processes, they now seem to be approached more as conditions with differing emphasis but with considerable overlap. In fact, very often, a diagnosis of depression/anxiety is made, or bipolar disorder in a person who variously demonstrates elements of both depression and "anxiety." Psychiatrists have rather strict criteria for making these diagnoses, with this approach particularly useful for research purposes. However, I would respectfully submit that just as with many other processes in life, we tend to box and categorize in an attempt to get clarity. Sometimes, and particularly with diseases or disorders of a structure as complex as the brain, it is acceptable to acknowledge the complexity and the frequent occurrence of hybrid conditions. What is absolutely unequivocal is that these conditions are extremely common, thus passing the prime litmus test for discussion in this treatise. What may not be so clearly appreciated is the marked disruption in life functioning, which may ensue from their appearance.

Depression and dysthymia have been mentioned in reference to barriers to effective medical care. We call that both conditions are common, with dysthymia being ubiquitous. Recall that dysthymia represents a very general feeling of discomfort or displeasure with life. It may play out as a deep-seated dissatisfaction, whereby life just seems to be out of balance. People experiencing this are prone to irritability and anger, leading to interpersonal problems. Nevertheless, many of them are able to function at a high level and may be financially and professionally successful.

In summary, with dysthymia, there appears to be an inability to "adjust" to the complexities of life, giving rise to the concept of an adjustment disorder.

Depression carries a heavier weight. People suffering with this condition feel deeply and basically distressed. Some feel as if there is something physically wrong with their brain. Many of them suffer first from the disease and second from shame of having this problem when on the surface they may appear to have everything that they need to be contented. They are often joyless. It is difficult for them to cope on a daily basis. They may have so called "vegetative" symptoms, with abnormalities in the realms of eating, sleeping, sexual activity, and general disengagement from others. It is very difficult for them to function well or even adequately in all domains of their life, including school, family, and work.

Anxiety also presents a heavy burden. This is much more than the type of feeling felt in reference to certain specific events deemed to be important, such as some type of performance, or interview, or engaging in some new activity. It is a deep-seated feeling of fearfulness and even terror, which surfaces off and on unassociated with the specifics of the day. At times, it can be chronic, present most of the time. Its bearers, who may be adults in positions of responsibility, may indicate that they cannot remember feeling differently all the way back to childhood. They too can have difficulty functioning in all realms of life.

As mentioned above, it is common for prominent elements of anxiety and depression to be present in the same person. Bipolar disorder is thought by many mental health professionals to be much more common than usually appreciated. This likely occurs because depressive manifestations tend to be much more persistent and dominant than the "manic" episodes, which may occur briefly and infrequently. Those in whom bipolar disorder is diagnosed often do poorly with antidepressant medications alone and often are seen by a number of health professionals over the course of years before the diagnosis is established.

Regarding treatment, those who consult with a physician are usually offered a medication of some type. On occasion, the results are dramatically positive, with the person feeling better than they have in many years, and often rather quickly. As noted before, however, often the results of medication alone are much less than dramatic, with the person stating, "I think I feel a little better." This is likely the case because of a change in appreciation of these mood disorders in the last ten to twenty years. At that juncture, with the appearance of a series of "second-generation" drugs utilized for depression and anxiety, the cause of the problem was thought to be likely a "biochemical imbalance" in the brain. Contemporary thinking holds that although chemical imbalances likely play a role, the cause of the mood disorder represents a complex blend of abnormal chemistry, childhood traumas, and the slings and arrows of the difficulties of living in a complex and highly competitive world. So, in these cases, as in many other realms of medicine, a pill cannot do it all.

So, what is left for the individual who "fails" treatment with a drug? Referral to a psychiatrist is likely in order at that time, with the hope that more skillful use of combination therapy, with or without psychotherapy or counseling, will be more helpful. In fact, "therapy" or counseling can be tremendously helpful. Its success, however, is dependent on the engagement of a skillful therapist and the need for the patient to consider the possibility of a long-term commitment to such therapy. Many medical insurance policies offer limited mental health coverage, sometimes adding a potential financial burden as well. Undoubtedly, with time, and patience and the efforts of a skilled therapist, the expectation is that this heavy burden of mental illness can be lightened.

This completes our survey of the nervous system. Any questions?

Section V

HEALTH OF THE MIND, INCLUDING THE SOUL'

GENERAL ELEMENTS OF SOUL HEALTH

In the context of this treatise, please note that the term "soul" is used not so much to describe an ethereal force or consciousness that proceeds and lives after the body but something at least slightly different. Soul health is a term which doctors and patients should use. We would all benefit to see it as a real entity, just as we see physical health as a real entity.

Soul health includes not only mental, emotional, and spiritual issues but much more than that. Soul issues are defined by their ineffability. They cannot be counted or measured, so in that sense, it does not include psychological or cultural disciplines, which are in a way too limited. Soul issues are transcultural. We as yet have not developed a distinct language to express soul issues. In essence, soul issues are intensely personal. They can be felt but not taught. Soul issues are intimately involved with the concept of relativity. Soul issues or soul awareness can be manifested by placing oneself in certain situations which are most likely to cause soulfulness to be felt.

When in everyday language, we say, "relatively speaking," or he or she or it is relatively such and such, we are in a way commenting about a sense of values. Built in to almost all of our thinking, and feeling, is a sense of "good" and "bad." In the language and feeling of soul, concepts of good and bad become muted. It is simply a way of acknowledging our inability to comprehend the very big picture and the effects of isolated events on such a picture. The far ends of the spectrum may remain definable… the murder of a child is "bad"… the giving of one's self to save another is "good." But most of what we experience and see and judge, in terms of relativity, becomes blurred and gray. We think or presume that we know the outcome of events. This seems obvious. But from the relative standpoint, it is only presumed, and it may be very wrong. The very long parable of the person who loses a leg early in his life, which many years later allows him to save his own life and the lives of others, is the cultural expression of our inability to accurately label an event as good or bad.

In fact, what emerges from the existing absolutism is no less than the parable of one person's garbage becoming the other person's treasure. We humans disagree on almost everything. We try harder and harder to find people who agree with us. And so, the number of people included in our absolutist family becomes proportionally smaller and smaller, and the number of our "enemies," or those who disagree with us, becomes larger and larger. Eventually, as stated by Gandhi, "an eye for an eye and the whole world goes blind." Alternatively, with relative thinking, we acknowledge our limitations. We acknowledge that we always emerge out of a cultural milieu, which is nothing more than an accident of birth.

So, another feature of soul is a sense of connectedness. However, it is not to the limited connectedness of our "tribe." We could try to take refuge in our tribe, naming it the United States of America, or China or country X, Y, or Z. We could name it Catholicism or Protestantism. Or Roman or Orthodox. Or Methodist or Presbyterian. Or Sunni or Shiite. Or the Smiths or the Jones. Or whatever! But it is nowhere near enough to describe any of this tribal allegiance or connectedness, as there are always more people and more things outside than inside. Those things outside eventually are conceived of as "enemies" on one level or another, out to get what we have and out to profit at our expense. In the existing paradigm, this inevitably becomes a self-fulfilling prophecy.

Connectedness in soul is connectedness to everything. Perhaps that sounds silly? However, all it takes is one simple acknowledgment, stamped deeply into one's heart and mind. "I don't know everything." In fact, "I am not sure that I know slightly more than anything."

Peculiarly, soul itself can be considered to be relative. There is not only one way to experience or partake in soul activities. Recall that the far ends of the spectrum remain relatively clear with regard to their basic positive or negative features. Soul is more easily encountered in a situation where sentient beings are not being injured. It is also more likely where so-called inanimate objects or places are not being injured (a strip mine or a strip mall). Many people around the world have for time immemorial considered rocks, monoliths, and countless geographic features to be holy places. Soul is more easily encountered where "beauty" can be found. My own bias informs me that quiet, if not silence, is an important element of beauty.

Ultimately, soul exists in the feeling of love—selfless love, giving one the feeling of heaven on earth. It can be nurtured and practiced in many different ways. For many people, looking into the eyes of a baby, person, or animal is enough. Experiencing the big rhythmic pulse of a city. Experiencing one of a multitude of natural places. Looking through a telescope.

A healthy soul is above all contented, is open and inquiring, is recognizing limitations, and is accepting complexity rather than the black and white of apparent cause and effect. It has unfettered self-inquiry and is feeling connected, even some of the time. Soul health as we define it is not dependent on physical health, and the reverse is true. Soul health, however, is by far the more potent of the two, with shortfalls making physical health much more difficult to achieve on a long-term basis. Certainly, one can imagine a person gifted with a naturally strong and balanced physiology. Even with severe soul sickness, that inherently strong constitution can function at a high level for a given period of time. However, such a situation is doomed to failure, with the premature emergence of poor physical health. Witness countless gifted athletes who falter or die prematurely.

So, wellness, to use a contemporary term—whether one looks at it for an individual or a group, a society, or even a species—must be appreciated in terms of a total global perspective. Will Rodgers stated that "I never met a man I didn't like," referring to the many famous people he had poked fun at. Similarly, I have never personally met a person with soul illness who was happy or contented. We simply cannot escape the pervasive issue of relativism. It is everywhere. Of all those legions of people, displayed before us in the mass media, with good looks, more money than they can count, more children than they know what to do with, and an adoring public, who of them are truly contented? It obviously depends upon which of them has a healthy soul. What is being displayed before us, because we the public ask for it, is their persona—the superficial qualities that they have, which allow them to fulfill the role that we have assigned to them. Which of them have soul health is rarely known.

Why is this? Why do we so pursue the trappings of "success" when it is abundantly clear that there is no correlation between that and health, and at the same time ignore these qualities which could lead us to deep health? Experiencing the presence of a person with deep soul health is far more intoxicating than anything having to do with superficialities. On the world stage, when such individuals emerge, they move history. They are extremely valuable to us for the function they serve, which is to alter our basic thinking of factors which limit freedom or promote dissention. They are always transcultural, standing above and beyond religious and tribal considerations. What is less well appreciated is that such individuals live right within our midst. They live and die unrecognized by history, but they are not less crucial than our greatest luminaries because they too move history. It is what Hegel called the "world spirit." Unfortunately, there are too few of such individuals in our midst, although we all hope that their ranks are growing. They can be identified as people whose presence endorses our highest callings of lovingness—and connectedness. It is possible that

Estimated Current Deficiency of People with Deep Soul Health		
World population	7,000,000,000	7 billion
Need for 5%	350,000,000	350 million
Current % 1%	70,000,000	70 million
Deficit	280,000,000	280 million

their numbers and influence could grow exponentially once a certain critical mass is reached, as their spoken and unspoken messages begin to take hold. Personally, I would guess that 1% of the people I have met are that way. I suspect the critical mass that would ignite the fire of the transformation of human consciousness and conduct is 5% to 10%. That is, we likely fall short by 280 million people right now. As huge as this number may seem, as will be mentioned in greater detail in the Epilogue, if hybrid states, combining neural factors and computer parts becomes widespread, this may be as close as we ever come to igniting an explosion of the higher consciousness of humans.

The clearly defining features of soul health are not obviously apparent due to the already stated ineffable qualities of soul. Whether sizing up one's own or speculating about another's soul health, recall that soul health does not deal with individual or tribal concerns. It is generalized, encompassing everything. When the fire of soul health is ignited, just as fire results in heat, soul health results in compassion. Compassion is simply a pervasive feeling of empathy, for everything. Not just for the person who has lost a loved one, but for all sentient creatures—all of whom struggle daily and all of whom are destined to die—and for the Earth itself, which also struggles and will eventually die with or without our meddling, when the light of the sun goes out four billion years from now. Likely, such information about a person will not emerge in a discussion at the check-out counter, and yet the person across from you in that venue may be the compassionate one.

The other feature which emerges from soul health is fearlessness, equally invisible at times. This quality has little to do with the startle response, which is a deep reptilian brain reflex, which may not be snuffed out even in the most fearless of us. Likely, our biggest fear is fear of death. Woody Allen's admonition that "I'm not afraid of dying! I just don't want to be there when it happens," says it well. Despite our intense fear of death, we have an incredible ability to imagine or fantasize that it is something that only occurs to other people. Our rhetoric attests to this. Our lack of rhetoric about death on an everyday basis also attests to it. The self-defeating belief is that if we do not talk about it, it is less likely to happen. Even doctors do not talk about death, and the results of this failure have tragic and avoidable consequences, which will be discussed later. Briefly, patients and families and desperately ill people assume that recovery is just around the corner. Recall the obvious constant that doctors are just people, embedded in culture, just like everyone else.

Please note another obvious fact. For most people who would define themselves as "religious," active members of an identifiable formal doctrine, the fear of death is unlikely to be less intense. Despite declining physical health spanning decades, interspersed with major problems requiring hospitalizations and surgery, and loss of body functions and even body parts, most individuals will choose to do it all again, if it prolongs their life. We have had to change our terminology to make such endeavors more palatable to all. Because of financial considerations, since many people are only allowed in the hospital "X" number of days following operation "Z," they are unable to go directly home, because of ongoing debility in early recovery. They used to go to the "nursing home" following hospitalization. Nursing home is actually a very good and appropriate name. It is a place where they interact primarily with nurses, who just like Florence Nightingale, are uniformly compassionate and caring, making them feel at home. Hence, "nursing, home." However, experiences in nursing homes have taken on an extremely negative connotation, as a trash heap where people go to die. So we changed the name to "convalescent home," a phrase still commonly used. However, for those of us who are really hip, we have moved beyond that static phrase to the newest moniker, the "rehabilitation hospital," or "rehabilitation unit." Nothing has changed regarding the physical plant; it is the same building. What have changed are the expectations. Both patients and families now expect that the overworked, underfunded, understaffed personnel at the "rehabilitation hospital" are going to turn things around for their 90-year-old loved one and will give them a new lease on life. Perhaps, this discussion regarding the nursing-home-to-rehabilitation-hospital transformation is redundant, having already been pointed out more eloquently and humorously by Andy Rooney.

In summary, nobody seems to be ready to die. Even those who say they are, change their minds from day to day. Fear of death remains a huge problem in modern day medical practice because of our ability to keep terribly ill people alive for very long periods of time, at unbelievably high costs, and with huge levels of chronic suffering. Recall the parable of the small group of people on the lifeboat, in the

562 | Dr. Barry Marmorstein

middle of the ocean, with dwindling resources and a dwindling chance of group survival. This parable beautifully illustrates the power of the presence of soul health. Recall that each of the unfortunate people on this boat has their own story. Each story is compelling. Each person is complex. One or several may be morally lacking. Perhaps, none of them deserved this fate. As the days go on, the situation becomes progressively more tense. Tempers flare. The fear factor rises. Finally, it is determined that if one person volunteers to go overboard, then the rest have a good chance of survival. The point regarding soul health is now obvious. The person who is truly compassionate for all sentient beings, even these morally weak or aggressive and ego-bound, and the person who is fearless will make it obvious to all that he or she is the one to go. So, in a sense, perhaps the goal of life is to be the one who obviously needs to be part of the raft group. That is, the person who may place group needs above their own and do so because it is unthinkable to do anything else. Recall that in the shocking loss of the supposedly unsinkable Titanic, the richest man on the boat, John J. Aster, lost his life alongside the hundreds of people in steerage. It did get him a huge funeral through the streets of New York.

Let us pause momentarily. What I have just described, i.e., going overboard for the group, bears some similarity to the activities of the present day scourge of suicide bombings. Human behavior, emanating from the depths of the most complex structure in the universe (our brains), is always a work in progress, jerking left or right as neural nets light up or turn off. Just as the preparation for a life of excellence and a life of winning (a societally accepted form of domination in our made-up world) may look the same for an indefinite time during their development, eventually, based on many factors, they diverge according to the dictates of the work in progress. So, the concept of martyrdom can superficially look the same for the Good Samaritan or the suicide bomber. The differences, however, are obvious. The Good Samaritan responds from a standpoint of non-judgment and compassion, while the suicide bomber responds from the standpoint of absolutism (strongly judgmental) and blind tribal xenophobia devoid of compassion. Simply stated, the response is generated by love in the Good Samaritan and by fear in the suicide bomber, clearly delineating the consequential results of love and fear.

Many of us fear loss of security only a shade less than fear of death. Please be advised that by carefully examining the solar system in which the Earth exists, and the earth itself, and the predatory nature of life on earth, there is no such thing as security. In essence, security is an illusion. Our lives could end in an instant. Multiple mass extinctions have attested to this, the last one 65,000,000 years ago, when our ancestors were still sightless creatures living in the sea. An earthquake through the center of a major city could eliminate security for occupants within a 100-mile radius of that city, in an instant.

Obviously, people also deeply fear loss of companionship. Although such is inevitable, we must be willing, if it seems appropriate, to reach out in any one of many ways to continue to feel integrated and appreciated. Humans want to feel relevant. Thinking out-of-the-box could easily provide one suffering loss of companionship, by replacing it with an ongoing deep-seated sense of relevancy, with avenues for a continued feeling of integration and relevance.

Working in medicine for many years does not allow one to easily escape dealing with death. It has been stated that people who choose health care as a profession have a fear of death which needs to be dealt with. Perhaps that is true. Long years in health care provide one with a somewhat unique perspective. Death is everywhere. It is just around the corner, even for the person with great physical and soul health. If it is feared, it permeates all areas of life with a bitterness and irritability.

A better option is to look straight at it. Do not flinch. You (and me) and death. Eye to eye. We should all consider ourselves to be running out of time. That is the truest truism. We should clean up our messes every day, so as not to leave a mess for someone else. We should finish every day with peace in our hearts and no known "enemies." We should harbor no anger towards anyone, recognizing that we daily create our own reality. In other words, we should act daily, as if this day were our last. Then, as George Burns quipped, when we awaken the next day without a row of candles on both sides, it is a great day!

CHRONIC ILLNESS

Life is fragile. Living organisms have remarkable powers of protection and self-repair. Which of these two statements would appear to hold the basic kernel of truth? Perhaps, it all depends on one's perspective. Both are true. Perhaps, one might speculate that to remain healthy is a matter of minimizing the former and maximizing the latter.

As is true with most health-related issues, we are presented with choices. Every choice can be weighed in terms of potential benefit and potential harm. Benefit and harm, of course, can both be looked at in terms of physical and mental *realms* (sole and Soul). As has been

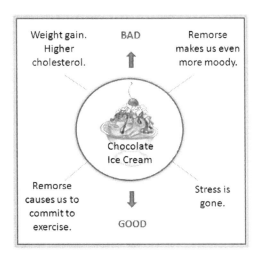

discussed, soul issues cannot be ignored and must be seriously considered. In fact, as has been mentioned, consideration is the crux. For instance, the overweight person with high cholesterol may be feeling so stressed out that he or she fears an imminent heart attack or nervous breakdown. A pint of the best chocolate ice cream sits in front of them, guaranteed to jeopardize one problem and relieve the other. What should they do? Taking this conundrum even further, to a much deeper level, which action is most likely to help or hurt which problem? Are we so sure about results that we presume to know the answer to that question? As is often the case, the result likely depends on the absolute uniqueness of the person's physiology and the unpredictability of actions taken or not taken. Despite all of the variability, as people move through life and into older age, their medical "problem lists" and thus their accompanying medication lists begin to look remarkably similar. It is as if each visit to the doctor's office is weaving the same kind of clothing. There is a handout available in the waiting room of my office whereby a recent study, published in the Archives of Internal Medicine pointed this out scientifically. The take-home message confirmed what had been long suspected. By (1) staying thin, (2) exercising 3½ hours a week, (3) never smoking, and (4) eating a healthful diet, the vast majority of chronic diseases do not appear.

So the ancient Greek dictum, to know thyself, ultimately must guide our actions. The paradox is that to know thyself is in fact a very difficult task, which requires us to be deeply self-reflective, in touch with our dark side, and ruthlessly honest. In other words, it is a place that most of us never want to go near and will do almost anything to avoid. What naturally follows is a more instinctive or impulsive response, perhaps not necessarily "wrong," but much less likely to hit the bull's-eye, where the action is based on self-knowledge.

Back to the point, philosophical complexities notwithstanding, our bodies are always trying to repair and reduce fragility. We really do not intellectually decide to turn on repair. It is built in. Alternatively, we do emotionally and spiritually decide to upgrade or downgrade our reparative capacity by our total engagement in life. In other words, the body does respond to subtle, if not unconscious, feeling states, which in turn acts through the autonomic nervous system and its sister system, the endocrine system to create a milieu conducive to or incompatible with repair.

Damage likely begins in utero. It is likely that within the next generation, we will learn a great deal about the factors that affect the mental and physical health of the fetus. Certainly, a great deal is known already, usually garnered by observing the effects of flagrant maternal physical and/or emotional illness on the offspring. However, it is likely that vast reservoirs of correlation exist regarding subtle or perhaps one-time negative effects on the fetus. One mistake in the kitchen can permanently alter the outcome of the meal. It is no different in terms of the uterine kitchen. How much and what types of events are most likely to permanently affect fetal development, particularly any one of a multitude of subtle, everyday type influences are very incompletely studied, will take long-term longitudinal studies, and may even then be difficult to interpret. However, ask any pregnant mother what she should do and should not do during her pregnancy, and no doubt a substantial list of "common knowledge" answers will emerge.

Damage certainly occurs during birth, as witnessed by the emergence of the screaming baby... obviously physically and likely emotionally traumatized. By the time of early childhood, various types of malignant processes make their appearance. Autopsies on young children may reflect the earliest beginning of arteriosclerosis. By teenage life and young adulthood, many of the chronic maladies which eventually bring us down are already well entrenched.

All through this, damage and repair, and more damage and more repair, are running parallel to each other. Simplistically, the magnitude of the problem progressing through adulthood depends on the extent of damage and the capacity for repair. Both of these processes are highly variable in any given individual. The balance of one against the other determines our fate in the last third of our lives.

ESSENTIALLY GOOD
OR ESSENTIALLY EVIL

How many of you, from time to time, experiencing daily life as it is, have questioned briefly or extensively the question as to the basic nature of the human animal? Philosophers, theologians, and others have published tomes on the subject, each with their own perspective, or biases, or wishes. Recall that each one of us at any point in time is a product of our life experiences. These experiences color our outlook and attitudes, in obvious and countless subtle ways. To look at the world with fresh eyes, baby eyes, is so very difficult and requires an enormous well of honest self-reflection.

The more deeply we look inward, the more frequently we encounter our so-called dark side. This concept too has been developed by many, most notably Carl Jung and his followers. What it appears to be is a closet full or perhaps a basement full of Negativity, with a capital N. Liken it to a severe representation of the "terrible twos," filled with anger, resentment, conflict, frustration, and with the constant threat of spilling over into an outburst which could be the trigger for WWIII. Countless wars and atrocities have left no doubt that the killer lurks in the depths of our dark side, in the majority of us, rational as we may be. We will go out of our way to never open that closet door or descend the steps to that basement.

No wonder it is so difficult for us to look at this. Most of us cannot, or can for only brief moments, face the horror that this beast lives in us. It is much easier to either project such capabilities on others or, at least, to imagine that the other feels this kind of aggression towards us. Please recall that labeling is endemic in our behavior. Categorization is part of the human psyche, part of the way our brains work. We are so curious, and so thirsty for understanding, that we naturally try to put things into boxes and smaller and smaller boxes, in the hopes that organization of all of this complex material in some way will allow us to understand it better. We, as a species, are desperate to understand. It is so intrinsic to us that we cannot imagine that it is not intrinsic to all living species. The wild animal, bottle fed by its "owner" since infancy, suddenly turns on its "master" and mauls him or her beyond recognition. This animal is clearly not evil, but doing what "wild" animals do when impulses from their potent "old brain" overwhelm restraints from their diminutive "new brain." Recall all the myriads of activities which we call "human nature," which may be an intrinsic part of our makeup but not of nature in general.

Labeling and categorization can safely be stated to be part of our nature. Both of these are products of limited knowledge and, as such, have limited accuracy and usefulness. Often, they inhibit rather than extend knowledge. This is a deep paradox. Be aware when labels are applied and activities are categorized by you and others. It is a very commonplace phenomenon, spawned by fear and meant to induce change. To the extent that we can free ourselves of the notion that these labels are factual, but rather perceptual on our part, we open the door to greater ease in dealing with our fellow species members.

What does all of this have to do with the good or evil of our species as a whole? Obviously, as we look around, there is abundant evidence for both types of activities. This is understandable and predictable from a simple morphologic perspective, recognizing that we as *Homo sapiens sapiens*, with a 200,000-year history, are relative newcomers on earth. Our distant ancestors emerged from the sea as predators, relying solely on our reptilian brain for survival. Over the eons, for reasons that are not completely clear, perhaps representing a self-perpetuating epigenetic phenomenon, we have developed this huge cortical brain, which has strongly influenced and modified the reptilian brain, but coexists with it in a tense standoff of dominance and submission. Our reptilian brain has been around forever. Although it is essential for survival, it is dense, cunning, unrelenting, and uncompromising. It is addressed and reinforced by cultural phenomena many times daily. It is survival personified.

Our neo cortex holds the keys to bliss. It weighs, and balances, and integrates, leading to a basket full of epiphenomena, including love, generosity, harmony, and beauty. Of course, it is also capable of indescribably astounding feats of comprehension and creativity. Remarkably, this part of our brain is much less often nurtured or explored by our daily activities. At its best, balanced brain function allows us to feel and express acts of selflessness and appreciation of beauty and rapture in all of its representations. At its worst, when the activities of the primitive brain are apparent, it can result in the most horrifying acts of humiliation and destruction as represented by the wars of the twentieth century.

We still have not answered the questions as to really good or really evil, but the answer is implicit. The answer, if one is so presumptuous to call it that, is that both are potentialities, alive and well in the hearts and minds of every one of us. So, is our future inevitably hopeless with development of better and better killing machines and deployment of weapons of mass destruction? Obviously, the answer is no, but changes are necessary to escape the living hell or Armageddon.

Think about this, and be very patient with it. Any individual at any given time is doing the best they can. It is not in the survival scheme of any species or individual to do poorly. From the survival standpoint, doing well is always advantageous. In recognizing this simple basic concept, the door opens towards a sense of compassion for those who are doing poorly, disallowing us to label them as inferior or "bad" and allowing us to generate a desire to help them instead.

By the way, who is doing poorly? What about selfish people? Angry people? Those who are covetous? Those who are rigid and closed? Those who are condescending? Those who presume to know all the answers? Most of all, those who are fearful of just about anything you can think of? These are the people whom Thoreau described as living "lives of quiet desperation" never contented, participating in a miserable death march to the grave.

Are there any of us doing well? These individuals are much more difficult to spot, but in fact, they are all around us, albeit the solid minority. You see them every day. Some of them have worked at being that way. Some were likely born that way. They are our living heroes.

PREDATION

As has been commented upon, our very distant ancestors, arising hundreds of millions of years ago, were sightless creatures living in the primordial sea. Not much is known about their nervous systems or their brain power, but it is a likely assumption that their cognitive capabilities were nearly nil. No one eyeing those small and helpless appearing creatures could possibly have imagined that two or three hundred million years later, they would be the only species to have ever physically reshaped the planet. So, with their innocent and fragile appearance, what could have allowed them to do that? It seems incredulous. As a sidelight and on the lighter side, what might be the next species to take over, as will inevitably happen? Are they already here with us, or are they as yet to emerge? Perhaps if they are here already, we should seek them out and befriend them, so as not to incur their wrath when they are finally in charge. (Perhaps we should all keep that in mind before we mindlessly squash a cockroach or a spider, or put a stick through a slug.)

Getting back to us, the exact mechanism of how we survived to become so absolutely dominant is not known. However, there would appear to be at least two safe guesses. First, there was always a niche, albeit changing, to be filled, and we needed to be able to adapt. Secondly, we knew how to get food, perhaps sometimes plant and often animal, but we knew how to hunt and gather.

We have a tendency to attach a negative perspective to species who co-exist with us now, whom we see as "predators." We state that nature is brutal and that they are simply part of this brutal scheme. This might include species all the way from the Venus flytrap to the polar bear, whom it is said is the only bear that will track a human in anticipation of a kill (do not worry about this naughty bear, who will be extinct soon anyway). The pejorative bent is another example of projection regarding the brutal aspect of nature, being exemplified by other species, but excluding us. In reality, with our 7 billion species membership, we are by far the most successful predator to have ever lived on earth, in terms of the amount of killing and eating presumed to be necessary to keep our species numbers intact. But it does not stop there. Our predatory behavior has physically reshaped the landscape to suit our needs, benefitting some species (dogs, cats, chickens, cattle), harming many others, and all done without a thought as to ethics and long-term ramifications of the activities and behavior of our species.

However, our predation in the modern world plays out in many other forms, even by vegetarians (even by vegans), against each other. Please note that we do not call this cannibalism, although the distinction is not always clear. Lately, in the wake of the 2008–2009 housing and banking crisis, we have heard the term "predatory lending." In fact, predation against each other occurs any time one of us interacts with another, with the express purpose to get something from you, for them. Perhaps the ultimate act of predation is to take another life. However, the interaction does not need to be physically violent. Domination over another can be economic, or sexual, or even spiritual, in the binding of another to you against their will. Recall that predation is a powerful survival mechanism lurking in the reptilian brain, often not even on a conscious level. We all need to be aware of its potential to rear up, so as to recognize it and choose not to act on it, as it truly has nothing to do with our own survival. The risk of predation is especially high in dealings of apparent unequals in power... parents and children, bosses and employees, landlords and tenants, men and women, women and men, teachers and students, rich people and poor people, etc. We must not carry our role playing to the point where it endangers the welfare of another person. We must simply be aware. It is essential that, for the good of all, we do not use other people for the express purpose of fulfilling our needs.

Consider the following philosophic conundrum. There is nothing that can be more apparent to us than the inevitability of the eventual death of all living things. Even the 3,000-year-old bristlecone pine must die. Observe please, in your own attitudes and in those of others, that there appears to be a pervasive blind spot. We find it relatively easy to discuss the death of others, but we seem to gloss over the absolute certainty that we will follow the same fate. The result is the notion as stated by the Rolling Stones, that "time... is on your side." If you knew for certain that today was your last day, would you behave badly? Recall that in its broadest form, behaving badly is doing harm to someone or something else. Despite our protestations and unwillingness to accept the certainty of our own death at any time, indeed we do behave poorly, often. When the total impact of a person's life is being examined after their death, in terms of whether or not they left the world a better (or worse) place, which of the following might carry the greatest weight—the very best thing they ever did or the very worst thing they ever did? Certainly, at countless eulogies given every day, we recount the multiple avenues of beneficence engineered by the individual. Obviously, we never hear about the dark side, be it big or little. A case can certainly be made for proposing that the worst thing can easily overrun the best. Obviously, a multitude of factors might play into determining this assessment. The point is that with our basic nature being so flagrantly bimodal, we must be constantly vigilant to tame the beast within, so as to not commit the one act which might turn the tide.

Good and evil are to a certain extent interchangeable. Certainly, they are relative and subject to bias. I cringe even using the terms as such, as they are so strongly culturally determined. Using religious metaphors, "say unto them 'as I live,' says the Lord God, 'I have no pleasure in the death of the wicked; but that the wicked turn from his way and live,'" (Ezekiel 33:11). In Buddhist tradition, all of life is thought to be a preparation for death. Redemption can occur up to the moment of death, so that the possibility of transmuting evil into good is always within a person's grasp. The purpose of a human life is to wake up and to see the whole picture.

As a segue to the next topic, I quote Paul Tillich: "The first duty of love is to listen."

SLOW DOWN AND LISTEN

The advantages of being alive in the twenty-first century as compared to ancient and even recent times are obvious. For most of human history, life expectancy was very short. Women have been particularly singled out for premature death. Currently in modern society with adequate medical care, maternal mortality in childbirth ranges from nine to thirteen per 100,000. Even in 1915, the figure was 600 per 100,000. In the eighteenth century, the figure was 1,000 to 1,200 per 100,000. Unfortunately, there are still a few pockets in the modern world where this latest figure is still the same, particularly sub-Saharan Africa and Afghanistan. In other words, one in a hundred women still die in childbirth, in these areas. In addition, it is estimated that in the seventeenth to nineteenth centuries, between three and five million women were burned at the stake as witches. In those times, given the wrong circumstances, if a woman loved animals too openly, or retired alone into a rural setting, that too could trigger accusations and a "trial." The same was true of course for alleged adultery. Men were subject to death in countless wars, where a common "flesh wound" could prove to be the initiating event of a fatal infection. Industrial accidents and fatalities were common. Both sexes were subject to death from childhood diseases, and recurring epidemics of plague, which repeatedly decimated large populations in urban centers for thousands of years.

For most of human history, food supplies have been subject to sudden severe disruptions. People have generally had to work long hours to provide themselves with basic food, shelter, and clothing.

(Incidentally, in the few remaining hunter–gatherer societies scattered around the globe today, people "work" an average of less than six hours per day! Check your local newspaper want ads.)

Lastly, access to books and other tools for learning has been extremely limited until very recent times. To say that there has been an explosion of knowledge and access to such knowledge in the last several hundred years is obviously true. In fact, over the same time frame, this has given rise to the science of epistemology. That is, what is knowledge, and how do we know it?

That is precisely the dilemma that we find ourselves in at this time. Particularly since the advent of the Internet, we are now swimming in a sea of information, affectionately called sound bites, blogs, twitters, and numerous other terms, all of which result in our being exposed to a limitless amount of information, be it factual or not. Recall a core belief that goes back at least to the time of Socrates, when he was acknowledged to be the wisest person in all of Athens. No one was more surprised than Socrates, who considered himself to be certain of almost nothing. In other words, the truly wise person, questions everything, ponders all possibilities, and listens to all opinions. Most of the sea of information currently available is unfiltered, non-digested, i.e., not "peer reviewed," and of little benefit to a seeker of true knowledge, let alone wisdom.

Perhaps we have gone too far in this Age of Information. Knowledge alone is not enough. Wisdom involves having factual data, but always being aware that the source of such data is people and that people are riff with biases according to their own backgrounds and level of introspection. In other words, "knowledge" must be always filtered and digested, and ultimately recognized as being possibly incorrect.

In recent years, we have been told that we suffer from noise pollution. More recently, there is data that we suffer from light pollution. Time will tell whether these influences are true, and whether or not an excessive amount of light and/or noise is actually harmful. After all, we have to be just as questioning of scientific data, as we are of data from the common blogger.

It does seem likely that in our modern societies as they are currently structured, we are not necessarily provided with enough built-in quiet time. Lack of such quiet time can have theoretical and some absolute detriments. It is no longer easy to avoid the kinetic nature and din of society. Just as the effects of poor sleeping can have powerful negative effects on us, so perhaps can the effects of too much stimulation negatively impact us. We seem to have a greater awareness about this in relationship to children, with recommendations to limit time with television, computers, video games, etc. I suspect that the same tendencies towards overstimulation persist throughout adult life. Note that we tend to emulate and reward people who are quick-witted and have the ability to speak quickly, as does the typical late-night talk show host. Doctors who specialize in sleep issues would likely attest to the possibility that such quick-footed banter does not often set the stage for restful sleep in those watching the display. They frequently enjoin their patients to participate in "sleep hygiene" behavior, in the hours leading up to bedtime, in the hopes of enhancing truly restorative sleep.

Time for another truism. We are much more likely to learn something, by listening, in contrast to speaking. In fact, although one can learn how others respond to your opinions as you speak, the opportunities for learning while speaking are very limited. But really, why should you care? Speaking invariably pulls into action the ego. Perhaps this is unavoidable, and harmless, as long as we recognize that it is occurring, and keep it in check. It is almost never appropriate to speak in absolute terms, which is the graveyard for being truly helpful. Speaking from a position of compassion and lovingness tends to minimize "egoism" and maximize connectedness. It is often simply much more pleasurable to allow another person to speak and share that part of themselves, while you, as the listener, sit calmly without overt threat of a quick interruption. (It has been noted that as a patient sits down with a doctor to recite a story, the doctor's first interruption on the average is eighteen seconds!) It is a great compliment to be described as a good listener, and one which comes frequently with such a person. It is also a great service to the relationship itself.

Now it is time for an opinion. Of course, I would not have made a note of slowing down and listening, unless I thought it to be an obstacle towards achieving soul health. How do we do this, and why? The opportunities for slowing down are limitless, all around us, and free. Spending time with animals, sitting with a book or magazine, going for a walk (or swim, or bike ride, or anything physical), being out in nature (including in traditionally considered inclement weather) listening to music (not rap), going to a religious sanctuary (even without a formal service), learning any one of a host of walking or sitting meditative processes, and many other venues would serve to slow us down. Importantly, do not be afraid to be alone. In fact, it is crucial to learn to be alone and to enjoy and relish such time. It pays dividends in obvious and many other not so obvious ways. All of these activities should nourish your body and your soul. Listening somewhat overlaps. Listen to the sounds of nature. Listen to the birds, which provide us with their sounds. Listen to your fellow travelers through life. Ask them questions. They want to and need to tell their stories. They may or may not want to hear your story at that moment. If not now, perhaps later. If never, it does not matter. You served them in your listening. It is difficult for me to imagine how slowing down and listening could be deleterious to you or others. However, recognizing that biases are impossible to escape from, it is possible that such activities, especially being alone, might not be good for you. Ultimately, one must trust their own inner knowing.

HAPPINESS, CONTENTMENT, AND THE CONCEPT OF GRACE

One could make a case for establishing happiness as a benchmark or litmus test for identifying the person with a healthy soul. We all have an inclination as to what happiness is, as most of us have experienced it at least once in our lives. One might hope, if not expect, that in a state of happiness, an individual might be inclined to be more generous and less fearful than at other times, thus being in a position to be more helpful to others. So, those of you who placed next to "goal in life" in your high school year book, "to be happy," do not necessarily have anything to be embarrassed about, as the years roll on.

Happiness it seems, however, is closely linked to external events... being acknowledged, being invited to the prom by the very person whom you desire, being elected, winning the lottery, passing your annual medical exam or, in my case, gaining acceptance into medical school. I can identify the moment I opened that envelope with the acceptance letter as being the single most happy moment in my life. External events are as changeable as the weather. Clearly, the vast majority of them are completely out of our control. As has been mentioned before, there are in fact only a very few core issues which are under our control. So, happiness by necessity is volatile and evanescent—here today, gone tomorrow.

So, perhaps those of you who indicated that "contentment" is your goal in the yearbook came closer to the mark of a truly healthy soul. Although there is obviously overlap between happiness and contentment, there is at least one fundamental difference. Contentment is essentially separated from daily (or hourly) events. Contentment is a deeply running current, flooding one's inner life with a feeling of gratitude and bounty, protected from the elements, and sustaining the physical body in the most basic of ways. Where does it come from? (In other words, where can I buy it?) Unfortunately, it is yet another of these illusive, ethereal features which seem to arise mysteriously and often unexpectedly. I have no problem calling its appearance an act of grace.

Grace is a stunningly beautiful and humbling concept. Intrinsic to its appearance is the inability to see even which direction it came from. It is almost as if it simply condenses from the ether, catching the person by surprise. It is the type of experience described by countless great religious leaders over the eons, but it is certainly not restricted to them alone. Is it given, or is it earned? Given by whom or what? Earned by doing what? Please recall that in dealing with elementary concepts such as these, we must be willing to give up our preconceived ideas of certainty. The emphasis is on please. If we are not able to do that, then we will never gain true compassion, never be truly humble (ignorant), and never see ourselves as all equal and deserving of respect.

To me, the appearance of grace remains inexplicable. I do not know the formula for "getting it." In my own rather extreme naïveté, I would hope that if the field is plowed, the harvest will follow. If we do the right things, we may be fortunate enough to perceive the workings of grace in our lives. May I caution those of you who are aware of this, not to try to describe it at the next cocktail party you attend, even with a generous supply of alcohol on board. Distilling it down to its essence (pardon the pun), perhaps the best single common word to describe the workings of grace is gratitude; tempered by deep humility.

"Doing the right things," meaning what? Very basically, avoiding intentionally harming another sensate being, physically, emotionally, mentally, or economically. Do as much as one can to support the efforts of these beings to experience their beingness. You may give advice, but only when requested. Otherwise, giving unsolicited advice is hubris, "outrageous arrogance" (Professor Rufus Fears)—the world according to you. Recall that you passively, daily advise by your character and by the conduct of your life. The biggest boost we can give another is supporting them in what they see as their life calling.

Just a word of caution: There are far too many of us, who appear to be "lost" in addictions, mental illness, or disengagement from all that nourishes health of the soul. Involvement with these people can test our mettle to the very core, trying to find the balance between support and enabling. There is no absolutely correct way to proceed. Just as the doctor must know that every person cannot be saved, there comes a point when reduction of suffering is more important than saving. These people suffer greatly. How to reduce their suffering? Start with, "I love you."

LOVESTREAM

If you were given the theoretical question as to what is the single most important factor that makes human life endurable, what would be your answer? Looking at it from the backside, the question would be: The loss of what experiential element would make life on earth unendurable? Given the multiplicity of human experiences and the obvious difference in people's nervous systems, many things would come up for consideration. Certainly, the answer could not be the same for everyone.

Individuals who have been incarcerated, particularly those who have been in solitary confinement, and those who have been so unfortunate as to have been in the most maximum of maximum security prisons, such as the unit south of Denver, Colorado, report the dehumanizing effect of severe reduction in human contact. Human contact appears to be a key element for most people. If we are nothing else as a species, we are social animals. We depend on each other, physically and psychologically. Perhaps, this may act to our detriment at times, in that our insecurity and our need for approval prevents us from spending time alone in contemplation and meditation, looking more and more deeply inward, until we have familiarized ourselves with, and thus neutralized our inner demons. As noted elsewhere with the construction of our everyday world which just happens to be completely "made up" by convention, rather than representing universal law, such introspection has become much more difficult.

The pressure to conform, to interact, to be accepted has become not just the means to an end, but the end itself. From every direction we are goaded to "be like Mike." In this milieu, those who stand out in even minor ways run the risk of incurring the crush of ridicule and marginalization. Review of the historical record confirms that there is "nothing new on heaven or earth." The same problems which torment us now have been replayed in striking similarities, cyclically going back thousands of years. As societal pressure builds around the issues of allocation of resources, insecurity, and the need for approbation, we run the risk of releasing the pressure in acts of egregious violence and greed, endlessly playing itself out until we collapse in an exhausted, post-orgasmic heap, and sign a peace treaty, again. If nothing else, acts of violence against one another have a strong element of intimacy. As we most treasure and protect our own lives, anything that is viewed as threatening such can seduce us into another round of conflict and brutality. So this intrusion into our privacy is not new. It is simply now more difficult than it has been before, as the ability to do harm to each other continues to grow.

So, the need for human contact appears to be rather universal. It seems that at its core, what we seek, and often fear at the same time is to experience love. Love, or lack of love, appears to be a crucial element in our social functioning and is a key to our physical and mental health. Lack of love at crucial times in the life of infants and babies can result in physical and psychic changes which can last a lifetime. Inability to freely experience lovingness is likely an integral part, if not a causative factor in the psychopathology of many mental disorders.

From whence cometh love? To me, the answer is simple, as it clearly comes from the same place from which Grace emanates. The answer is that we do not know and cannot know where either comes from. More importantly, we should not want to know and should not even contemplate looking for the answer. The greatest miracle of all is that these twin blessings are apparently epiphenomena of neural networks of living creatures likely emanating from our "new brain," the neo cortex. We never asked for them, but we have them anyway, free of charge, and available to the vast majority of humans. That is, the miracle of miracles, a blessing of incredible value.

Why then, with these pervasive forces supportive of life and so readily available, is life so obviously difficult? Is "evil" built in to the structure of the universe? What is the opposite of love? (Hatred?). Or, the opposite of grace? (Bad luck???) In fact, there are no truly opposing forces, no epiphenomena of doom, per se. However, the concept that most clearly blocks the appearance or action of love and grace is ego. Please note that it is necessary to separate "the ego," an identification of self, and value neutral, from "ego," which represents survival of me above all costs, representing the essence of the reptilian brain. Ego thus defined is the end stage or full development of the vastly inflated sense of self importance. Such ego, I would speculate is never beneficial, even in modest development or expression. The greater the development, the less likely that love or grace can weave through the life of a person.

Great religious traditions have all tried to deal with issues of good and evil, the sources of happiness and misery, with varying levels of success. Within any given religious tradition, the discerning critic can find sublime expressions of truth, and preposterous expressions of xenophobia, side by side. Hence, the desire of many to lump these "religions," which can separate us, into the term "wisdom traditions, " which can bind us together, and to cull out the uplifting and drop the primitive fearfulness into a new paradigm, which can unite us.

In the daily examining of our life, we need to constantly watch our ego relentlessly, until we recognize it quickly in all of its guises.

Ego can appear to be generously concerned for others, such as in the giving of charity. However, it is still ego unless the charity is given anonymously (ego needs recognition and appreciation). Eventually, we come to realize that we are all connected. We all came from the same slime pit. Our station in life is an accident of birth. Our belief systems are a product of the interplay of mysterious intrinsic forces and our own life experiences. We are all doing the best we can do at any moment. We all need help. We all need, and thrive on love. In fact, we die without it.

With constant awareness of ego at work, we can tame it. The inevitable outcome is that we increasingly see the other as self. Something cannot be good for me, if it is clearly harmful for someone else. For me to be truly contented, I must think about the contentment of the people with whom I interact. Using a modern-day idiom, I must constantly think about win–win interactions. This all obviously raises questions about the notion of competitiveness and winning, which appears to be endemic in human interactions. We act competitively to experience the bliss of tribal kinship, at the cost of the majority of those who are not in our tribe. In fact, they are. They emanate from individual and collective ego. Can we really ever tame ego to allow for development of a sane and supportive world population? On the surface, it appears to be an incredible pipe dream. On the other hand, scientists have recently discovered that the development of the dog from the wolf occurred in the space of fifty years or less. Since then, dogs have prospered abundantly, and wolves have been repeatedly pushed to the brink of extinction. If dogs can do it, perhaps human competitors can become kinsman as well. The emphasis is on perhaps.

To the extent that ego is tamed, love and grace make increasingly greater protrusions into a person's life. The lovestream begins to flow and support life. Without it, life would not be sustainable. Love is difficult, very, very difficult. As stated so well by Woody Allen, "To Love is to suffer. To avoid suffering one must not love. But then one suffers from lack of love." As we become removed from the lovestream, our sense of angst can become unendurable, and will ensure the life of "quiet desperation" (Thoreau); "solitary, poor, nasty, brutish, and short" (Thomas Hobbs). As we become fully immersed, we feel bliss. Many of us are fearful of putting our toe into the stream. Love always carries with it the threat of loss, although this is a frighteningly realistic illusion. The ability to love grows on itself. Only ego is fearful of loss.

So how to begin, for those of us who are so timid (a less pejorative term than fearful)? Most of us already have started. I think that abstract love of beauty, of truth, is not the answer for most of us but a dry river bed. We need to love living things, including Gaia, the earth. Baby animals are safe. Who among us cannot feel warm and fuzzy looking at, or even better, engaged with a baby cat or dog? Almost any baby animal will do. (Watch out for baby rattle snakes, which are fully venomous). A simple step-up in difficulty would be an adult animal. They are beautiful and have an aura of animal power or security or knowingness. And, they are generally safe because they would not break our hearts, unless they die.

It is far more difficult to love humans, so few of whom are members of our tribe. They have the ability to hurt us, deeply and repetitively. The safest start here is a baby. Who cannot look at the innocence and frailty of a baby, and not feel a sense of loving warmth? Recall that Jesus never said anything about being born sinful. That came from early followers of Jesus, trying to organize and clarify parables. In fact, consider the possibilities that babies came into the world to give us reoccurring opportunities to experience unconditional love. More about conditionality later.

As children grow into young adults and fully mature adults, the task of loving, even members of one's own family can become really difficult. Our ego and their egos can clash. We want them to please us and vice versa. Ego at work, overtly and covertly, is easy to discern multiple times daily, in the interaction with these individuals.

What about loving people outside of one's tribe? This is very difficult and takes courage. In order to experience widespread lovingness, one must break free of tribal confines. The tribe gave us our first taste of orientation in life. It gave us a reference point. It gave us our first taste of love. We cling to tribal values with a death grip. Beyond a certain point, however, it stands as a perpetual barrier between us and all other living creatures.

And what about the mythical concept of unconditional love? Actually it does exist, in the real world, and it is attainable by anyone who works towards it. It involves reducing ego to the point whereby the welfare of the other is on equal footing and is indeed indecipherable from one's own welfare. In simple terms, it is nothing more and nothing less than accepting the person as they are, relinquishing all attempts to mold them into what you might want them to be. It involves supporting them in their efforts to grow, in the way that they feel the need to grow. Standing in opposition to these concepts, passively or actively, is not only unloving, but in a broader sense, is immoral.

In the early stages of such a process, ability to love unconditionally can be enhanced by a few simple tools. Study pictures of the individual as a child. Look at their face and how they hold their hands. Keep these images in your mind's eye. In the present, look at them in their more vulnerable states, such as sleeping. Look at them when they are engaged completely in something else, noting especially the back of the head, the way they hold their shoulders.

Can everyone have a soulmate? Does everyone need a soulmate? Can a soulmate develop over time? Perhaps these questions arise because of the potential for experiencing the deepest type of adult connectedness and the greatest sense of oneness in the setting of a soulmate. Certainly, pursuit of one's soulmate can be ego-driven, ego once again looking for maximum safety and support. Everyone who wants or needs a soulmate can experience it. It seems that the route getting there has a few basic characteristics. Of course, ego must be quieted. It may be very long in development such that patience is necessary. Finally, a little bit of grace may be necessary. Recall, that having done the groundwork, grace arises spontaneously, and often quietly and without fanfare. So, finding a soulmate is an evolutionary process, during the process of waking up. Look upon it more as a reward than a necessity. The most graced of all have multiple soulmates. Frosting on the cake.

COMPETITION AND WINNING/ THE CONCEPT OF EXCELLENCE AND HUMILITY

At times the extremism of the optimist, let alone the perfectionist, could be construed as excessive, intrusive, and laughably unnecessary. In this discourse, some aspects of the competitive instinct are questioned, certainly risking questions about the sanity of the questioner. The competitive instinct is obviously not simply a human trait but in fact is widespread throughout the animal kingdom. Although more difficult to perceive in the plant kingdom, as plants do not emanate intent in a way that we can easily perceive it as such, it is likely present there as well. Something so very widespread cannot possibly be changed or altered, and perhaps attempts to do so should not even be tried. Right?

The only "new" feature having to do with competitiveness is that at least on this, our earthly home, and perhaps nowhere else in the history of the universe, has a creature with the intellectual prowess of modern humans been an active player. Ever since the cosmology of the Big Bang concept began to take hold sixty or perhaps eighty years ago with technological advancements allowing us to peer progressively more deeply into space and with the growing awareness that the universe is vast beyond comprehension, expanding, and with countless billions of stars, and who knows how many planets, it has been accompanied by a sister presumption. Along with this inundation of awareness and expletives, the sister presumption is that the statistical likelihood that there have been and/or are millions of places in the universe which advanced species could inhabit is high.

Thus, arises the concept, deeply and widely held (at least in the scientific community), that we are not alone. The first SETI (Search for Extra Terrestrial Intelligence) conference occurred in 1961, and scientists have been looking for it ever since. Well, guess what? At the same time that our knowledge about the universe has dramatically increased, thus far, we have found zero evidence for the presence of extraterrestrial intelligence to match that of ours.

The amazing thing is that there has evolved so little speculation about the possibility that after all is said and done... we are alone! It seems that the "we are not alone" notion is very important to us, for whatever reason. At this point in time, although the possibility of finding evidence for extraterrestrial intelligence equal to ours is still within the realm of possibility, the longer we go with improved tools looking for our distant brethren, and not a peep is heard nor seen with all our listening devices, maybe we really are alone. Why is this so important? It seems to me that the issues confronting us here and now are so compelling, and so urgent, that for the moment, our attention is best directed here.

This brings us back to the "... end of all our exploring... to arrive where we started and know the place for the first time." (T.S. Eliot) We are the most advanced intelligence ever to have existed. Obviously, the concepts of being advanced and being perfected are not the same. We are obviously advanced and non-perfected. We all know that. So now, as the time has come to steady the head beneath the guillotine, let us try to nudge the non-perfected index slightly towards the perfected side.

Our competitive drive appears to be misdirected and excessive. Lord Acton issued a restatement of an idea that has been similarly expressed into the distant past. In 1887, he noted that "Power corrupts. Absolute power corrupts absolutely." Although there are always exceptions to the rule, this simple statement stands as a warning to those seeking power. Basically, it seems that to avoid falling victim to corruption, one can avoid attempts to achieve power. This runs antithetically to what most of us would like or try to achieve most of the time. The alternative is to achieve power, in whatever context, but somehow manage to escape the shoals of corruption. Recall that the ancient Greek philosophers alluded to this, and it was later so clearly stated by Edmund Burke (d. 1797) that "those who don't know history are destined to repeat it." The challenges involved in avoiding the repetition are daunting.

So what is power? It certainly is more than being the absolute dictator of the most powerful nation in the world. It exists in myriads of forms, whereby one person or one group has some type of dominion over another. Such dominion would enable that entity to dictate terms to another entity, based on what is best for the stronger of the two. It exists in the myriads of interpersonal relationships which we encounter every day. To avoid behaving in a domineering way takes continuous, conscious attention. Our competitive nature is so deeply woven through the human psyche that we do not even question it or look upon it as being possibly destructive. So, we repeat.

Competitiveness, trying to "beat" the other, is easily discernable in the play activities of young children, in both their verbal and physical displays. It is easy to see this pattern in people of all ages in the darkest of times. It is more difficult to see it in other times, but it is there if you look for it. It is like the pictures presented to us with the "six hidden animals"—easy to miss, but once we pick them out, that is all we can see!

Our competitiveness is seen in almost all sporting encounters. It has been speculated that sporting activities are beneficial because they allow us to burn off our aggression, without physically killing each other. Needless to say, this beatific concept has never been proven. Perhaps the opposite is true, in that it allows us to practice aggressiveness. This is where sports and many other performing activities (music, dance, theater) diverge. All of these activities are at least partially pursued for the intense sense of connection and camaraderie that a successful performance creates. Recall that the purpose of life is to awaken to the big picture. In so doing, we realize that as ego is tamed, we emerge as a small (but important) part of a huge mosaic. We begin to see the subtleties of life everywhere, and the pattern of connectedness begins to emerge as the illusion of separatism dissipates. If one could capture, bottle, and dispense the kind of intoxicating connectedness that emerges between performers, and between performers and their audience, and between audience members that arises during a performance, to be imbibed whenever needed, then oh happy day!

Recall that our activities are best directed towards the emergence of win–win situations… good for me and good for you. That is what the contents of this bottle are. For whatever reason, if we must settle for a lesser outcome, we can rework it at another time. What we need to avoid at all costs is to be part of the creation of lose–lose situations. Unfortunately, these experiences occur frequently, and can be spotted easily by the unmistakable feeling at the end of an engagement with another person, that you or they have been rendered diminished.

Many of our engagements create win–lose situations, this being a direct result of our competitiveness. The same feeling of diminishment may be felt and is the bellwether signal of an interaction which could have gone better. In this case, however, at the conclusion, both parties are likely to recognize the shortfall and can correct it promptly.

Is an athletic event always win–lose? Or is it always lose–lose? The second question deals with the fact that the loser lost. However, it raises the question about the winner, supremely competitive and aggressive who "won," but now becomes the party with the power and subject to the corruption of the soul that goes almost hand-in-hand with power. I am not so naïve as to foresee the end of competitive athletics. The "ratings" for this year's Super Bowl was apparently the highest in the history of television ratings ever. With that having been said, it was interesting to hear a sport commentator on ESPN the next day, voicing his shock that only 35% of television viewers watched it, whereas 65% did not! We tend to live in our own little cubby holes, with our cubby-hole companions being just another tribe to whom we belong.

Continuing on with competitive sports, there are a number of baby steps which could be invoked immediately, to move away from the otherwise win–lose or lose–lose situation. Easiest of all would be to avoid the egregious displays of domination, such as fist pumping, chest thumping, towering over a downed opponent, etc. Such a radical departure would need to be a top–down phenomenon, starting with the principal (high school), regents (college), and owners (professional), bought into by coaches, ancillary staff, parents, and… yes… you, the fans (short for fanatics). Egregious displays of physicality, with intent to stun, or injure, or punish another player, should be handled with decisive and arbitrary action by referees and umpires, with consequences that really matter. At the end of the contest, all contestants could meet, congratulate each other, and celebrate having had the opportunity to experience and generate this deep connection. That was the original intent of the ancient Olympic Games, almost 2,700 years ago, presented in the context of a religious ceremony, with the assistance of sculptors, poets, and other artisans, and intended to foster peace and harmony.

HUMILITY

Humility is an outstandingly attractive and desirable personality trait. What is the opposite of humility? Opposites are sometimes difficult to discern. Philosophically, the opposite of love is not hate but indifference. The opposite of humility may be bravado or conceit. Or, just maybe, insecurity. I think that insecurity, a sense of a deeply fractured self, calling upon the ego to paste it back together is the cause of much of our negative behavior. On the surface, this seems like a great tragedy, as it seems as if it would be so simple to fix. On the other hand, it is so endemic, so likely to have penetrated our DNA after a millennium of competition and conflict with one another, that obviously, such is not the case. To the extent that we can raise our humility index, we have a better chance of effectively communicating with each other and developing true, automatically triggered empathy.

There is a viable, healthful alternative to competitiveness and aggressiveness, in this scenario leading to win–win conclusions. That is, each person could be challenged by others or by their own inner drive to pursue excellence. Although the training activities leading to excellence or winning may be the same, the motives are radically different. Those who pursue excellence do not intend to subdue others. We owe it to each other to do our work, and to walk our walk excellently, no matter what that walk may be. It is the least we can do for each other. It sets the stages for the coveted win–win situations.

Even if it appears that you have gone unnoticed, you have given your best and have likely benefitted countless souls with whom you have come into contact. They, of course, are blessed by your attention and concern. If you are exceptionally blessed, sixty years later you may get a note of appreciation and a small sum of money, as are the common people supported by the Foundation for the Righteous, for having risked their lives to shield people during the years of the Nazi persecution.

Even within the context of the sports milieu, it is often stated that the best "teammate" is the participant who lets the game come to them. In other words, prepare yourself for excellence. Listen for the call. Perform excellently.

SECTION VI

DOCTOR, DOCTOR TELL ME WHAT TO DO!

HOW TO STAY WELL, WHEN STAYING WELL SEEMS IMPOSSIBLE

Twin studies have been particularly useful, with substantial explanatory power, in terms of isolating nature and nurture. Whenever I have been in a tight spot, it has always been possible for me to blame it on my twin brother. Separated at birth, we remain alarmingly alike but disarmingly different. For instance, who could have imagined that both would have found their way into medical school? On the other hand, the route after graduation was so different. Me, the very traditional medical pathway, with a brief sojourn into the army, drafted but allowed to complete internal medicine training before serving during the Vietnam war. Military service for me was a combination of tension, over the possibility of needing to take my pacifist leanings to Vietnam, joy day by day for not having to do that, wonderment over making my first prolonged sojourn in the South, surprised that I felt quite at home, and gratitude for the ability to experience the real world of clinical medicine during my prodigious "moonlighting" experiences.

Yes, this involved doing civilian work as a doctor, while an active duty member of the US Army Medical Corps, without their knowledge—commonly done, conveniently ignored but not really legal. It proved to be immensely enjoyable and a continuation of my medical training program. I became the only doctor for a group of a hundred nursing home residents, way out in the country. Most of them were black—very black, and beautiful, and with heavy accents, making me grateful for my formative training program at Cook County Hospital in Chicago. On weekends, I covered the enormous practice of a small town GP, as he flew his plane off on various junkets, grateful to have me as his willing standby. It was a remarkable experience, which could not be replicated now. I found myself delivering babies and doing minor surgery in his old mansion, converted to his own private 12-bed hospital. The insurance broker who sold to me my first malpractice policy for $29 said, "Son, there's never been a successful law suit against a doctor in the state of South Carolina." (Unbelievable, but perhaps true.) After the army, it was back to my final formal training in pulmonary medicine, rigorous and challenging, before hanging up the shingle.

Brother Leon embraced the military in a different way. He chose the Marines. Swept up into the mystique of the military at war, and leapfrogging in as a doctor at the level of captain, soon to be major, he devised a track never before done. In so doing, he had re-written military history and changed the lives of thousands of young men. After a stint in Vietnam, Major Leon Marmorstein surrendered his commission, becoming the first physician-trained drill sergeant in the Marine Corps. With the help of his superior officers, his personal charisma, and his own prescient views about health, he was given permission to try to create a generation of young men who were to become his own private database. This was a win–win situation. Brother Leon was allowed to bring his theories and philosophies to a group of "captive" young men, and the Marine Corps received a continuing infusion of dedicated soldiers and leaders.

They said of him that he could have done anything he wanted to. He could have been Commandant of the Marine Corps. His intensity and commitment were contagious. His fledglings, as well as his supervisors, listened to him. He bubbled with plans and ideas. He was reminiscent of the ancient Greek philosophers, more interested in doing things in the here-and-now and getting results, rather than publishing data, receiving accolades, and looking for the limelight.

Basic training with Drill Sergeant Marmorstein was something the military had never seen before, requiring it to be kept under wraps, until its value could no longer be ethically kept secret. The program evolved slowly. First, the emphasis was on the physical body and then on the mind. Brother Leon was the perpetual student, always seen buried in a book, even if only for five minutes. His interests were very eclectic but did not much encompass Japanese issues. Nevertheless, several people commented to him that he appeared to be resurrecting a Samurai code. His response was usually a genuinely surprised, "Really?", or "No kidding?" He always felt that it was evolving from forces working inside of him.

Eventually, there were didactic and experiential activities which could only be seen as an attempt to round out the complete man—a kind of Übermensch. He was relentless. Where did he get these ideas back in 1969? That was his genius. If there were a Nobel Prize for development of the complete person, he would have won it going away.

Emphasis on the body began in the context of basic training and progressed from there. There was Marine Corps basic training, and basic training the Drill Sergeant Marmorstein way. The thinking was—that left on their own—these young men would do their brief military stint and then return to their previous ways, becoming middle-aged couch potatoes, dissolving into oblivion just like all the other John and Jane Does. It did not happen that way. His impassioned and repeated teachings about the undisturbed path of the family pedigree got their attention. Strenuous physical exertion became a pattern so deeply entrenched that to slack off on a day of feeling sub-par created such a sense of giving up and fear of backsliding, as to negate the possibility. Done within the confines of a highly supportive group, the daily strenuous activity "vaccine" took place. Long after basic training, these troops carried on their daily routine of one hour or more of outdoor activity. Out of doors, because that is where the human animal evolved and, in a sense, belongs. In the elements, experiencing life as the predatory animal that he is. He had a strong conviction that there existed a distinct benefit in experiencing the change of seasons and changes of weather, and interacting with the natural elements and creatures. It also seemed to nurture a kind of toughness or resiliency, not experienced in the confines of the gym.

Participants began to hear about the "50,000 mile" topic, at first somewhat veiled in mystery. However, eventually it became clear that what seemed absurd at one time, became a possibility after the physical routine was entrenched. Could an average person actually circumnavigate the globe at the equator, by walking or running twice in a lifetime?

The meditation experiences appeared to have a subtle but powerful effect in terms of controlling or muting aggressive or predatory tendencies. Beginning with short sessions, easily taught, and easily learned, the value of this daily activity became gradually apparent to the trainees, so as to eventually require no prompting. The form of meditation was flexible and varied greatly with the individual and their respective backgrounds, all helping to shape the quiet time of reflection in the midst of the regimented training of a military organization.

"Let your food be your medicine, and your medicine your food." This aspect of training took considerable convincing of the military cooks, but Sergeant Marmorstein was a persuasive man and knew how to pull rank. His contingent began with a high protein, low carbohydrate diet, with emphasis on healthful fats, vegetables, fruit, and absence of traditional desserts. Simple carbohydrates were singled out as the enemy and picked off one by one. No cakes, sugar, breads, pastas, or white foods. Surprisingly, this was the toughest battle, year after year. Sergeant Marmorstein thought of himself as a visionary, whereby others considered him to be verging on a madman. He would then stop them in their tracks by simply proclaiming, "You eat what you like! I eat what is good for me!"

This was the vaccine which appeared to be the most likely to fail and yet was such a key component. But he would not let that occur. More lectures and discussions with the victims of this outrage. Having grown up on a farm, he had observed what he interpreted to be intense fear, frozen into the bodies of animals at the time of slaughter. He imagined a pouring out of stress hormones, contaminating the flesh, making it unsuitable as nourishment. Gradually, during his tenure, data came forth in bits and pieces, always aggressively denigrated by the powers to be and hidden whenever possible. Nevertheless, many studies confirmed the negative medical effects of a meat-based diet. Later, further studies of an environmental nature confirmed beyond any controversy the enormous stress on the global environment generated by the meat industry. He admitted to believing in the theory that there was a conspiracy lurking in every corner, invariably driven by the two-headed, money-greed monster, with people willing to ignore data completely, if their livelihood or power base depended on it ("Me first, and to hell with the rest"). His trips to a variety of factory farms illustrated this clearly, as the daily suffering of unfortunate animals was obviously enormous. He could not begin to relate to the often quoted concept that a certain degree of animal suffering was an unfortunate intrinsic by-product of producing food for people. He so deeply believed that animal rights were equal to human rights that it pained him to realize that most people thought that to be absurd.

More pep talks with the cooks to do better. Make those wheat berries tastier. Make those lentils more savory. Figure out a better way to make soybeans taste "meatier." In fact, the meat so dearly loved despite its negative effects on the goals of the program was gradually phased out. Chicken was phased out… too many hormones, and stress-induced toxins, and fats, let alone the massive suffering forced on living creatures treated like nothing but a commodity. A field trip to a factory farm, to observe firsthand the environmental stress, and the suffering of the "bird victims" was helpful in convincing them that expecting this "food" to be beneficial to them is an impossibility. Fish were the last to go, when it was appreciated that all that was needed from them was the omega 3 fatty acids, readily available from other food and commercial sources. Growing up on the farm, he had read about the massive erosion of topsoil which had occurred over the preceding century. To try to compensate for this, he watched as huge amounts of chemical fertilizers were dumped and sprayed on the land. He imagined that depletion of topsoil equated with depletion of nutrients from the food chain. He reasoned that at least a few essential vitamins and supplements were needed.

His visionary ideas spilled over into more ethereal areas. He was fascinated by concepts of intention and consciousness which were beginning to emerge. He felt strongly that an element of the sacred needed to be brought into everyday experience, rather than being relegated to a 1½ hour time slot at a religious service on Sunday. The contemplation–meditation work helped with that. He taught the need to make this an everyday and ultimately as an every moment experience. He saw the act of eating as a sacred one, taking in the bodies, elements, and consciousness of plants and animals into one's own body, reflecting the connectedness of all of nature and its ability to transform and strengthen us. Eating was carried on in a quiet environment, with attention directed to the food and what it represents. Conversation was subdued. The act of eating was slowed. Sitting, and no standing or walking. Overall, very much like a religious service.

The results have spoken for themselves. Weight came off. The body became strong and supple. The minds were simultaneously sharp and calm. Many of the trainees went on to Officers Candidate School and became respected career officers. They have been followed for almost forty years. The results have been impressive. All of the commonly seen degenerative diseases which have swamped society since then are rarely seen. More than 75% of these men, many now sixty-plus years of age, are taking no prescription medications. Most have never since been hospitalized. The vast majority is still physically active and psychologically sound, with a very low incidence of anxiety and/or depression. The scores are high in contentment, on psychological testing. Many have had leadership roles in their communities. Every year many more are added to the 50,000 mile club.

What about the leader himself, Doctor Drill-Sergeant Marmorstein? Some have thought of him as a fanatic. Most considered him to be different. He saw it differently. He thought of himself as a lucky guy who did everything he wanted to do and even helped the world be a better place. People said that he would never quit and that he would die leading his troops while on a walking meditation. He surprised them again by stepping down at normal retirement age. He could still pass the same physical tests that his eighteen-year-old recruits had to pass. Easily, in fact. It was just time to leave.

A few people have loved him unconditionally, so I guess he cannot be all that strange. I feel that way about him. So does his wife. It only takes one unconditional love to change a life. He knew this from his own personal experience. He received it and passed it on to all of his troops who would accept it. He reports occasional vivid dreams of alienation and just not quite fitting in. He dreams of being invited to lecture a group of doctors, and no one shows up.

He is still doing things his own way, retired to a small rural community, tending a small farm—animal sanctuary—and a menagerie of previously homeless or unwanted critters, living out their lives in safety and expressing their individual animal nature. He has recently mentioned the possibility of writing his memoirs. He insists that he is not withdrawn and certainly not depressed, but simply living the quiet life which seems appropriate to him at this time. He has a guesthouse to accommodate the stream of visitors from the ranks of the young men he first met as an impassioned physician/drill sergeant, who come to be in his presence again, after all these years.

Somehow, I have a persisting feeling that we have yet to see his final expression. He may still have one more gig to go. We will see.

(See the The Message in the Bottle)

SECTION VII

EPILOGUE

YOU CAN'T ALWAYS GET WHAT YOU WANT (GETTING WHAT YOU NEED)

Who could argue with the concept that it is better to be a giver than a taker? A giver, by implication, senses abundance. A taker by implication needs assistance. The fact that the taker may "deserve" the thing offered does not detract from the fact that somebody, somewhere has given, so that the taking is possible. Who would argue with the concept that "you cannot always get what you want?" It is a truism for everyone. What most of us really want is to be cared for lovingly, unequivocally respected for who we are, and in constant recognition of connectedness, so that we will never have to feel lonely or abandoned. On the dark side, the reptilian side, what we really want is to be able to do whatever the hell we want to, whenever the hell we want to.

The above sets of "wants" quite clearly describes taking. Big time taking. Every step requires the presence of a giver—of care, of love, of respect, of availability, and of license to run wild. As stated above, all of this taking requires the energy of givers. It disenfranchises the taker, even if he or she wears a real crown or possesses a source of power such as a huge bank account. It is a losing proposition.

Getting what you need is far better. All that entails is accepting the basics as enough, which in turn places oneself in a position to be a giver, to those in need, of whatever. In my opinion, even in dealing with sick people for almost fifty years, the glass is half full for 95% of these people, 95% of the time. Perhaps that in turn means that you make do with a little less money. If you follow your bliss, that will not matter. Now you might ask, "What in Sam Hill does this have to do with health?" The answer is "everything." Recall the image of the brain as a big powerful battery, the seat of your memory, your consciousness, and your soul. These differing elements of brain animate the world around you. With depression, anxiety, anger, and disappointment comes a shutting down of brain power. The lights begin to dim, and the entire complexity of the immune system begins to disintegrate into an inert glob of cellular debris. The lights of your reptilian brain flicker out last, so that your last brain state might involve "Me, me, me. I want…" Having these types of brain states as a major portion of your totality is incompatible with a state of good health. Everything you do needs to support contentment rather than disenchantment. Following your bliss, setting yourself up to be a giver, thinking about other people (and animals, plants, rocks, soil…) is a good start.

THE SECOND CURVE

It is not so difficult to predict the near-term future; that is the first curve. The material outlined in this treatise is likely to be relevant to a substantial degree for ten to twenty years. Some of it may be relevant for hundreds of years. The future of big chunks of it, over the next twenty to fifty years is in doubt. What we know as a fact is that the rate of scientific understanding of our world is increasing at a logarithmic rate. For a non-mathematician like me, this means that knowledge and understanding are occurring at a faster pace each year. Making predictions about the next twenty to fifty years (that is the second curve) seems more difficult at this point in history than ever before because of two enormous forces approaching—Earth from "outer space" and the minds of all inhabitants of this, our home.

The first Big Fact is that we are approaching the possibility of an absolutely unprecedented explosion of knowledge. Applications of this have startling possibilities, which at this point in time, as near as they may be, would still strike most people as science fiction, if not science fantasy. But it is very easy to point backwards, perhaps 150 years, and note that life as it is lived today could not have been imagined by the vast majority of people on earth, with only a few visionaries thinking beyond the railroad and the telegraph. The speculations put forth at this time, although seeming to be preposterous, in some ways are no more revolutionary than a description of air travel, computer operations, or wireless communications would have been to inhabitants of the mid-1800s.

Briefly, speculation posits that we are now on the threshold of being able to control and mold expressions of genes to produce whatever proteins are needed to switch on and off receptors, which will greatly delay programmed cell death. This is the so-called genetic revolution, already in full swing. The details of how to do this are being worked out as a computer model. Mastery of this technique opens many doors, including the possibility of creating young tissues in an older person by using one type of cell "programmed" to function as a different type of cell, thus giving rise to the potential to grow new organs. Cloning technologies raise the possibility of creating meat in a factory, without animals. In fact, much of this can already be done. However, the incidence of genetic mistakes creating errors of one type or another is still prohibitively high to be openly endorsed.

Following along with the evolution of genetic mastery may come stunning breakthroughs in nanotechnology, that is, the creation of and utilization of "gadgets" roughly the size of red blood cells and thus capable of going to every cell in the body, to accomplish re-programming. So-called nanobots could then carry computer programs to any cell or organ targeted, to clean up, fix up, and rejuvenate that cellular structure (heart, liver, etc.). Computer scientists and engineers are already debating the possibilities of installations of these types of nanobots and, at the same time, beginning to anticipate problems in design and implementation. The doctors at the hospital at which I work were recently given a presentation about nanobots by a scientist from the University of Texas. The creation of structurally new materials is giving us a glimpse of their potential usefulness in many areas, including the potential to function as external batteries, using solar power. Successful implementation is predicted by some optimists to have the potential for enormously extending life expectancy.

The third revolution, intersecting with the first two, involves robotics and particularly artificial intelligence. When combined with nanotechnology and the likelihood that artificial intelligence will exceed human intelligence by a factor of hundreds to thousands of times in the near future, the questions about the integration of neural elements and implanted computer parts arise. It seems that should this occur, the ultimate Brave New World will have arrived. Personally, thoughts of "beings" having a "brain" which is part neuronal and part computer cause me to shiver with fear, while it causes others to shiver with excitement. The expansion of brain power might be so vast as to be impossible for many to resist, somewhat like cocaine. To me, however, it appears that if that did occur, we *Homo sapiens sapiens* will have ended our sojourn on earth, having thus accomplished the first ever mass suicide of a species. Imaginary scenes of the debates between brains, computers, and hybrids of such are chilling. So while the most optimistic of the futurists see this new brain power as having the potential of solving all worldly problems, the world as we know it would have already ended.

This leads to the second Big Fact which seems to be fast approaching. Unfortunately, it appears to be approaching like a tsunami, giving us no warning until minutes before its arrival. This is the crisis of overpopulation of the world by humans and the crisis of global warming. We are by far, the most successful predator in the history of our planet. Too successful. Too many of us. Too much stress on the planet. Massive global climate changes, with floods, droughts, and rising sea levels to put the likes of much of coastal Southeast Asia and Florida under water. Disruption of human populations would be so great, as to make creative solutions in the midst of massive food and fresh water shortages very unlikely.

So, which will come first? Will it be the solution of all human problems by enormously enhanced brain power or a fall into global anarchy? As mentioned, these are issues of such enormity, as to make predictions about the second curve almost impossible. Please note that the purpose of the discussion was not to predict the "End of Days" or the Apocalypse but to suggest the possibility that the face of human biology and medicine may change as much in the next twenty to fifty years, as it did in the previous 2,000.

DEATH

Unless the most optimistic of the futurists are correct, and the ensuing years do give us the opportunity or at least the option to live as long as we desire, without having to do anything about it except to authorize the installation of an army of nanobots into our bodies, to patrol and repair our cells "on the fly," the wisdom of Benjamin Franklin will prevail—"In this world, nothing is certain except death and taxes."

I wish to take a brief sojourn, as we get progressively closer to the end of this document which you have so patiently reviewed. As a matter of fact, this will be our last such diversion. Being the Libran, I find it necessary to balance everything, on the fly. I also wish to preserve my reputation for anyone who might read this stream of consciousness in the future.

Regarding the "futurists" recently mentioned, in fact they are brilliant people. They are not naïve. They have done their homework, particularly regarding the mathematical and scientific portions of their projections. As a respectful critic of their work, what I see lurking, perhaps, is the application of a rigorous ethics to accompany the math and science. The conclusion regarding brain function recently traversed is that we need to use our whole brain. That itself is likely the panacea which can pull us back from the edge of the abyss. Recall that much of what bombards our senses goes directly to our reptilian brain, so that we will buy more, eat more, consume more, look better, and be hipper, slicker, and cooler than anyone else on the block. The appeal is to our deep-seated sense of insecurity and inferiority, with the lure of bringing us to the promised land of domination. The ultimate expression of this occurred in Nazi Germany, when highly educated, romantic people were sucked into a national psychosis and depravity.

On paper, being a quasi-scientist myself (clinical doctors are quasi-scientists, whereas research doctors are the real thing) and being a student of history, or at least intellectual history, I truly believe that the predictions of the futurists are not only possible but likely, unless a very serious ethical debate scuttles full implementation of what is possible. For a person interested in intellectual history, the debates and discussions surrounding issues such as bringing back the dead (Yes! That is part of the promise), including beloved pets that have passed, species that have long since passed (like dinosaurs, ala Jurassic Park), and yes human loved ones, gives me the least excitement about sticking around as long as I can. If we think that debates regarding stem cells and abortion have been heated, wait until these issues are debated! The Tasmanian tiger became extinct seventy years ago, when the last member of the species died in a zoo in Hobart, Tasmania. Genetic material extracted from that animal has been revived in a mouse's body. There is an abundance of bodies of woolly mammoths, extinct for 10,000 years, frozen in ice and permafrost. Part of the genome of these animals has been mapped. These technologies are rapidly advancing.

However, the excitement about these possibilities is quickly tempered if not dashed when we deeply explore questions debating whether our "ability" to do these things means that we "should" do them. After all, we can kill any other person. Yet almost every civilized culture extending back to the beginning of the historical record has had at least some restraints or prohibitions against this type of activity, often with very severe penalties for transgressions. Using our whole brains, which pulls in our capacity for empathy and compassion about bringing facsimiles and loved ones back into an already crowded world, radically different from what they know and with no reference point to hang on to, does it truly seem acceptable to bring loved ones back?

Finally, I mentioned (jokingly, of course) that I needed to protect my reputation. Recall my dedication to the proposition that 98% of life is gray, with the rest black or white. It is very dangerous to be absolutely arbitrary and to say this or that is impossible. Great minds have made statements about topics timely for their age, which appear to us to be so quantifiably absurd as to be laughable. Up until the last 100 years or so, it was widely appreciated by most people that animals were sophisticated machines and thus without a soul. Nietzsche's rescue of a horse being beaten on the street was not deemed an act of conscience but part of his madness, representing another reason to confine him. Nowadays, attempting to soften the hardness of heart of this nascent human approach, the response might be "Well, I guess they never spent time with my dog," or cat, or bird, or whatever. Every episode of ethnic cleansing has hinged on the same precepts, that the people being cleansed are subhuman, i.e., animals, i.e., soulless. So, although I believe that currently unbelievable events regarding biologic phenomena may begin to unfold in the near future, I cannot help but believe that there will be prohibitions on what parts of the scientific possibilities are allowed to proceed.

THE POLST FORM

Physician Orders for Life-Sustaining Treatment (POLST)

FIRST follow these orders, **THEN** contact physician, nurse practitioner or PA-C. This is a Physician Order Sheet based on the person's current medical condition and wishes. Any section not completed implies full treatment for that section. Everyone shall be treated with dignity and respect.

Last Name /First/Middle Initial

Date of Birth _____   Last 4 #SSN _____   Gender ☐ M ☐ F

A
Check One

CARDIOPULMONARY RESUSCITATION (CPR): Person has no pulse and is not breathing.
☐ CPR/Attempt Resuscitation   ☐ DNR/Do Not Attempt Resuscitation (Allow Natural Death)
When not in cardiopulmonary arrest, follow orders in **B**, **C** and **D**.

B
Check One

MEDICAL INTERVENTIONS: Person has pulse and/or is breathing.
☐ **COMFORT MEASURES ONLY** Use medication by any route, positioning, wound care and other measures to relieve pain and suffering. Use oxygen, oral suction and manual treatment of airway obstruction as needed for comfort. **Patient prefers no transfer:** EMS contact medical control to determine if transport indicated to provide adequate comfort.

☐ **LIMITED ADDITIONAL INTERVENTIONS** Includes care described above. Use medical treatment, IV fluids and cardiac monitor as indicated. Do not use intubation or mechanical ventilation. May use less invasive airway support (e.g. CPAP, BiPAP). **Transfer** to hospital if indicated. Avoid intensive care if possible.

☐ **FULL TREATMENT** Includes care described above. Use intubation, advanced airway interventions, mechanical ventilation, and cardioversion as indicated. **Transfer** to hospital if indicated. Includes intensive care.

Additional Orders: (e.g. dialysis, etc.) _____

C
Check One

ANTIBIOTICS:
☐ No antibiotics. Use other measures to relieve symptoms.
☐ Determine use or limitation of antibiotics when infection occurs, with comfort as goal.
☐ Use antibiotics if life can be prolonged.

Additional Orders: _____
_____

D
Check One

ARTIFICIALLY ADMINISTERED NUTRITION:
Always offer food and liquids by mouth if feasible.
☐ No artificial nutrition by tube.
☐ Trial period of artificial nutrition by tube.
(Goal: _____
_____)
☐ Long-term artificial nutrition by tube.

Additional Orders: _____
_____

E MEDICAL CONDITION/GOALS:

F SIGNATURES: The signatures below verify that these orders are consistent with the patient's medical condition, known preferences and best known information:

Discussed with:	PRINT — Physician/ARNP/PA-C Name	Phone Number
☐ Patient ☐ Parent of Minor		
☐ Legal Guardian	Physician/ARNP/PA-C Signature (mandatory)	Date
☐ Health Care Agent (DPOAHC)		
☐ Spouse/Other:	Patient or Legal Surrogate Signature (mandatory)	Date

Use of original form is strongly encouraged. Photocopies and FAXes of signed POLST forms are legal and valid

THE POLST FORM—
GETTING WHAT YOU NEED

Back to death. I am a medical doctor. I have always considered that my first mission was to alleviate suffering. After all, that is written into the Hippocratic Oath regarding the welfare of the patient and to do no harm. During medical training, one sees so much death, and suffering leading up to it, that it early on crystallizes the connection between suffering and death. Recall the philosopher who labored over the issues of the pleasantries of life, and the glories of the life to come, but the difficulty in getting from one to the other. The "getting from one to the other" is the gap where the doctor can be tremendously helpful. For a patient with intact mentation, the choice of how aggressive to be with treatment should be theirs. This should include a statement from the doctor about the possibility of suffering, if no limitations are set. In a patient felt by doctors and/or family to be incapable of understanding the subtleties of difficult questions, it is up to the family, and in particular to the "power of attorney," that is the one having legal authority, once again with the help of the doctor.

Up until very recently, unfortunately the formal document that we had to deal with was the so-called living will. This document created by attorneys and written substantially in legalese had only one vague medical reference having to do with two doctors agreeing that so and so is terminally ill (actually we are all technically terminally ill), that so and so does not want heroic measures, whatever the heck that means. The bottom line is that doctors reading that document had no idea what the person wanted.

For the last four or five years, with a revision one year ago, we now have a much improved form, with input from doctors, whereby the person is now able to state quite precisely what they want or do not want, in the case of serious and/or life-threatening illness. This is called the POLST form, an acronym for Physicians Orders for Life Sustaining Treatment. Table P is the actual "working page" of the form. The instructions for completing the form are on the back side. Section A asks what should be done, should a cessation of cardiac function and breathing occur. The two options are to proceed with full cardiopulmonary resuscitation (CPR) by lay or professional personnel or not (allow natural death). The physician should make it clear that the decision is up to the person. However, there are a number of things they need to know. First of all, are there comorbid conditions which would either make successful resuscitation very unlikely or impossible? Examples of this might include severe pulmonary hypertension or severe cardiomyopathy. Similar but slightly different is whether or not the person has an illness which is in its final stages, such as end-stage renal disease or advanced cancer. Thirdly, the person needs to know that with CPR, very forceful compressions of the chest are administered. Some people, particularly those who are elderly, frail, and with known bone loss or certain types of chest deformity, have a high likelihood of experiencing multiple rib fractures and/or sternal fractures with resuscitation attempts. These are extremely painful for weeks afterwards. Certain types of chest deformity also would tend to minimize the chances of a good result. They also need to know that a tube is placed through the mouth and into the windpipe. During placement of this tube, damage can be done to the teeth, mouth, throat, or voice box. They need to know that they will not be able to speak during the duration of the time that the tube is in place. This procedure, called intubation, is uncomfortable (recall that this is doctor terminology for "painful"). Need for the tube could be only a few hours or as long as weeks to months. Lastly, they need to understand that during the early resuscitation procedure, because of the possibility of very low blood pressure and blood oxygen levels, brain damage from mild and temporary to severe and permanent may occur. Based on all of this, the doctor can and should give the patient advice. "If this were me, I would…." The patient may or may not agree with the advice.

Section B implies that complete stoppage of cardiac and respiratory functions does not ensue, and the person obviously ill makes it to the hospital. The three choices at that point are more or less self-explanatory. There is even the option of not transporting the person to the hospital. Otherwise, they can request comfort measures only, such as oxygen, and pain medication. They may quickly improve and be able to leave the hospital, or they may remain due to emergence of other problems. They can ask for limited treatment, such as addition of antibiotics, breathing assistance, and intravenous fluids. Or they can ask for full treatment, which includes everything including resuscitation, should it be needed because of progressive respiratory failure or because of full-blown cardiac arrest.

Section C could actually have been included under limited or full treatment of section B. Antibiotic treatment is relatively safe and painless, and is not likely to be turned down under appropriate circumstances unless the person is not invested in being "saved" and wants comfort measures only.

Section D represents a much stickier topic. Once the sick person arrives in the hospital, with or without a breathing tube in place, there are a host of reasons that could make eating either very unsafe or impossible (endotracheal intubation). A common scenario is the person with a stroke, which either causes a person to be obtunded (very sleepy) or with interruption of the swallowing mechanism. People can make a complete recovery from stroke, over days to months, no recovery, or worsen and die. If the sick, stressed body is not fed within three to five days, catabolism (breakdown of tissue) will commence and ensure a negative outcome. Therefore, the window of opportunity for improvement is relatively short, before tube feedings become essential to support recovery. The tube is inserted via an endoscopic approach. The endoscope goes through the mouth and into the stomach. Its intensely bright light is directed up at the abdominal wall and can be seen through the skin. After appropriate local anesthetic to the skin, a one-inch incision is made over the area of light, and after several clever exchanges, the tube is drawn through the abdominal wall and secured. It can stay in indefinitely and is basically not painful. Full nutrition can be provided. The procedure takes about fifteen minutes. The answers to the use of the tube are "no," "short-term trial" (to see if recovery is occurring), or "yes."

That is the POLST form. In people who are seriously ill, and even those who are not yet ill, it is an essential document. You may need to schedule an appointment with your doctor to ask as many questions as you need to understand the ramifications of the answers. All of this is an attempt to ensure that you indeed get what you need, rather than what you (or someone else) think you want.

THE FINISH LINE

Continuing along the discussion of death, it is not a question of if, but when. We all feel differently about life and death. We feel pain differently. We experience suffering differently. We are afraid of or unafraid of death. We see it as a termination of everything personal about us, or we see it as a transition to a "better place." We are so individually immersed in self that to try to imagine the world without self is numbing. The three major religions throughout most of the "industrialized West," Christianity, Islam, and Judaism all subscribe to an afterlife, held out to be a vast improvement over our earthen quagmire. Yet when it comes right down to it, nobody seems to want to go there.

I can assure you having been a witness to this more times than I care to recall, the process of dying can appear to be a very difficult challenge. With generic "discomfort," defined as a kind of pervasive restlessness, with or without frank pain, high-level mental functioning begins to fade. Recall the concurrent emergence of the big brain and language, and the intellectual debate regarding which provoked which. It is easy for me to imagine, and perhaps that is as far as we will ever be able to take it, that input to our higher brain function may remain intact as the body weakens and death draws near. There is no doubt that output drops off, and sometimes completely ceases, with eyes closed, passionless facies, and non-responsiveness. Anecdotal reports of people who appeared to be near death and survived, frequently attest to an out-of-body experience which includes enhanced auditory function and a complete understanding of the dialogue surrounding them, despite the inability to respond. In other words, in that particular mind–body state, it seems that perhaps it is much easier to receive than to give. So, it would seem very appropriate to quietly speak to the person, saying everything you want them to hear, as they prepare to leave. It would seem equally appropriate to remove other conversation to a different room, and to speak it quietly, if you deem it as something to be kept from the dying person. Although I have never been present at this time at the passing of one of my most intimate family or friends, I have been present during the passing of many beloved pets, speaking to them as if they were children, telling them how good and how loved they are, and what a wonderful gift they were for me.

All of this can be beautiful and inspiring, and life enhancing for those left behind. The problem is that the body has a mind of its own. Perhaps that mind is reptilian brain energy, whose function is not to evaluate and integrate the big picture. Its purpose always was and still is "survival." So this can create a huge problem in allowing a person or animal to die naturally, as suffering can rise to a level that is unacceptable.

In my opinion, we tend to hang on too long and, in some cases, way, way too long. Back to the Hippocratic injunction to relieve pain and suffering. When I see a dying person, I do not have the desire to prolong their moment of death, until relative x, y, or z arrives from wherever. I want to stop that person's suffering. A frequently encountered problem is that the doctor may be able to sense the process of what is paradoxically called "actively dying" (in other words, having passed the point of no return) weeks to months before friends or family have come to grips with this. If the doctor is correct, and if the loved ones are steadfast in going full steam ahead with the treatment, this can result in months of continuous, high-level suffering before death. Of course, the doctor is not always correct in this assessment. At that point, a second doctor can be pulled in to give an opinion. If this doctor agrees with the first, we then have fulfillment of the antiquated "living will," whereby the person has indicated that he/she does not want to be kept alive under that circumstance. If there is no resolution between doctor's opinion and the loved ones' opinions, the loved ones (almost) always win. In the meantime, in the two months before the person dies, there may be another operation, fifty more blood draws, five more MRIs, a feeding tube, and more intravenous devices and tubes, all of which hurt. As stated at the beginning of this long paragraph, in my opinion, having watched this play out countless times, most often we delay the moment of death far too long, far too often.

This person upon whom all of this attention and consideration has been brought to bear, like all of us through our lives, made daily decisions or non-decisions about their own healthcare, whether it be diet, how much or how little professional health care, tobacco, alcohol, mental stresses and attitudes, and many other issues. Now they find themselves at the brink. This is not the time to become suddenly repentant about poor health habits, as there is really nothing to be done about it at that time. At the time of death, ideally one should be accepting and unrepentant. They lived their lives making choices. They take responsibility for their choices—good or bad. The workings of the world are just too complex to expect that every choice we make will always be the right one.

WAKING UP

For the majority of us who are given enough time to make it into adulthood, the whole purpose of this life is to learn to make conscious choices. "Waking up" is what it is all about. Recognizing and uniting the divergent notions that we are infinitely small and feeble, yet vitally important and powerful. Grace at some point may intervene and make it suddenly apparent that separateness is a tenacious illusion of the reptilian brain, but an illusion nonetheless. We are all connected. Waking up illuminates the fact that every one of us is given a load to carry. Look at the load. Where did it come from? Do I want to get rid of it? If so, how do I do that? Look at the dark side. It's only you. And everyone else. Do not run from it. Integrate it, embrace it, and transform it into a creative force, which is one of the greatest gifts of waking up. The dark side is dark only so long as it is not noticed and integrated. Once this is accomplished, the gifts of fearlessness, lovingness, and fullness arise naturally, signaling the appearance of balanced brain functioning. With this entourage, you can spring across the finish line with panache.

For the last time, the purpose of life is to awaken. Look around, and you quickly note how very difficult this is to pull off… lives of quiet desperation are seen everywhere. You need not worry about the integrity of your reptilian brain. It is pandered to and seduced from every corner, every day. It does not need this goading. It has been part of us for many millions of years. It is our ignition system, lighting the fire that animates us. It is the higher brain which is neglected in most of contemporary society. It is stimulated here and there, but stimulation must be pursued and allowed to wash over us. It provides us with the blessing of balanced brain function, resulting in patterns of passionate and radical lovingness and acceptance. It allows us to be non-judgmental, living in the gray and eschewing the black and white. It allows us to embrace our dark sides, fearlessly. It allows us to transform predation into commitment and determination. Finally, it allows us to finally understand that something cannot be good for me, if it causes another living creature, human or otherwise, to suffer or feel diminished. It encourages us to pursue excellence in place of winning, as winning too often spurs losing. It allows us to be generous to the point of sacrificing ourselves for the betterment of those less fortunate. It fosters giving rather than taking, listening rather than lecturing. It opens the portals so that any passing wisps of grace, idly drifting by, may find its way to us.

Soul work requires courage. It requires the ability to feel deeply alone at times, taking on the load of sorrow in the world, carrying it off, and purifying it. The finished product is lovingness—the power that sustains all in the world.

By the way, there are isolated reports that Dr. Maurice Goldstein has been sighted! These reports are as yet unconfirmed. It could be true, and that could be a great benefit to you. It could even help you to wake up. But that is another story.

Until then, take care of yourself. Make conscious choices, with no regrets.

AUTHOR: DR. BARRY MARMORSTEIN

I have been witness to fundamental changes within the healthcare system during the time of my chosen career path. I see the emergence of problems in the delivery of healthcare which perhaps are still value neutral, but which I believe are trending toward negative outcomes. After all, what doctors are supposed to do is deliver healthcare. I am disturbed by what I see, and I wish to bring this to the awareness of you, the consumer. Aha! A timely example of change! Doctors are no longer termed doctors. We are now "providers." You are no longer termed "patients." You are now "consumers."

So, as my career drifts relentlessly towards its dusk, I wish to share some thoughts with you and give you a distillation of what I have learned during the past 46 years since I was anointed with an "MD" degree.

Author Barry Marmorstein, M.D. specializes in Internal Medicine and Pulmonary Diseases. He received his medical degree from the University of Illinois in Chicago and completed his residency in Internal Medicine at the University of Iowa in Iowa City. He completed a fellowship in Critical Care and Pulmonary Disease at the University of Colorado in Denver.

Dr. Marmorstein had a solo practice in Pulmonary Diseases and Internal Medicine in Bellevue, Washington for 36 years. He was then given an offer which he could not turn down. This would allow him to complete the journey "home", in the image of Dr. Goldstein, to work as a PCP in a small town in the mountains 70 miles east of Seattle. Married and with two children, he lives on a lake on the edge of a national forest, able to pursue his other interests including running, exploring the natural wonders in his back yard, and especially pushing steadily to "wake up."

THE MESSAGE IN THE BOTTLE

Deceptively easy, but most people fail.

(According to Yogi Berra, 90% is mental and the other half is physical)

1. Recognize that your health status is largely up to you, determined by the choices and decisions that you make moment to moment.

2. Staying well requires focus and a plan.

3. Engage in regular, strenuous physical activity, at least five days per week.

4. Never smoke, nor use any tobacco products.

5. Stay trim, using high school graduation weight as a barometer.

6. East the best diet—low in calories, with vegetables, fruits, and nuts as the cornerstone; very low in animal fat, and very low in processed foods.

7. Recognize your doctor for what she or he is—an advisor.

8. Listen to the messages from your body (symptoms) and consult your doctor-advisor when appropriate.

9. Mental-emotional health is essential to the flourishing of physical health.

    a) Strive for excellence rather than winning.

    b) Live fully in the present.

    c) Knowledge is always fragmentary.

    d) The world is almost always gray, with black and white exceptional.

    e) Knowledge of C. and D. opens the door to humility, compassion, and forgiveness.

    f) Each of us is doing the best we can at any given point in life.

    g) Never think never, and never think always.

    h) Come to recognize that the glass is almost always half full.

    i) Strive to be a giver.

    j) Always push to awaken to the connections, between all of us and everything.

CPSIA information can be obtained at www.ICGtesting.com
Printed in the USA
BVOW011449021212

307065BV00003B/24/P